Cutting Edge Preclinical Models in Translational Medicine

Cutting Edge Preclinical Models in Translational Medicine

Special Issue Editor
Chiara Attanasio

MDPI • Basel • Beijing • Wuhan • Barcelona • Belgrade • Manchester • Tokyo • Cluj • Tianjin

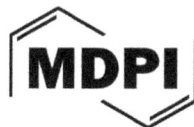

Special Issue Editor
Chiara Attanasio
University of Naples Federico II
Italy

Editorial Office
MDPI
St. Alban-Anlage 66
4052 Basel, Switzerland

This is a reprint of articles from the Special Issue published online in the open access journal *Journal of Clinical Medicine* (ISSN 2077-0383) (available at: https://www.mdpi.com/journal/jcm/special_issues/translational_medicine).

For citation purposes, cite each article independently as indicated on the article page online and as indicated below:

LastName, A.A.; LastName, B.B.; LastName, C.C. Article Title. *Journal Name* **Year**, *Article Number*, Page Range.

ISBN 978-3-03936-138-0 (Hbk)
ISBN 978-3-03936-139-7 (PDF)

Cover image courtesy of Antonio Palladino & Isabella Mavaro (C. Attanasio Lab).

© 2020 by the authors. Articles in this book are Open Access and distributed under the Creative Commons Attribution (CC BY) license, which allows users to download, copy and build upon published articles, as long as the author and publisher are properly credited, which ensures maximum dissemination and a wider impact of our publications.

The book as a whole is distributed by MDPI under the terms and conditions of the Creative Commons license CC BY-NC-ND.

Contents

About the Special Issue Editor vii

Chiara Attanasio and Mara Sangiovanni
Preclinical Models: Boosting Synergies for Improved Translation
Reprinted from: *J. Clin. Med.* 2020, 9, 1011, doi:10.3390/jcm9041011 1

Laura Lossi, Claudia Castagna, Alberto Granato and Adalberto Merighi
The *Reeler* Mouse: A Translational Model of Human Neurological Conditions, or Simply a Good Tool for Better Understanding Neurodevelopment?
Reprinted from: *J. Clin. Med.* 2019, 8, 2088, doi:10.3390/jcm8122088 5

Francesco Urciuolo, Costantino Casale, Giorgia Imparato and Paolo A. Netti
Bioengineered Skin Substitutes: The Role of Extracellular Matrix and Vascularization in the Healing of Deep Wounds
Reprinted from: *J. Clin. Med.* 2019, 8, 2083, doi:10.3390/jcm8122083 41

Aurelio Salerno, Giuseppe Cesarelli, Parisa Pedram and Paolo Antonio Netti
Modular Strategies to Build Cell-Free and Cell-Laden Scaffolds towards Bioengineered Tissues and Organs
Reprinted from: *J. Clin. Med.* 2019, 8, 1816, doi:10.3390/jcm8111816 69

Antonio Palladino, Isabella Mavaro, Carmela Pizzoleo, Elena De Felice, Carla Lucini, Paolo de Girolamo, Paolo A. Netti and Chiara Attanasio
Induced Pluripotent Stem Cells as Vasculature Forming Entities
Reprinted from: *J. Clin. Med.* 2019, 8, 1782, doi:10.3390/jcm8111782 95

Federico Salaris, Cristina Colosi, Carlo Brighi, Alessandro Soloperto, Valeria de Turris, Maria Cristina Benedetti, Silvia Ghirga, Maria Rosito, Silvia Di Angelantonio and Alessandro Rosa
3D Bioprinted Human Cortical Neural Constructs Derived from Induced Pluripotent Stem Cells
Reprinted from: *J. Clin. Med.* 2019, 8, 1595, doi:10.3390/jcm8101595 113

Adele Leggieri, Chiara Attanasio, Antonio Palladino, Alessandro Cellerino, Carla Lucini, Marina Paolucci, Eva Terzibasi Tozzini, Paolo de Girolamo and Livia D'Angelo
Identification and Expression of Neurotrophin-6 in the Brain of *Nothobranchius furzeri*: One More Piece in Neurotrophin Research
Reprinted from: *J. Clin. Med.* 2019, 8, 595, doi:10.3390/jcm8050595 127

Alessia Montesano, Elena De Felice, Adele Leggieri, Antonio Palladino, Carla Lucini, Paola Scocco, Paolo de Girolamo, Mario Baumgart and Livia D'Angelo
Ontogenetic Pattern Changes of Nucleobindin-2/Nesfatin-1 in the Brain and Intestinal Bulb of the Short Lived African Turquoise Killifish
Reprinted from: *J. Clin. Med.* 2020, 9, 103, doi:10.3390/jcm9010103 143

Veronica Rey, Sofia T. Menendez, Oscar Estupiñan, Aida Rodriguez, Laura Santos, Juan Tornin, Lucia Martinez-Cruzado, David Castillo, Gonzalo R. Ordoñez, Serafin Costilla, Carlos Alvarez-Fernandez, Aurora Astudillo, Alejandro Braña and Rene Rodriguez
New Chondrosarcoma Cell Lines with Preserved Stem Cell Properties to Study the Genomic Drift During In Vitro/In Vivo Growth
Reprinted from: *J. Clin. Med.* 2019, 8, 455, doi:10.3390/jcm8040455 165

Daniele Dondossola, Alessandro Santini, Caterina Lonati, Alberto Zanella, Riccardo Merighi, Luigi Vivona, Michele Battistin, Alessandro Galli, Osvaldo Biancolilli, Marco Maggioni, Stefania Villa and Stefano Gatti
Human Red Blood Cells as Oxygen Carriers to Improve Ex-Situ Liver Perfusion in a Rat Model
Reprinted from: *J. Clin. Med.* **2019**, *8*, 1918, doi:10.3390/jcm8111918 . . . . **185**

Maria Felicia Fiordelisi, Carlo Cavaliere, Luigi Auletta, Luca Basso and Marco Salvatore
Magnetic Resonance Imaging for Translational Research in Oncology
Reprinted from: *J. Clin. Med.* **2019**, *8*, 1883, doi:10.3390/jcm8111883 . . . . **201**

Ernesto Forte, Dario Fiorenza, Enza Torino, Angela Costagliola di Polidoro, Carlo Cavaliere, Paolo A. Netti, Marco Salvatore and Marco Aiello
Radiolabeled PET/MRI Nanoparticles for Tumor Imaging
Reprinted from: *J. Clin. Med.* **2020**, *9*, 89, doi:10.3390/jcm9010089 . . . . **231**

About the Special Issue Editor

Chiara Attanasio, veterinarian by background, currently serves as an assistant professor at the Department of Veterinary Medicine and Animal Productions of the University of Naples Federico II, Italy, where she is mainly active in animal tissue characterization and preclinical model development. She leads a research group—focused on the design and validation of tissue-engineered constructs, as an affiliated researcher at the Center for Advanced Biomaterials for Health Care—Istituto Italiano di Tecnologia (CABHC-IIT). She is also an adjunct professor of Animal Anatomy and Histology at the Magna Graecia University of Catanzaro. During the first part of her career, at the Center of Biotechnologies of Cardarelli Hospital in Naples, she was involved in studies aiming to control ischemia/reperfusion injury in liver, kidney and islet cell transplantation, and to improve the performance of AMC-bioartificial livers. During this period of time, she spent nearly one year at Harvard Medical School Transplant Center, Boston, MA, USA, where she explored novel mechanisms to maintain islet cell function and improve transplantation outcome. In 2013, at CABHC-IIT, she started to integrate this background into the field of bio-logic materials, by designing and validating bioengineered constructs and smart interfaces. From 2016 onward she also drives the Intravital Microscopy Lab of the Interdepartmental Center for Research in Biomaterials of University Federico II.

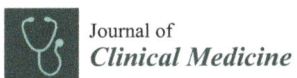 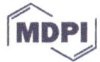

Editorial

Preclinical Models: Boosting Synergies for Improved Translation

Chiara Attanasio [1,2,3,*] and Mara Sangiovanni [4]

1. Department of Veterinary Medicine and Animal Productions, University of Naples Federico II, 80137 Napoli, Italy
2. Center for Advanced Biomaterials for Health Care—Istituto Italiano di Tecnologia, 80125 Napoli, Italy
3. Interdepartmental Center for Research in Biomaterials (CRIB) University of Naples Federico II, 80125 Napoli, Italy
4. Stazione Zoologica "Anton Dohrn", 80122 Napoli, Italy; mara.sangiovanni@szn.it
* Correspondence: chiara.attanasio@unina.it

Received: 24 March 2020; Accepted: 1 April 2020; Published: 3 April 2020

The field of preclinical models is a very vast arena, in which finding connections among groups acting in apparently very distant research areas can sometimes prove challenging. An osmosis of mindset and competencies (methodologies, techniques, models), along with a comparison of different standpoints, is always an opportunity to reflect on where one's work stands in a wider scenario. The goal of this Special Issue is to collect information, and ultimately share ideas and foster debate about different approaches to translational model research. The eleven papers composing this issue will be of interest to researchers looking for an update of the currently heterogeneous panorama of preclinical models and to those in search of inspiring ideas in the field.

Figure 1 shows a visual representation of the connections among the papers here presented. Each colored ribbon relates a paper with a topic. It is immediately apparent how many topics are addressed and how many relationships exist among the different research areas. Multidisciplinarity, which is intrinsic to the very nature of preclinical models, emerges at first sight as a relevant feature.

Out of eleven papers, six are based on animal models [1–6], highlighting that these models still play a crucial role in translational medicine, even in a historical moment in which the need to find alternative methodologies is increasingly pressing.

In this context, the issue raised by some authors about the translational validity of a certain animal model, in this specific case the Reeler mouse, is very timely. Central to the debate is the rare occurrence of the very conditions for which mice homozygous for the Reeler mutation have been created, and the objective difficulty of fully validating the mice expressing the heterozygous genotype as a translational model for more frequent diseases such as autism and schizophrenia [2].

After all, animal models are often suspended "halfway" between being widely accepted as good tools for basic research and being recognized for their translational potential. Therefore, this issue should always be considered when somebody, whether experimenter or modeler, decides to work with them. In this regard, one paper focuses on the improvement of cellular and animal models of chondrosarcoma. The authors [4] provide four cell lines, displaying tumorigenic and invasive features suitable to be used as valuable alternatives to veteran endless passaged cell lines. They also detail the genetic drift that these cells underwent as an adaptive response to in vitro and in vivo expansion.

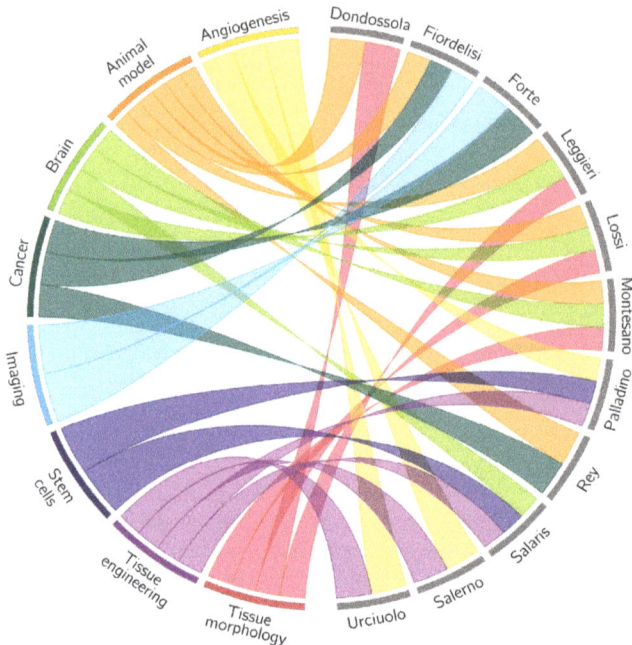

Figure 1. A visual representation of the connections among the papers presented in this Special Issue. Several topics were defined by widening the keywords specified in each paper (colored sectors on the left side of the image). Papers (gray sectors on the right side of the image) are identified by the first author's name. Colored ribbons connect papers with the topics treated. The figure was made with the Circos software [7].

Cancer, and more specifically the usage of nanoparticles (NP) both for multimodal imaging and as contrast agents (CAs), is the topic of a review [8] which highlights the advantages of using NP-based PET/MRI multimodal imaging in tumor diagnosis and characterization. Additionally, these nanosystems can be applied to theranostics in the very prominent scenario of personalized medicine. The authors point to multidisciplinarity as an essential requisite to deeply understand the possible applications and the underlying biomolecular processes of the targeted diseases.

The centrality of interdisciplinary synergies is further highlighted in a paper [6] specifically focused on the high potential held by MRI imaging in translational oncology. By analyzing several disease models and cancer types, the authors present their approach to reduce the gap from preclinical applications to clinical practice.

The "from bench to bedside" path is also the leitmotif of an article [9] addressing several issues related to the use of human-induced pluripotent stem cells (iPSC). More specifically, the paper analyses the potential of iPSC-endothelial cells in accelerating tissue regeneration and their suitability to enter progressively more clinical trials. The most represented research field in this Special Issue is tissue morphology [1–3,5] followed by tissue engineering [9–11] and neuroscience [1–3], with one article intercepting both these areas of expertise [12]. This latter work reports, indeed, a method to generate a three-dimensional neuronal system composed of cortical neurons and glial cells derived from iPSCs, suitable for drug screening and disease modeling.

Good news from the field of skin regeneration: the work on bioengineered skin substitutes has been selected by the editorial board as the cover story of the issue of December 2019 (www.mdpi.com/2077-0383/8/12). The article, presented by a group active in the field of dermal substitutes [13] and three-dimensional tissue-like models [14], is focused on the analysis of the most modern strategies to overcome the scarring process and promote skin regeneration, by implanting an engineered dermis capable of recapitulating the architecture and presenting molecular signals similarly to the native dermis [10].

The essential role of tissue-engineered constructs in mimicking extra-cellular matrix morphology and function is also highlighted in another work, in which the authors analyze the most promising fabrication technologies in the field. In particular, the paper reports the real effectiveness of the "bottom-up" approach for cell-free and cell-laden scaffolds in tissue and organ bioengineering [11].

Passing to the fascinating and complex field of neuroscience, two original research articles contributed to this Special Issue. It is worth noting how they both witness the increasing value of the short-lived African turquoise killifish *Nothobranchius furzeri* as an emerging vertebrate model in aging research. In particular, one paper describes, for the first time, the expression of neurotrophin-6 in different brain areas in both young and old animals [1], while the other one provides the first evidence of nucleobindin-2/nesfatin-1 expression and its role as a food intake regulator in vertebrate aging [3].

Finally, very high translational potential arises from a work proving the effectiveness of human red blood cells to act as oxygen carriers for graft preservation in liver transplantation. In particular, the study is aimed at enhancing the potential of normothermic machine perfusion, a modern methodology applied to organ preservation [15]. In view of the crucial role of transplantation for patients with end-stage disease and the consequent increasing demand for the inclusion of marginal donors, new methods to improve organ preservation and, eventually, induce graft repair are undoubtedly relevant to the clinical setting [5].

An important contribution might come from *in silico* modeling, a field that has unexpectedly been neglected in this Special Issue despite being a constitutive piece of the puzzle. In fact, *in silico* models prove to be useful at several stages of the process from research to clinical application, in a vision that aims at a deep digital transformation of all the production steps. This might be accomplished either with data-driven approaches, such as in omics or materiomics simulations, or with mechanistic modeling (e.g., bioreactors process) in tissue engineering [16]. Another interesting avenue is the development of *in silico* models capable of exploiting patient-specific data to build personalized medical treatments, such as three-dimensional mathematical models of tumors [17]. The urgency of an integrated approach merging *in vivo* experiments and *in silico* representations to obtain more powerful descriptive and predictive models is also emerging: for instance, the integration of microfluidic devices and computational modeling to better study vascularization dynamics in cancer [18].

The harmonization of data coming from different fields [19,20] and the exchange of expertise at several levels are fundamental parts of an essential strategy whose final aim is to accelerate the translation and the design of more precise preclinical models, in a true accomplishment of the "from bench to bedside" paradigm.

Author Contributions: Both the authors wrote the manuscript. Both the authors have read and agreed to the published version of the manuscript.

Acknowledgments: The authors thank Giulia Iaccarino and Debora Capece for fruitful discussion.

Conflicts of Interest: The authors declare no conflict of interest.

References

1. Leggieri, A.; Attanasio, C.; Palladino, A.; Cellerino, A.; Lucini, C.; Paolucci, M.; Terzibasi Tozzini, E.; de Girolamo, P.; D'Angelo, L. Identification and Expression of Neurotrophin-6 in the Brain of Nothobranchius furzeri: One More Piece in Neurotrophin Research. *J. Clin. Med.* **2019**, *8*, 595. [CrossRef] [PubMed]
2. Lossi, L.; Castagna, C.; Granato, A.; Merighi, A. The Reeler Mouse: A Translational Model of Human Neurological Conditions, or Simply a Good Tool for Better Understanding Neurodevelopment? *J. Clin. Med.* **2019**, *8*, 2088. [CrossRef] [PubMed]

3. Montesano, A.; De Felice, E.; Leggieri, A.; Palladino, A.; Lucini, C.; Scocco, P.; de Girolamo, P.; Baumgart, M.; D'Angelo, L. Ontogenetic Pattern Changes of Nucleobindin-2/Nesfatin-1 in the Brain and Intestinal Bulb of the Short Lived African Turquoise Killifish. *J. Clin. Med.* **2020**, *9*, 103. [CrossRef] [PubMed]
4. Rey, V.; Menendez, S.T.; Estupiñan, O.; Rodriguez, A.; Santos, L.; Tornin, J.; Martinez-Cruzado, L.; Castillo, D.; Ordoñez, G.R.; Costilla, S.; et al. New Chondrosarcoma Cell Lines with Preserved Stem Cell Properties to Study the Genomic Drift During In Vitro/In Vivo Growth. *J. Clin. Med.* **2019**, *8*, 455. [CrossRef] [PubMed]
5. Dondossola, D.; Santini, A.; Lonati, C.; Zanella, A.; Merighi, R.; Vivona, L.; Battistin, M.; Galli, A.; Biancolilli, O.; Maggioni, M.; et al. Human Red Blood Cells as Oxygen Carriers to Improve Ex-Situ Liver Perfusion in a Rat Model. *J. Clin. Med.* **2019**, *8*, 1918. [CrossRef] [PubMed]
6. Fiordelisi, M.F.; Cavaliere, C.; Auletta, L.; Basso, L.; Salvatore, M. Magnetic Resonance Imaging for Translational Research in Oncology. *J. Clin. Med.* **2019**, *8*, 1883. [CrossRef] [PubMed]
7. Krzywinski, M.I.; Schein, J.E.; Birol, I.; Connors, J.; Gascoyne, R.; Horsman, D.; Jones, S.J.; Marra, M.A. Circos: An information aesthetic for comparative genomics. *Genome Res.* **2009**. [CrossRef] [PubMed]
8. Forte, E.; Fiorenza, D.; Torino, E.; Costagliola di Polidoro, A.; Cavaliere, C.; Netti, P.A.; Salvatore, M.; Aiello, M. Radiolabeled PET/MRI Nanoparticles for Tumor Imaging. *J. Clin. Med.* **2020**, *9*, 89. [CrossRef] [PubMed]
9. Palladino, A.; Mavaro, I.; Pizzoleo, C.; De Felice, E.; Lucini, C.; de Girolamo, P.; Netti, P.A.; Attanasio, C. Induced Pluripotent Stem Cells as Vasculature Forming Entities. *J. Clin. Med.* **2019**, *8*, 1782. [CrossRef] [PubMed]
10. Urciuolo, F.; Casale, C.; Imparato, G.; Netti, P.A. Bioengineered Skin Substitutes: The Role of Extracellular Matrix and Vascularization in the Healing of Deep Wounds. *J. Clin. Med.* **2019**, *8*, 2083. [CrossRef] [PubMed]
11. Salerno, A.; Cesarelli, G.; Pedram, P.; Netti, P.A. Modular Strategies to Build Cell-Free and Cell-Laden Scaffolds towards Bioengineered Tissues and Organs. *J. Clin. Med.* **2019**, *8*, 1816. [CrossRef] [PubMed]
12. Salaris, F.; Colosi, C.; Brighi, C.; Soloperto, A.; de Turris, V.; Benedetti, M.C.; Ghirga, S.; Rosito, M.; Di Angelantonio, S.; Rosa, A. 3D Bioprinted Human Cortical Neural Constructs Derived from Induced Pluripotent Stem Cells. *J. Clin. Med.* **2019**, *8*, 1595. [CrossRef] [PubMed]
13. Mazio, C.; Casale, C.; Imparato, G.; Urciuolo, F.; Attanasio, C.; De Gregorio, M.; Rescigno, F.; Netti, P.A. Pre-vascularized dermis model for fast and functional anastomosis with host vasculature. *Biomaterials* **2019**, *192*, 159–170. [CrossRef] [PubMed]
14. Corrado, B.; Gregorio, V.D.; Imparato, G.; Attanasio, C.; Urciuolo, F.; Netti, P.A. A three-dimensional microfluidized liver system to assess hepatic drug metabolism and hepatotoxicity. *Biotech. Bioeng.* **2019**, *116*, 1152–1163. [CrossRef] [PubMed]
15. Ceresa, C.D.L.; Nasralla, D.; Coussios, C.C.; Friend, P.J. The case for normothermic machine perfusion in liver transplantation. *Liver Transpl.* **2018**, *24*, 269–275. [CrossRef] [PubMed]
16. Geris, L.; Lambrechts, T.; Carlier, A.; Papantoniou, I. The future is digital: In silico tissue engineering. *Curr. Opin. Biomed. Eng.* **2018**, *6*, 92–98. [CrossRef]
17. Karolak, A.; Markov, D.A.; McCawley, L.J.; Rejniak, K.A. Towards personalized computational oncology: from spatial models of tumour spheroids, to organoids, to tissues. *J. R. Soc. Interface* **2018**, *15*, 20170703. [CrossRef] [PubMed]
18. Soleimani, S.; Shamsi, M.; Ghazani, M.A.; Modarres, H.P.; Valente, K.P.; Saghafian, M.; Ashani, M.M.; Akbari, M.; Sanati-Nezhad, A. Translational models of tumor angiogenesis: A nexus of in silico and in vitro models. *Biotech. Adv.* **2018**, *36*, 880–893. [CrossRef] [PubMed]
19. Attanasio, C.; Latancia, M.T.; Otterbein, L.E.; Netti, P.A. Update on Renal Replacement Therapy: Implantable Artificial Devices and Bioengineered Organs. *Tissue Eng. B Rev.* **2016**, *22*, 330–340. [CrossRef] [PubMed]
20. Antonelli, L.; Guarracino, M.R.; Maddalena, L.; Sangiovanni, M. Integrating imaging and omics data: A review. *Biomed. Signal Process. Control* **2019**, *52*, 264–280. [CrossRef]

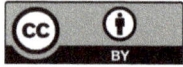

© 2020 by the authors. Licensee MDPI, Basel, Switzerland. This article is an open access article distributed under the terms and conditions of the Creative Commons Attribution (CC BY) license (http://creativecommons.org/licenses/by/4.0/).

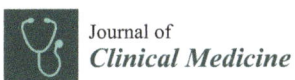
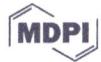

Review

The *Reeler* Mouse: A Translational Model of Human Neurological Conditions, or Simply a Good Tool for Better Understanding Neurodevelopment?

Laura Lossi [1], Claudia Castagna [1], Alberto Granato [2,*] and Adalberto Merighi [1,*]

1. Department of Veterinary Sciences, University of Turin, I-10095 Grugliasco (TO), Italy; laura.lossi@unito.it (L.L.); claudia.castagna@unito.it (C.C.)
2. Department of Psychology, Catholic University of the Sacred Heart, I-20123 Milano (MI), Italy
* Correspondence: alberto.granato@unicatt.it (A.G.); adalberto.merighi@unito.it (A.M.); Tel.: +39-02-7234-8588 (A.G.); +39-011-670-9118 (A.M.)

Received: 9 October 2019; Accepted: 28 November 2019; Published: 1 December 2019

Abstract: The first description of the *Reeler* mutation in mouse dates to more than fifty years ago, and later, its causative gene (*reln*) was discovered in mouse, and its human orthologue (*RELN*) was demonstrated to be causative of lissencephaly 2 (LIS2) and about 20% of the cases of autosomal-dominant lateral temporal epilepsy (ADLTE). In both human and mice, the gene encodes for a glycoprotein referred to as reelin (Reln) that plays a primary function in neuronal migration during development and synaptic stabilization in adulthood. Besides LIS2 and ADLTE, *RELN* and/or other genes coding for the proteins of the Reln intracellular cascade have been associated substantially to other conditions such as spinocerebellar ataxia type 7 and 37, *VLDLR*-associated cerebellar hypoplasia, *PAFAH1B1*-associated lissencephaly, autism, and schizophrenia. According to their modalities of inheritances and with significant differences among each other, these neuropsychiatric disorders can be modeled in the homozygous ($reln^{-/-}$) or heterozygous ($reln^{+/-}$) *Reeler* mouse. The worth of these mice as translational models is discussed, with focus on their construct and face validity. Description of face validity, i.e., the resemblance of phenotypes between the two species, centers onto the histological, neurochemical, and functional observations in the cerebral cortex, hippocampus, and cerebellum of *Reeler* mice and their human counterparts.

Keywords: reelin; LIS2; ADLTE; autism; schizophrenia; translational models; GABAergic interneurons; dendritic spines; forebrain; cerebellum

1. Introduction

Neuronal migration and precise setting during neurogenesis depend, among others, on reelin (Reln), a 388 kDa glycoprotein secreted by certain neurons within the extracellular matrix [1,2]. The name was given to the protein after the detection of its coding gene, and the acknowledgement that its lack was causative of the mouse *Reeler* mutation [3], which was described, about half a century before, consisting in a form of ataxia [4]. The mutation is autosomic and shows recessive transmission. Consequently, only homozygous recessive *Reeler* mice ($reln^{-/-}$) are totally devoid of Reln and have a definite phenotype. Behaviorally, the latter consists of dystonia, ataxia, and tremor; structurally it primarily affects the design of the cerebral cortex, hippocampus, and cerebellum [5,6]. Contrarily to the mutants, the phenotype of heterozygous *Reeler* mice ($reln^{+/-}$) is normal, but, interestingly, these animals may be translational models of certain human neuropsychiatric disorders [7].

Shortly after the original discovery, it became clear that the mouse gene (*reln*) had a very high homology to that in humans (*RELN*) [8]. Then, a few years later, it was shown that autosomic recessive mutations of the *RELN* gene were linked to a form of lissencephaly with cerebellar hypoplasia (LCH) [9], with associated findings suggested that *RELN* was linked to some neuropsychiatric conditions [10], and *RELN* was demonstrated to be reduced in the cerebellum of autistic patients after Western blotting and immunodetection [11].

Determining a good translational mouse model for a neuropsychiatric condition needs construct, predictive, and face validity [12]. Rigorously, construct validity only relates to transgenic mice, but, in a broader definition, it also comprehends the syndromic models and the spontaneous DNA mutations linked to the phenotype under study. In other words, this factor defines the similarity of the disease between the mouse and the human disorder in terms of the causal gene(s) as e.g., deducted from gene association and linkage analysis. As mentioned above, LCH is a human monogenic condition caused by a mutation in *RELN*. Therefore, the *Reeler* mouse fully meets the criterion of construct validity for the condition. There is also evidence for genetics to be associated with the etiology of several neuropsychiatric conditions, such as autism and schizophrenia, but, as the result of their multidimensional clinical symptoms, causal gene(s), if any, persist to be undiscovered [13]. Nonetheless, there are numerous genes associated with the human autistic pathology after analysis of Mendelian disorders (syndromes), rare mutations, or association studies; see e.g., [14].

Predictive validity, i.e., the similarity of the response to cures in humans and mice is difficult to establish, in the nonexistence of a recognized therapy in humans [14]. Thus, in the context of this discussion, face validity, i.e., the resemblance of the model phenotype to that of the human disorder, is the most important parameter to consider.

Assessment of face validity in neuroscience translational studies requires a careful consideration of their behavioral and structural phenotypes. Broadly speaking, there are contradictory opinions as regarding the repetition in mouse of the human behavioral neuropsychiatric changes. This was, to some extent, predictable, as only a few trials, such as e.g., pre-pulse inhibition (PPI), which records sensory-motor responses, are highly comparable with only minimal modifications in the two species [15]. Notably, the issue has been the subject of several reviews on rodent models of autism, e.g., [16]. The conclusion of these surveys was that, although most of the models that have been used in drug discovery display behaviors with face validity for the human symptoms (i.e., deficits in social communication and restricted interests/repetitive behaviors), many drugs that were found to be useful in ameliorating these autism-related behaviors in mice were ineffective in humans.

Therefore, it becomes imperative to compare the structural alterations of the brains in the two species to substantiate or invalidate the models. We here summarize the state-of-art knowledge on the translational validity of homozygous ($reln^{-/-}$) and heterozygous ($reln^{+/-}$) *Reeler* mice with reference to the most common neuropsychiatric conditions directly or indirectly related to *RELN*. Because of its importance, we will primarily focus onto the brain structural modifications at magnetic resonance imaging (MRI) and histopathology in the two species.

2. The Reelin Gene and Protein

In humans, *RELN*, which has 94.2% homology with the mouse orthologue [8], is in chromosome 7q22 [17] and encodes for REELIN (RELN), a large glycoprotein of the extracellular matrix. The murine gene (*reln*) that also encodes for Reelin (Reln) was originally identified as the mutated gene in the *Reeler* mouse, which displays, among others, irregular lamination of the cerebral and cerebellar cortices, with an inversion of the regular 'inside-out' design observed in mammals [3,18]. The mouse and the human proteins have a similar size of 388 kDa. The structure of the protein recalls that of certain cell adhesion molecules, which specific cell types produce during brain and spinal cord development.

In the neocortex, the Cajal–Retzius cells synthesize the glycoprotein and secrete it into the extracellular space [19]. Then, in post mitotic migrating neurons, Reln activates a specific signaling pathway that is required for proper positioning of these neurons. Northern blot hybridization showed that other areas of the fetal and postnatal brain also express the protein, with levels particularly high in cerebellum.

Reln is part of a signal transduction pathway that includes the apolipoprotein E2 (ApoER2), the very low-density lipoprotein receptors (VLDLR) and the cytoplasmic protein Dab1 [20]. Notably, the brain phenotype of mice with disruptions of *mDab1* or of both *apoER2* and *vldlr* closely resemble the brain of the *Reeler* mouse [21]. Another gene that interacts with the components of the Reln signaling pathways is platelet-activating factor acetyl hydrolase IB subunit α *(PAFAH1B1)*, also referred to as *LIS1* [22].

3. *RELN*-Related Human Neurological Conditions and Their Mouse Counterparts

Several human neurological conditions have a direct or indirect link with *RELN* and its encoded protein, as well as with the components of the RELN signaling pathway (Figure 1 and Table 1). We will briefly describe these conditions below, aiming to put in the better perspective those features that may be useful for well understanding the translational relevance of the *Reeler* mouse.

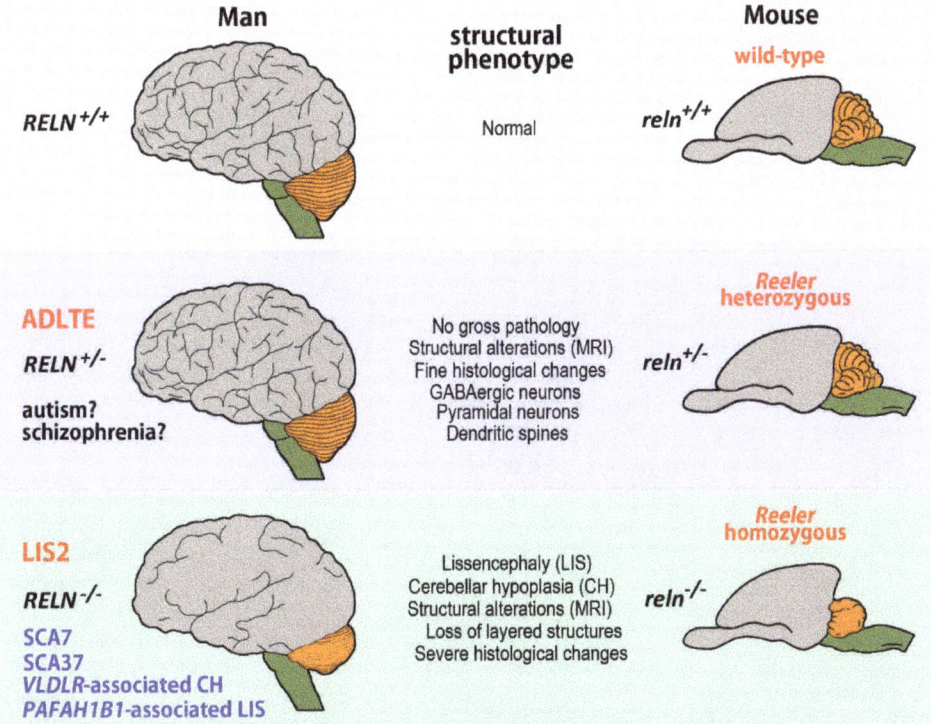

Figure 1. Summary of the most relevant human pathologies modeled in the *Reeler* mouse. The monogenic conditions provoked by the *RELN* gene, i.e., ADLTE and LIS2, are in red, those related to genes encoding for the proteins of the Reln intracellular cascade or only tentatively linked to RELN are indicated in blue. Autism and schizophrenia, which have a complex multifactorial etiology, are in black with an interrogative mark to underline the still tentative association of the two disorders with *RELN*. Abbreviations: ADLTE autosomal-dominant lateral temporal epilepsy, LIS2 lissencephaly 2, PAFAH1B1 platelet-activating factor acetyl hydrolase IB subunit α, *RELN* reelin gene (human), *reln* reelin gene (mouse), SCA37 spinocerebellar ataxia type 37, SCA7 spinocerebellar ataxia type 7, VLDLR very low-density lipoprotein receptor.

Table 1. Summary list of the human neurological conditions related to the *RELN* gene.

Disease	Transmission	Causative Gene(s)	*Reeler* Mutants of Translational Interest	Other Mouse Models
LIS 2	Autosomal recessive	*RELN*	Homozygous	see text
ADLTE	Autosomal dominant	*RELN* (in 17.5% of cases)	Heterozygous	*LG11*-mutated
VLDLR-associated cerebellar hypoplasia	Autosomal recessive	*VLDLR*	Homozygous	*VLDLR* knock-out
SCA37	Autosomal dominant	*DAB1*	Homozygous	*DAB1* knock-out *apoER2* knock-out
PAFAH1B1-associated lissencephaly	Autosomal dominant	*PAFAH1B1*	Homozygous	*Lis1*$^{+/-}$
SCA7	Autosomal dominant	*ATXN7*	Homozygous	SCA7 knock-in
Autism	Isolated cases Multifactorial	see https://omim.org # 209850	Heterozygous	see text
Schizophrenia	Autosomal dominant	see https://omim.org # 181500	Heterozygous	see text

Note that only LIS2 and autosomal-dominant lateral temporal epilepsy (ADLTE) have a demonstrated link with *RELN*. *RELN* may be relevant for *LIS1*.

3.1. Neurological Conditions Caused by RELN Mutations

Several diseases are based on mutations of *RELN* or of genes encoding for proteins associated with the RELN signaling pathways. Among these, lissencephaly 2 (LIS2) and autosomal-dominant lateral temporal epilepsy (ADLTE) are of relevance to the present discussion as they have a clear genetic link with *RELN*.

3.1.1. Human Lissencephalies and the Homozygous *Reeler* Mouse

Human lissencephalies are a group of cortical malformations that are consequent to neuronal migration disorders. Broadly speaking, the structural phenotype in lissencephalies ranges from a thickened cortex and complete absence of sulci (agyria) to a thickened cortex with a few, shallow sulci (pachygyria) [23]. The main feature of classic lissencephaly, formerly referred to as type I lissencephaly but today named lissencephaly 1 (LIS1), is a marked thickening of the cerebral cortex with a posterior to anterior grade of severity. An anomalous neuronal migration in the interval between the ninth to the thirteenth week of pregnancy causes LIS1, resulting in an assortment of agyria, mixed agyria/pachygyria, and pachygyria. An abnormally thick and ill ordered cortex with four highly disorganized layers, diffuse neuronal heterotopia, enlarged cerebral ventricles of anomalous shape, and, often, hypoplasia of the corpus callosum are typical of LIS1 [24]. The basal ganglia are normal, except that the anterior limb of the internal capsule is usually not noticeable, and, most often, the cerebellum is normal as well.

Lissencephalies are now classified based on brain imaging results and molecular investigation [25], as they have been associated with mutations in several genes such as *LIS1* (*PAFAH1B1*; MIM#601545), *DCX* (Doublecortin; MIM#300121), *ARX* (Aristaless-related homeobox gene; MIM#300382), *RELN* (Reelin; MIM#600514), *VLDLR* (MIM#224050) and *TUBA1A* (αtubulin 1a) [26]. Some rare forms of lissencephaly (LCH) are associated with a disproportionately small cerebellum.

Lissencephaly 2

a) Humans

Lissencephaly 2 (LIS2) also referred to lissencephaly syndrome, Norman–Roberts type or Norman–Roberts syndrome (OMIM #257320) is associated with *LIS1* but displays several specific clinical features. In 2000, Hong and colleagues were the first to describe an autosomal recessive form of lissencephaly that, at MRI, also exhibited severe alterations of the cerebellum, hippocampus, and brainstem. More specifically, these alterations consisted of a thickening of the cerebral cortex with a simplified convolutional pattern that was particularly evident in the frontal and temporal lobes, whereas the parietal and occipital lobes were almost normal. The hippocampus was unfolded and flattened, lacking definable upper and lower blades. The corpus callosum was thin and the lateral ventricles enlarged. The cerebellum was clearly smaller than in the normal brain, hypoplastic, and devoid of folia. Authors also showed that the responsible gene mapped to chromosome 7q22 and that the condition was associated with two independent mutations in *RELN*, resulting in low or undetectable amounts of RELN after Western blots analysis of the patients' serum [9]. Two other unrelated groups of patients, later, presented the same type of LIS2 [27]. They were children that, at MRI, displayed a 5–10 mm thick cerebral cortex, a malformed hippocampus and a very hypoplastic cerebellum, almost completely devoid of folia. As LIS2 is a rare disease, there are very limited histopathological data on the condition. To our knowledge, the only post-mortem description of a male fetus with Norman–Roberts syndrome reported the occurrence of a four-layered cerebral cortex (Figure 2A,B), a well-developed cerebellum with organized folia, and heterotopia of the dentate nucleus [28].

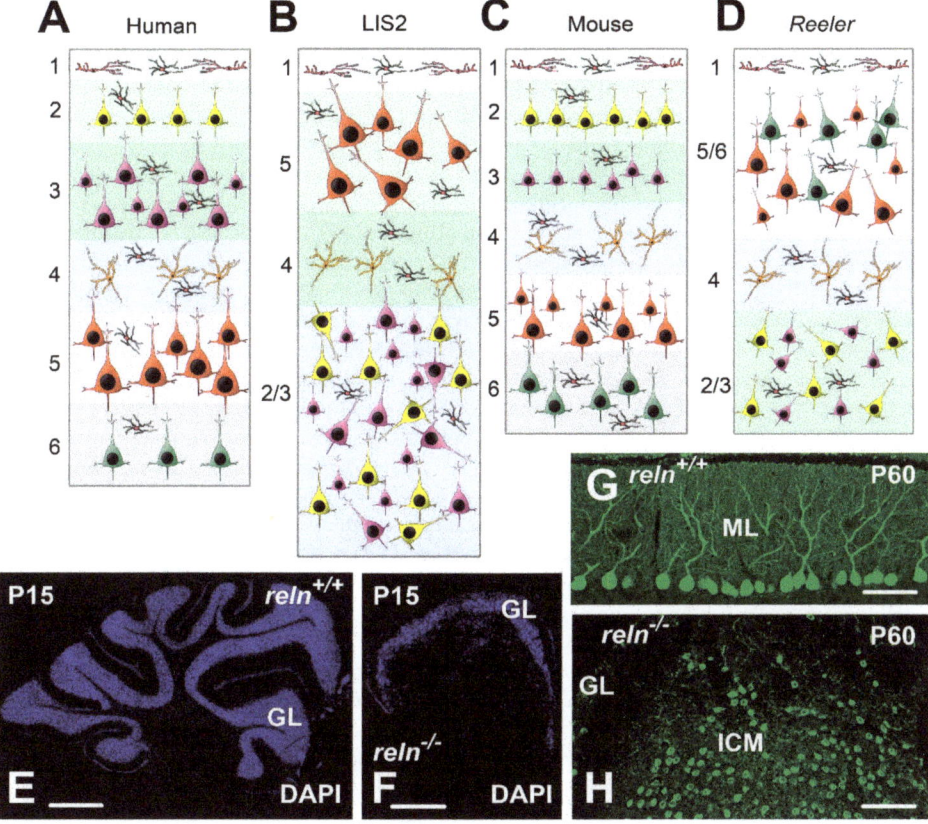

Figure 2. Structural alterations in human, LIS2, and homozygous *Reeler* mouse (**A–D**); modifications of the neocortex architecture in human LIS2 (**B**); and *Reeler* mutation (**D**); compared to healthy controls (**A**,**C**). After MRI imaging, the human LIS2 cortex is thicker than normal, whereas there are apparently no thickness changes in mouse. Note that in both species the pathological neocortex only consists of four layers, with an upside-down layer disposition mainly affecting the pyramidal neurons that are also irregularly oriented compared to their usual positioning in normal individuals/mice. Pyramidal neurons are in different color and sizes according to their position in cortical layers. Stellate spiny cells of layer 4 are orange. Inhibitory interneurons are black with a red nucleus. Cajal-Retzius cells of layer 1 are red.

(**E–H**): Structural alterations in the *Reeler* mouse cerebellum; (**E**) sagittal sections of the P15 cerebellum in a normal *reln*$^{+/+}$ mouse; and (**F**) a *Reeler reln*$^{-/-}$ mouse: the *Reeler* cerebellum is much smaller and devoid of folia, with a smooth surface. (**G**) Misalignment of the Purkinje neurons in the P60 cerebellum of the *Reeler* mouse. After calbindin 28 kDa immunostaining, the Purkinje neurons are well aligned in a monolayer below the molecular layer in *reln*$^{+/+}$ mice. They, instead, form a large internal cellular mass within the white matter in *reln*$^{-/-}$ mutants (**H**). Abbreviations: DAPI = 4′,6-Diamidine-2′-phenylindole; GL = granular layer of the cerebellar cortex; ICM = internal cellular mass; ML = molecular layer of the cerebellar cortex; P = postnatal day.

b) *Reeler* Homozygous Mice

Alterations in *Reeler* homozygous recessive mice fully recapitulate those in human LIS2 (Figure 1). Due to obvious technical and practical reasons, the amount of MRI data in mouse is by far less abundant than in patients, whereas mice have provided extensive histopathological information. The first MRI description of the neuroanatomical phenotypes in homozygous (and heterozygous) mice using morphometry and texture analysis, led to conclude that the structural features of the *Reeler* brain most closely copied the MRI phenotype of LIS2 patients [29]. Indeed, the *reln*$^{-/-}$ mice had a smaller brain, but larger lateral ventricles compared to wild-type littermates. Sharp differences existed in the olfactory bulbs, dorsomedial frontal and parietal cortex, certain districts of the temporal and occipital lobes, and the ventral hippocampus where gadolinium-based active staining demonstrated a general disorganization with differences in the thickness of individual hippocampal layers. The cerebellum also resulted profoundly affected by the mutation and appeared strongly hypoplastic. A subsequent study, based on the use of manganese-enhanced MRI (MEMRI) to better detect the cortical laminar architecture, compared the MEMRI signal intensity in the cerebral cortex of normal and mutant mice. The authors of this survey observed that signal was low in cortical layer 1, increased in layer 2, decreased in layer 3 until mid-layer 4, and increased again, peaking in layer 5, before decreasing through layer 6. In *Reeler* there were, instead, no appreciable changes in signal intensity, an observation consistent with the absence of cortical lamination after histological examination [30]. A more recent and very elegant study has employed diffusion tractography imaging (DTI) to perform an in vivo origin-to-ending reconstruction of the mouse somatosensory thalamo-cortical connections and demonstrated an extensive remodeling in *Reeler* mutants because of the highly disorganized cortical lamination [31].

In keeping with the results of imaging studies, at gross anatomical examination the *reln*$^{-/-}$ mouse brain was atrophic, as total volume in mutants decreased of about 19% when compared to normal mice [29]. Such a reduction was particularly evident in the cerebellum (Figure 2E,F) that also displayed a very limited degree of foliation. Therefore, also the gross anatomy of the *Reeler* brain closely resembled that of the LIS2 human brain.

In general, it seems that the histological anomalies in mutants depended on an abnormal migration of neurons, rather than an alteration in cell fate determination or axonal guidance. Among these anomalies, the most distinguishing ones are that the cerebral and cerebellar cortices lose their layered structure, in accordance with the MEMRI observations [30]; numerous neuronal nuclei disappeared or, at least, became hardly recognizable in several brain regions; and neurons often displayed an ectopic position. Table 2 summarizes the most important structural anomalies of the *reln*$^{-/-}$ CNS without taking into consideration the histological alterations in the cerebral cortex, hippocampus and cerebellum, as we will analytically discuss the phenotype of these brain areas in the following sections. Detailed descriptions of the morphological phenotype of the *Reeler* mouse CNS can be found e.g., in [29,32].

Table 2. Main histopathological changes in the homozygous *Reeler* mouse.

Division of CNS	Region/Division	Subdivision/Nucleus	Type(s) of Alteration	Ref
Forebrain	Olfactory bulb		• Slight disruption of the glomerular layer. • Numerical reduction and clustering of granule cells	[33,34]
	Striatum		• Decreased PV-immunoreactivity	[35]
	Diencephalon		• Misrouting of GnRH neurons to the cerebral cortex	[36]
		Mammilary bodies	• Alteration of projections to hippocampus	[37]
Midbrain	Rostral colliculus		• Loss of individual limits in the three more superficial layers • Spread of corticotectal projections • Anomalies of retinotectal projections	[38]
	Mesencephalic nucleus of V		• Spread of neurons along their route of migration	[39]
	Substantia nigra		• Anomalous clustering lateral to the ventral tegmental area	[40]
	Medulla oblongata and pons	Dorsal cochlear nucleus	• Partial loss of layered organization	[41]
		Inferior olivary nucleus	• Loss of folding - Swelling	[42]
		Somatic motorneurons (Nucleus ambiguous, facial and trigeminal)	• Slight displacement and loss of somatotopic organization (muscolotopy)	[6,43]
		Pontine nuclei	• Ventral shift	[44]
Spinal cord	Dorsal horn (laminae I-II)	Nociceptive	• Abnormal neuronal positioning	[45]
	Lateral horn	Preganglionic sympathetic and parasympathetic neurons	• Abnormal neuronal positioning	[46,47]

The Table does not list the histopathological observations on cerebral cortex, hippocampus, and cerebellum.

Very early observations demonstrated the occurrence of dendritic anomalies in cortical and hippocampal neurons of *Reeler* mice [48,49]. The discovery of *Reln* confirmed the dendritic pathology, as not only Reln but also the molecules of its signaling pathway resulted to be necessary for the correct maturation and differentiation of the dendritic branches and spines in hippocampal and neocortical pyramidal neurons [50,51].

Due to the complexity of the phenomena involved in dendritic maturation, one can argue that dendritic anomalies represented a consequence of the deep cytoarchitectonic derangement occurring in *Reeler* mice rather than a primary effect of the lack of Reln, but observations on heterozygous mice were not supportive of this interpretation [52,53]. Interestingly, the block of the Reln signaling by means of specific antibodies resulted in an increased complexity of branching in the apical dendrites of layer 2/3 cortical pyramidal neurons, whereas their basal arborizations remained unaffected [54].

There are many important issues related to the structure and role of the dendritic tree of neocortical and hippocampal pyramidal neurons that make the *Reeler* mouse an important tool for the study of (forebrain) neurodevelopment. Inputs to layer 5 neurons are processed by separate compartments, with the basal dendrites receiving bottom-up information and the apical dendrite being the recipient of a feedback input from higher cortical areas, see e.g., [55]. This framework is, however, even more complex because apical dendrites span most cortical layers before reaching layer 1, where the apical tuft is located [56]. Today we know well that the type and distribution of ion channels at the neurolemma ultimately determine the electrophysiological properties of a neuron.

Essential to the function of the long apical dendrite of the pyramidal neurons is the progressively increasing density of hyperpolarization-activated cyclic nucleotide–gated (HCN) channels, proceeding from proximal to distal segments [57]. Such a gradient critically contributes to the functional distinction between dendritic compartments. Although Reln signaling specifies this gradient [58], 17β-estradiol, which stimulates Reln expression, promoted the enrichment of HCN1 in the distal dendritic compartment of CA1 neurons without the intervention of Reln [59]. The evidence that Reln was involved in the trafficking and targeting of ion channels in cortical and hippocampal neurons suggested that their intrinsic electrophysiological properties could indeed be different in the *Reeler* mouse. However, an early study by Bliss and Chung [60] demonstrated that, despite the layering derangement, the basic synaptic organization of the hippocampus was largely unchanged in mutants.

More recently, Silva et al. [61] carried out an accurate survey dealing with the intrinsic electrophysiological properties of cortical neurons in *Reeler* mice. These authors showed that the firing pattern and synaptic responses of the pyramidal neurons were normal, but with an inverted radial distribution. Notably, these authors concluded that, although mispositioned, neurons maintained the membrane properties appropriate to their function.

The apparent discrepancy between the data demonstrating the role of Reln in the modulation of ion channels and the relative lack of anomalies in the intrinsic properties of cortical neurons in mutant mice might have several explanations. Other factors, such as neuronal activity [62] could be more effective than Reln for the modulation of membrane channel targeting. Furthermore, the complex machinery of the long apical dendrite is required when layer 5 neurons settle appropriately but might be useless for the same neurons displaced to more superficial cortical layers. Finally, future investigations based on refined electrophysiological techniques, such as direct dendritic recordings, will help to establish if indeed the cortical neurons in *Reeler* mice display subtler changes of their firing/intrinsic properties that those so far ascertained.

Reln signaling is also able to modulate key molecules of the cascade leading to synaptic plasticity, such as the NMDA receptors [63,64]. Therefore, several studies concentrated on the changes of synaptic plasticity in *Reeler* mutants. Ishida et al. [65] reported that the induction of long-term potentiation (LTP) was impaired in the CA1 region of the hippocampus, claiming that the malpositioning of some neuronal populations could account for such an alteration. On the other hand, both the overexpression of Reln in transgenic mice [66] and Reln supplementation strongly increased LTP [67]. Later, a defective LTP was observed in the hippocampus of *vldr*-deficient mice, but slice perfusion with Reln was able to enhance LTP in CA1 [68].

Most cortical neurons are spiny, glutamatergic pyramidal cells, whose migratory path during prenatal development follows an inside-out radial pattern from the ventricular zone to the final position [69]. Reln signaling is essential for the localization of pyramidal neurons to appropriate cortical layers, as reviewed in [70]. Consequently, the lack of Reln caused a disruption of the layered cortical organization, including abnormal positioning [71,72], as well as an increased percentage of inverted pyramidal cells [73,74] (Figure 2C,D).

Inhibitory GABAergic interneurons represent a minority population within the neocortex. Yet, their morphological, neurochemical and functional diversity likely plays a key role for the cortical function, see e.g., [75]. Unlike pyramidal neurons, interneurons originate in the ganglionic eminence of the ventral telencephalon and follow a tangential migratory path to the cortex [69]. While the malpositioning of the pyramidal neurons in *Reeler* mice is evident, it is not clear if the Reln signaling cascade also affects the migration of the interneurons. An answer to this latter issue came from observations on *Reeler* mutants crossed with mice expressing the green fluorescent protein (GFP) in inhibitory neurons. Thus, the results of these observations confirmed that also the cortical interneurons displayed an abnormal laminar position and morphology [76]. However, we still do not know whether interneurons' ectopy directly depends from Reln signaling or is rather the consequence of the malpositioning of principal pyramidal projection neurons. The debate on this issue is still open, as contradictory views exist in the literature. Namely, while some observations [77,78] argue against a direct role of Reln,

Hammond et al. [79] showed that only early-generated cortical interneurons were misplaced as a consequence of the ectopy of the pyramidal neurons, whereas the correct layering of late-generated interneurons seemed to be directly modulated by Reln signaling.

Other basic neurodevelopmental features, such as cortical [80] and cerebellar neurogenesis, seem to be as well regulated by the glycoprotein. Consequently, the minicolumnar organization of the cerebral neocortex appeared to be deeply affected by Reln deficiency [81] and some physiological counterparts of cortical connectivity, such as trans-synaptic signal propagation, were also impaired [82]. However, the outcome of Reln deficiency on the microcircuitry sustaining the cortical machinery is controversial and, surprisingly, the deep architectonic disorganization that follows the lack of the protein occurs in the absence of dramatic functional anomalies. Both early and more recent studies point out that the absence of Reln did not prevent the development of functionally appropriate cortical connections and maps [31,83–86]. In addition, when studied at the fine-scale electron microscopic level, the basic synaptic organization of misplaced cortical neurons was unchanged [87]. Therefore, although the laminar organization is thought to be critical for cortical computation [88,89], evidences obtained in *Reeler* mice led Guy and Staiger [90] to challenge the importance of cortical lamination, affirming that "future studies directed toward understanding cortical functions should rather focus on circuits specified by functional cell type composition than mere laminar location".

Macroscopically, the cerebellum of the *Reeler* mouse is smaller than that of age-matched littermates (Figure 2E,F); it is club-shaped with the main axis transverse to the mid plan of the body, and has an almost completely smooth surface, with just a few superficial grooves [91]. The architecture of the *Reeler* cerebellum is profoundly different from the normal pattern, firstly because of the impairment in the complicated series of migrations made by neurons to reach their destination in the mature organ. Trajectories of migrating neurons follow two opposite directions from the surface to the depth of the cerebellum and the other way around, depending from the species, the type(s) of neurons and the developmental stages (for details see e.g., [92]). Eventually, disturbances in the migration of the cerebellar neurons make that *Reeler* mice display a cerebellum that retains several features of immaturity.

The area of the cerebellar cortex in mutants was analyzed quantitatively during postnatal (P0–P25) development and resulted to be reduced compared to age-matched controls [93]. Reduction in the extension of the cortex was particularly evident in the molecular layer and the (internal) granular layer. Physiologically, as the cerebellum matured, the molecular layer became more and more populated by the parallel fibers, but, at P25, its increase in size was about one third in the mutants compared to $reln^{+/+}$ mice [93]. Post-migratory granule cells, which are born in the temporary subpial external granular layer, progressively populate the (internal) granular layer during normal cerebellar development. This process was disturbed in *Reeler*, to the extent that, from P0 to P10, the granular layer of $reln^{+/+}$ mice increased about five-folds in size, but only 2.6-fold in $reln^{-/-}$, where it was significantly reduced in size to 0.62-fold that of normal mice after P10 [93]. In a different way from the cortex, the medullary body was larger in the mutants than in wild-type mice. Its progressively increasing area mainly reflected the ongoing myelination of the axons of the Purkinje neurons that abandon the cortex moving across the white matter to reach the cerebellar nuclei, as well as the expansion of the incoming afferent and departing efferent fiber systems. The mass of the medullary body augmented in relation to postnatal age irrespectively of the lack of Reln ($reln^{-/-}$ 2.59, $reln^{+/+}$ 1.93-fold), but, at P25, *Reeler* mice had a larger medullary body than normal mice (1.88-fold) [93]. In brief, *Reeler* mice had a reduced cerebellar cortex but a bigger medullary body than their $reln^{+/+}$ littermates. The cerebellar hypoplasia was thus a consequence of a reduction in cortical magnitude and cellularity and the latter, in turn, resulted to be associated to measurable differences in the degree of cell proliferation and apoptosis, as well as imbalances in the timing of postnatal cortical maturation [93]. The same study led to conclude that density of proliferating cells was the most significant predictive factor to determine the cortical cellularity in *Reeler* [93]. Therefore, beside the well-defined consequences onto neuronal migration, the lack of Reln also caused a calculable deficit in neuronal expansion. Ultrastructurally, the cerebellar neurons underwent several different forms of programmed cell death during postnatal development and the deficit of Reln affected the kind and grade of neuronal death [94].

Perhaps the most striking histological feature in mutants is the lack of alignment of the Purkinje neurons to form a discrete intermediate layer in the cerebellar cortex (Figure 2G,H). Thus, in *Reeler*, only about 5% of the Purkinje neurons were in a normal position, 10% were still inside the cortex but in the granular layer, and the remaining 85% formed an internal cellular mass intermixed with the white matter [95–97]. Ultrastructurally, in *Reeler* there was a reduction in the density of the contacts between the Purkinje neurons and the parallel and climbing fibers, from P5 onward [98]. Functionally, both the normally placed Purkinje neurons and those ectopically dislocated in the granular layer displayed a 0–1 response to stimulation, indicating that, as in normal mice, they received a synaptic contact by a single climbing fiber. The Purkinje neurons in the internal cellular mass, instead, showed intensity-graded responses to electrical stimulation, as several climbing fibers provided them with a convergent input [95], likely as a failure of physiological pruning to occur [99]. Neurochemically, there were no obvious variations between normal mice and the mutants in the temporal expression of some widely diffused neuronal and glial markers (NeuN, vimentin, calbindin, GFAP, Smi32, GAD67) during postnatal development [93], but the Bergmann glia was misplaced in *Reeler* [100].

To conclude, the histological and electrophysiological observations in *Reeler* mutants suggest that similar structural and functional alterations may also occur in LIS2 patients, particularly in relation to the postnatal growth retardation, severe intellectual disability, and spasticity observed in affected subjects (see also https://www.orpha.net/).

Lissencephaly 3

TUBA1A mutations [101,102] cause lissencephaly 3 (LIS3), another human condition that has a mouse counterpart. TUBA1A chiefly occurs in cortical, hippocampal, cerebellar and brainstem post-mitotic neurons, with expression falling soon after birth but persisting through adulthood [103]. The mouse phenotype consists, among others, in a failure of the cerebellar Purkinje neurons to migrate, so that, similarly to *Reeler*, they remain entrapped into the medullary body, where they form a series of streaks intermingled with the neurons of the cerebellar nuclei [104]. Several other mutations of *TUBA1A* exist in humans. They give rise to a predominant phenotype of LCH, which also shows irregularities of the corpus callosum and the basal ganglia/internal capsule [105].

3.1.2. Autosomal-Dominant Lateral Temporal Epilepsy and the Heterozygous *Reeler* Mouse

ADLTE, also referred to as autosomal dominant epilepsy with auditory features, partial epilepsy with auditory aura or partial epilepsy with auditory features, is a genetic epileptic syndrome, clinically showing typical focal seizures in response to specific sounds. ADLTE is genetically heterogeneous, and mutations in the leucine-rich, glioma inactivated 1 gene (*LGI1*) account for fewer than 50% of affected families. Very recent observations demonstrated that heterozygous *RELN* mutations give rise to a classic ADLTE syndrome, clinically identical to that associated with mutations of *LGI1*. Seven different heterozygous missense mutations in *RELN* were, in fact, described in some unrelated families of Italian ancestry with familial temporal lobe epilepsy-7 (ETL7–OMIM #616436) [106]. Incidence was 17.5% over the total number of families studied that were specifically suffering by lateral temporal lobe epilepsy [106]. By three-dimensional modeling, the same authors anticipated that the outcomes of these mutations would be protein structural defects and misfolding. Some of the affected individuals displayed a reduction up to 50% of their serum levels of the 310 kDa RELN isoform in comparison to healthy subjects and thus, very likely, the mutations also resulted in a loss of function. In a subsequent study on the same patients, 1.5 T MRI scans were not useful in detecting structural anomalies of the brain [107]. Similarly, in a very recent study on an 18-year old ADLTE patient, 3T MRI brain scans could not provide relevant information on indistinct grey-white matter connections, voxel-based morphometry, and cortical thickness [108]. However, analysis of functional connectivity with high-density electroencephalography (HdEEG) revealed greater local synchrony in the left temporal (middle temporal gyrus), left frontal (supplementary motor area, superior frontal gyrus), and left parietal (gyrus angularis, gyrus supramarginalis) regions of the cerebral cortex and the cingulate cortex (middle cingulate gyrus) as compared to normal subjects [108].

As the discovery of RELN mutations in ADLTE is a quite recent finding, there are, at present, no observations on heterozygous *Reeler* mice focused to ascertain possible similarities with the human phenotype. Like ADLTE patients, $reln^{+/-}$ mice display a 50% reduction of Reln in their serum. Therefore, it would be interesting to investigate whether sound-triggered epileptic manifestations also occur in these animals. A very recent study has demonstrated that optogenetic stimulation of the parvalbumin (PV) immunoreactive GABAergic neurons of the mouse basal forebrain can modulate the cortical topography of auditory steady-state responses [109]. As the regional distribution of these neurons displayed relevant differences in $reln^{+/-}$ mice compared to wild-type animals [110,111], any phenotypic alteration may be of interest to shed additional light onto human ADLTE. Finally, a very latest report has provided proof of concept that HdEEG can be used to record electrical activity from the mouse brain in a model of juvenile myoclonic epilepsy [112]. Therefore, one can envisage applying such an approach to analyze the brain electrical pattern in $reln^{+/-}$ mice aiming to collect data for translational comparison with ADLTE.

3.2. Human Conditions Caused by Mutations of Genes of the Reln Intracellular Pathway and Their Mouse Correlates

In general, the brain phenotype of the human monogenetic conditions that are consequent to mutations of the genes coding for the proteins of the RELN intracellular signaling pathway is similar to that of the $reln^{-/-}$ mouse brain, except that, in certain cases, differently from *Reeler*, the human cerebellum is normal at MRI and gross anatomical observation (Figure 1). We will briefly describe these conditions below.

3.2.1. VLDLR-Associated Cerebellar Hypoplasia

VLDLR-associated cerebellar hypoplasia is an autosomal recessive genetic form of non-progressive congenital ataxia [113]. The main clinical symptom of the condition is a predominantly truncal ataxia with retarded ambulation, so that children either learn to walk after six years of age or never walk without aid. Dysarthria, strabismus, moderate-to-profound intellectual disability, and seizures are other features of the disorder. MRI findings comprise hypoplasia of the inferior portion of the cerebellum, affecting both the vermis and the hemispheres; pachygyria of the cerebral hemispheres with a negligibly but uniformly thickened cortex in the absence of a neat anteroposterior gradient, reduction is size of the brainstem, particularly the pons. The condition is monogenic, and due to mutations in *VLDLR*.

Vldlr only knock-out mice did not show the drastic brain phenotype that can be seen in double knock-out mice devoid of *vldlr* and *apoER2*, which, instead, recapitulate in full the phenotypic alterations of *Reeler* mutants or *dab1* knock-out mice [21,114]. As Reln interacts with both Vldlr and ApoER2, clear functional differences in how these two receptors transduce the glycoprotein signal have been postulated [114]. That the interaction of Reln with Vldrl occurs with much lower affinity than with ApoER2 [115] could explain the less severe phenotype of the *vldlr* knockout mice compared to *Reeler*. Remarkably, alterations that in mouse followed the knocking-out of *vldlr* were particularly noticeable in cerebellum and consisted in failure of the Purkinje neurons to form a well-defined monolayer and reduction of their dendritic arbor [114]. They thus recall in full the human MRI phenotype of *VLDLR*-associated cerebellar hypoplasia.

3.2.2. Spinocerebellar Ataxia Type 37

Spinocerebellar ataxia type 37 (SCA37) is a late onset syndrome that affects adults, with dysarthria, slowly progressive gait and limb ataxia, severe dysmetria in the lower extremities, mild dysmetria in the upper extremities, dysphagia, and abnormal ocular movements. In most cases, the first clinical signs encompass tumbles, dysarthria, or stiffness followed by a typical cerebellar syndrome. The early presence of altered vertical eye movements is a characteristic clinical feature of SCA37 that foregoes the symptoms of ataxia. The progression is slow and affected individuals usually become wheelchair bound between ten and thirty-three years after the onset of the disease [116]. At MRI, there is an initial atrophy of the vermis. Later, atrophy rapidly affects the entire cerebellum, without alterations of the brainstem [117]. Molecular analysis has shown that an unstable repeat insertion in *DAB1* is the cause of the cerebellar degeneration and, on the basis of the genetic and phenotypic evidence, the mutation has been proposed as the molecular basis for SCA37 [118].

Notably, the *dab1* deficient mice that derived from a spontaneous mutation called *Scrambler* or from gene knockout were phenotypically indistinguishable from the homozygous *Reeler* mice [119].

3.2.3. PAFAH1B1-Associated Lissencephaly/Subcortical Band Heterotopia

PAFAH1B1-associated lissencephaly/subcortical band heterotopia, also referred to as *LIS1*-associated lissencephaly/subcortical band heterotopia, encompasses Miller–Dieker syndrome (MDS), isolated lissencephaly sequence (ILS) and, infrequently, subcortical band heterotopia (SBH) [120]. MRI findings for lissencephaly are the absence or the abnormal broadening of cerebral gyri, and the aberrant thickness of the cerebral cortex. Less frequently, it may be possible to observe an enlargement of the lateral ventricles, mild hypoplasia of the corpus callosum and of the cerebellar vermis. In *PAFAH1B1*-associated SBH, just beneath the cortex of the parietal and occipital lobes there are subcortical bands of heterotopic gray matter separated from the superficial cerebral cortex by a thin layer of white matter. Histologically, the cerebral cortex in LIS1-associated lissencephaly consists of four layers: a poorly defined marginal zone, which, however, has a very high cell density; a superficial neuronal layer with diffusely scattered neurons; a deeper neuronal layer with relatively sparse neurons; and a deepest neuronal layer with neurons arranged in columns.

The architectural alterations of the human cerebral cortex and hippocampus can be somewhat recapitulated in genetically engineered mice. For example, the overexpression of *pafah1b1* disturbed neuronal migration and layer formation in the developing cerebral cortex [121], whereas *lis1* deficiency in homozygous mice resulted in early embryonic death and in heterozygous mice led to a derangement of the normal hippocampal organization with ectopy of the granule cells [122]. Of note, Lis1, the protein encoded by *Pafah1b*, is part of the Pafah1b complex and binds, downstream of the Vldlr receptor, to Dab1 that becomes phosphorylated in response to Reln [123].

3.3. Human Conditions Possibly Related to RELN Mutations and Their Mouse Correlates

3.3.1. Spinocerebellar Ataxia Type 7

Spinocerebellar ataxia type 7 (SCA7) is an autosomal-dominant neurodegenerative syndrome that outcomes from polyglutamine expansion of ataxin 7 (ATXN7). Remarkably, although ATXN7 has a widespread expression in SCA7 patients, the pathology primarily hits the cerebellum and the retina [124]. A recently published paper suggested that RELN might be a formerly unidentified factor accountable for the tissue specificity of SCA7 [125].

3.3.2. Autism and the Heterozygous Reeler Mouse

The disorders of the autistic spectrum (ASD), which are characterized by social, behavioral, and language insufficiencies, comprise Asperger syndrome, autism, and pervasive developmental disorder-not otherwise specified (PDD-NOS). Less than 20% of these disorders, acknowledged as "syndromic autism", derives from monogenetic diseases, most commonly fragile X syndrome and tuberous sclerosis. The remaining 80% of ASD cases are classified as "non-syndromic autism" and are widely investigated to find candidate genes that may contribute to pathology [126].

Genetics

At present autism cannot be considered, strictly speaking, a genetic disease, as one or more causative gene(s) has (have) not been found yet. The first gene association study implicating *RELN* in autism dates to 2001 [127]. However, subsequent gene population surveys yielded contrasting results [128–131]. Nonetheless, a more recent meta-analysis showed that at least one single nucleotide polymorphism (SNP) in *RELN* could be significantly associated with the risk of autism [132]. Therefore, results of SNP analysis appear to be compatible with the idea that heterozygous mutations in *RELN* may contribute to the onset of the disorder. Genetic studies on autism led to two main outcomes: 1. the more predominant existence of rare or de novo inherited mutations of a number of genes in autistic patients; 2. the discovery of certain common gene variants that contribute to the risk of autism but are also present, albeit at lower frequency, in the normal population [133]. When more than two de novo mutations occur in a gene, the latter becomes a very likely causative candidate of a disorder. There are four unique documented de novo mutations of *RELN* associated with autism [134–136], thus implicating *RELN* as a possible cause of ASD. However, although nonsense mutations are more frequent in autistic patients than in controls after whole-exome sequencing, there is not a striking gross increase of de novo mutations in the former [135]. To study autism heritability, one can also employ a different approach that distinguishes total narrow-sense heritability from that due to common gene variants. By this method, it was concluded that narrow-sense heritability of autism is ~52.4%, and that the main contribution heritability was due to common gene variants, whereas rare de novo mutations contribute only for about 2.6% of cases, but substantially influence individual liability to the condition [137]. Thus, *RELN* may primarily have a role in the individual *predisposition* to manifest autism rather than being one of the contributory causes of the disorder.

Further support for a RELN involvement in autism derived from the detection of reduced expression of the *RELN* transcript and protein in autistic individuals. Decreased RELN levels were apparent in the superior frontal cortex [10] and cerebellum of autistics as compared to controls [10,11,138]. In these areas, the levels of *RELN* mRNA were lower, as was the *DAB1* transcript, whereas *VLDLR* mRNA levels augmented.

Imaging

Imaging findings in autism have been recently reviewed [139]. Numerous observations join to prove that there is an atypical development of the brain in autistic children. Early cross-sectional studies demonstrated that the brain of these children had a higher volume than that of regularly developing subjects. However, growth curves in the two groups eventually met at later childhood. More specifically, in the 6–35-year interval, there was an initial period of brain overgrowth, and then growth slowed down or even stopped during early and late infancy to which a phase of fast reduction of the brain volume eventually followed [140]. Neuroimaging data also indicated that differences in the brain of autistic people started to be detectable within the first two years after birth, *before* clinical symptoms became obvious. There are conflicting views about the probability that an accelerated growth rate of the brain in this postnatal window goes together with the occurrence of early neurodevelopmental perturbations [139]. In relation to this, it is relevant that we still do not know when the initial neuropathological signs of autism occur, also from the paucity of studies on autistic children during the first year of life.

The mechanisms at the basis of the abnormal growth of the autistic brain are also unclear. Although most imaging studies have focused onto the gray matter of the cerebral cortex, there are data indicating that an increased amount of cerebrospinal fluid in the subarachnoid space [141] and/or a greater volume of the white matter [142] occurred in parallel to the enlargement of the autistic brain. As regarding the cerebral cortex, its surface, but not thickness, increased in the autistic brain [143].

To summarize, that an initial brain overgrowth may be a reliable biomarker for autism remains highly questionable. Thus, it seems more profitable to focus onto regional brain structural differences in a more effective search for new neuroanatomical findings of clinical relevance [139].

Before entering the description of regional MRI investigations in autism, it is important to stress that, at present, there are no specific and/or causative objective findings for the condition, but, instead, the very same regions altered in autism may be interested in other psychiatric conditions.

The individual constituents of the neural circuitries causal of ASD are well defined. They include regions of the fronto-temporal, fronto-parietal, and dorsolateral prefrontal cortex (PFC); parts of the limbic system; the fronto-striatal circuitry, and the cerebellum. Neuroimaging studies on these regions have employed different approaches such as the definition of a region-of-interest (ROI), voxel- or vertex-vise methods. Traditional ROI studies have reported atypical findings in brain areas that participate to social cognition such as the medial PFC, the anterior cingulate cortex (ACC), the inferior frontal cortex, the superior temporal sulcus, the amygdala, and the anterior insula.

The cerebellum was larger than in controls in several MRI studies on autistic patients older than three years [144], but not in younger children [143]. Differently from the cerebellum, the size of the vermis was smaller [145–147] or larger [146] or did not display any relevant difference [147], and such discrepancies possibly depend from the different clinical presentations of the condition [147,148]. It is also unclear whether there are differences in size of individual vermal lobules, as claimed by some authors [145], but not others [147]. Similarly, there were no differences between cerebellar hemispheres in one study [147], whereas another group has found the hemispheric size as the only significant structural dissimilarity between verbal and nonverbal subjects [149].

The still fuzzy picture emerging from the imaging studies onto the autistic brain makes it very difficult to compare the human and mouse data in the search for common biomarkers. To our knowledge, there are only two MRI studies on the brain of the heterozygous *Reeler* mouse. In the first, Badea and co-worker [29] reported that the total volume of the brain, the ventricular volume and the hippocampal volume correspondingly raised of about 6%, 82%, and 7% compared to normal control mice. However, after statistical analysis, they showed that these volumes were like those of $reln^{+/+}$ normal mice. They also measured the areas of different parts of the brain in comparison with wild-type mice and found no differences in hippocampus and cerebellum, but an enlargement of the lateral ventricles. A more recent paper confirmed the ventricular enlargement, but found a reduction of the cerebellar volume, whereas the volume of the motor cortex as well as its thickness was unchanged [150]. Therefore, given the paucity of data in mouse and the still unclear MRI pattern in human autistic subjects, one can only conclude that, at present, the cerebellum could be a part of the brain deserving further imaging investigations for translational purposes.

Histopathology

A series of histological alterations of the whole brain occur in the autistic brain. In the first histological surveys, the only cortical area showing qualitative structural abnormalities was the ACC that, in autistic patients, lacked architectural refinement and had only a coarse lamination [151]. However, in the following decades substantial amounts of data have been collected and the list of cerebral structures displaying histopathological changes in ASD has grown substantially to include a series of cortical regions, the amygdala, the cerebellum and the brainstem, see e.g., [152,153]. Below we will briefly summarize the most significant histopathological findings in human patients and compare them to those in the heterozygous *Reeler* mouse. However, the interpretation of both human and mouse finding needs often much caution, because not all studies used sound quantitative approaches and/or proper stereological procedures.

a) Changes Affecting the Whole Brain

The diffuse alterations observed in the brains of autistic subjects at postmortem included cortical dysplasia and neuronal heterotopia, with the formation of aggregates of neuronal cell bodies in anomalous positions [154]. Other alterations, i.e., differences in size of the neuronal nucleus and perikaryon, occurred at the cytological level. These differences started being evident in young children and became more apparent in adults, but then tended to re-equilibrate with time [155].

Remarkably, there might be some compensations between different areas, as in some parts of the brain neurons were bigger, but smaller in others.

In the autistic brain there was also an increase of the neuropil extension in certain but not all cortical areas that have been investigated so far [156]. It is unclear which neuropil component(s) is (are) responsible of these volumetric variations. Fewer dendrites were, in fact, immunostained for microtubule-associated protein 2 (MAP2) in the PFC [157] and a reduction of dendritic spines was reported in hippocampus [158], but other studies reached completely opposite conclusions after examination of the pyramidal neurons from layers 2 and 5 in the frontal, temporal, and parietal cortex [159]. The issue of dendrite and dendritic spines density is quite important in the general framework of this discussion, because these parameters have been widely investigated, primarily aiming to validate the heterozygous *Reeler* mouse as a translational model.

Alterations in neuronal differentiation and migration may also occur in the autistic nervous system and, thus, the consequences of a dysregulation of these processes may be at the basis of whole brain changes in autism [154]. In spite of this, there are only a few investigations on the expression of RELN in the brain of autistic patients and, after quantitative analysis, there was no alteration in the density of layer 1 RELN+ neurons in the superior temporal lobe of the autistic brain, although these neurons represent about 70% of the total layer 1 population [160].

b) Brain Regional Changes

Forebrain

Most of the histopathological observations on the brain of autistic patients focused on the cerebral cortex and hippocampus and, broadly speaking, alterations were almost exclusively restricted to neurons. The parameters considered have been size, number, and density of the different neuronal populations, often in relation to the cortical layers or the hippocampal subfields. A point of attention in considering these studies is that, in several cases, comparative brain volume evaluations between autistic patients and controls are missing, while they are, instead, essential to settle whether modifications in cell density reflect true differences in total cell counts.

Cerebral Cortex

The autistic pathology affects several regions of the cerebral cortex.

The PFC, which plays a major role in cognitive control, displayed a general overgrowth with an increase in the number of neurons, whereas glial cells were apparently unaffected. Among the GABAergic interneurons, there was a numerical increase of the PV-immunoreactive chandelier neurons, whereas the calbindin- and calretinin-expressing neurons were unaltered [153,161–163]. However, after qRT-PCR, the levels of the RELN and GAD67 mRNAs diminished in the post-mortem PFC from autistic patients in comparison to healthy controls [164].

In the inferior frontal cortex, changes affected the small-sized pyramidal neurons that did not display numerical alterations but were of smaller size [163].

The fusiform gyrus, which intervenes in facial recognition and social interactions, had a reduced neuronal density in layer 3, whereas neurons in layers 2, 5, and 6 were less numerous, being also smaller in layers 5 and 6 [165], but these alterations were not confirmed in [166].

In the frontoinsular cortex and ACC, both intervening in emotional regulation and self and others awareness, lamination was rudimental. In the former, von Economo neurons (VENs) of layer 5 increased in number [167–169], whereas in ACC neuronal density augmented in layers 1–2 of area 24a of the left hemisphere but diminished in layers 5–6 of area 24c; size, instead, diminished in all layers of area 24b [151,170].

The anterior midcingulate cortex also displayed a numerical increase of VENs, as well as of the pyramidal neurons of layer 5 that, however, were of smaller size [171].

Lastly, the entorhinal cortex, which has a role in memory, navigation and perception of time, displayed characteristic terminal swellings, referred to as spheroids [172] that were also observed in all hippocampal subfields (see below).

Another issue of interest is the possibility that there are alterations in the minicolumnar organization of the cerebral cortex in early age onset autism [156], as it might be the case in *Reeler* mice. Specifically, it appeared that minicolumns were smaller, more numerous and with lower neuronal density in several cortical areas of autistic (and Asperger's syndrome) patients, although these observations still need to be confirmed in full [156]. Under this perspective, it may be useful to here recall some of the results on the localization of the neural cell adhesion molecule 2 (NCAM2) in the *Reeler* mouse because the molecule has also been proposed as a predisposition gene for the development of autism [173]. In mutants, NCAM2 immunopositive and negative patches formed a mosaic filled with dendritic aggregates originating from two different populations of neurons in a fashion suggestive of a minicolumnar organization [174,175]. However, one must consider these findings with much caution, as that minicolumns are indeed the fundamental modular units of neocortical organization is currently still a matter of debate, see e.g., [176] for review.

Whereas the human cerebral cortex has been widely investigated in autism, investigations on the cerebral cortex of the heterozygous *Reeler* mouse have been relatively few but reported a reduction in the levels of GAD67 [53,177] like that observed in humans. Since the studies on hippocampus led to highly comparable results in the two species, it would be of importance to undertake rigorous investigations on the number and density of the cortical neurons in $reln^{+/-}$ mice, with attention to the different neurochemical populations of inhibitory interneurons. The results of these studies will be relevant, from one side, to validate the mouse model and, from the other, to confirm some numerical observations in humans that, as mentioned at beginning of this section, need validation using approaches more reliable than those often employed at histopathology.

Hippocampus and Amygdala

In humans, beside the widespread occurrence of spheroids, other general changes in hippocampus [151,158,172,178,179] consisted in a reduction of neuronal size and dendritic arbors, and these smaller neurons appeared to be more densely packed. There were also a series of specific modifications affecting the excitatory pyramidal neurons that were more numerous in CA1, but less abundant in all other adjacent hippocampal regions. The GABAergic inhibitory interneurons, instead, displayed a higher density, specifically the calbindin-immunoreactive neurons in the dentate gyrus, the parvalbumin-immunoreactive neurons in CA1 and CA3, and the calretinin-immunoreactive neurons in CA1 [151,158,172,178,179].

In the heterozygous *Reeler* mouse the hippocampus displayed reduced levels of GAD67, [53,177] that could be somewhat restored after stereotaxic injections of Reln [67,180]. These experiments indicated the existence of a causal link between the decrease in GAD67 expression and Reln haplodeficiency. In keeping with such a possibility, Reln supplementation could, at least partly, reverse such a decrease. Other experiments, in line with this interpretation, have confirmed that the decrease in the levels of GAD67 in heterozygous mice can be overturned, e.g., after administration of nicotine, which reduces the GAD67 promoter methylation and increases its transcription [177].

In heterozygous mice, pyramidal neurons displayed a reduction in the average length and width of their apical and basal dendritic spines [52], consistent with the decrease in the spread of the dendritic arbor of the same population of neurons in humans. Additionally, Reln supplementation was effective in promoting a full (apical) or partial (basal shaft) spine recovery [180]. These morphological observations are in line with a previous report showing that, in the forebrain, spines were hypertrophic in mice conditionally overexpressing Reln [66]. At electrophysiological recordings CA1 pyramidal neurons displayed reduced spontaneous inhibitory postsynaptic currents [181], an observation that was fully coherent with the reduction of the inhibitory input from the GABAergic interneurons observed histologically.

Synaptic plasticity is fundamental for hippocampal function. In CA1 of heterozygous mice, LTP was impaired [182] as well as long-term depression (LTD) [181], which returned to normal levels after the administration of Reln [180]. Additionally, in $reln^{+/-}$ and $reln^{-/-}$ mice, post tetanic potentiation (PTP), a form of short-term plasticity that depends on neurotransmitter release, was reduced in CA1 [180,183] and could be reversed by Reln [180].

Collectively these data indicate that the experimental administration of the glycoprotein was able to reverse the morphological, neurochemical, and physiological hippocampal deficits consequent to a reduction of brain Reln. Translationally, they are very important because they offer some cues for further investigations onto the autistic brain. It would be of interest to map the post-mortem distribution of hippocampal RELN in patients compared to healthy controls, to ascertain whether the pattern of immunoreactivity will be consistent between humans and mice.

In the autistic patients, several studies reported that the amygdala, which is involved in emotional learning, increased in size and displayed an augmented density of neurons within the medial, central, and cortical nuclei [151,184–187]. Neurons were, however, less numerous, although numerical variations could be age dependent. To our knowledge, Boyle et al have investigated in detail the amygdala of the homozygous *Reeler* mouse with a marker-based phenotypic approach [188], but there are no data on heterozygous mice.

Cerebellum

Analysis of cerebellar alterations in autism has attracted many efforts of the basic researchers and clinicians. The most consistent anatomic findings in autistic patients were a reduction in size of certain lobules of the cerebellar vermis (but see 3.3.2b Imaging) and a decrease in the number [186,189–192] and size [193,194] of the Purkinje neurons. The inhibitory GABAergic basket and stellate interneurons that connect with these neurons did not show quantitative differences compared to normal cerebella [195]. This observation is indicative of a late developmental death of the Purkinje neurons, as they differentiate well before the interneurons. In addition to structural observations, Western blots demonstrated a reduction of about 40% in the level of expression of RELN in autistic patients related to age and sex corresponding controls [11]. Quantitative RT-PCR also showed a drop of RELN and GAD67 mRNAs in the post-mortem autistic brain [164].

Notably many of the histological alterations in the human autistic cerebellum are like those described in $reln^{+/-}$ mice. These animals displayed a progressive loss of Purkinje neurons already during the first weeks of life [35], and inferior numbers of these cells were observed in adult subjects as well [196]. Human MRI studies did not allow, at present, to ascertain whether the cerebellar vermis is hit by the pathology in its entirety or, rather, only at specific lobuli. Therefore, our group has, at first, focused its attention on five different lobules, which receive diverse types of afferent functional inputs, to analyze the number and topological organization of the Purkinje neurons in $reln^{+/+}$ and $reln^{+/-}$ adult mice of both sexes [197]. We have thus shown that the Purkinje neurons: 1. Displayed a lower density in $reln^{+/-}$ males (14.37%) and $reln^{+/-}$ females (17.73%) compared to $reln^{+/+}$ males; 2. Were larger in $reln^{+/-}$ males than in the other phenotypes under study, and smaller in females (regardless of the *reln* genetic background) than in $reln^{+/+}$ males; 3. Were more messily arranged along the YZ axis of the vermis in $reln^{+/-}$ males than in $reln^{+/+}$ males and, except in central lobule, $reln^{+/-}$ females.

Very recently, as many observations have associated a number of synapse-related genes in the genesis of autism and other neuropsychiatric conditions [198,199], we have examined the expression of synaptophysin 1 (SYP1) and contactin 6 (CNTN6) in the vermis of $reln^{+/-}$ and $reln^{+/+}$ adult mice of both genders [200].

SYP1 is a pre-synaptic marker and CNTN6 is a marker of the synapses made by the parallel fibers onto the Purkinje neurons' dendrites. Notably, there is evidence, although still to be validated in full, that SYP1 is involved in the structural alterations of the autistic synapses [189,201], and very recent observations have shown that copy number variations [202] or a truncating variant [203] of

CNTN6 are found in autistic patients. In addition, *CNTN6* mutations may be a risk factor for several neurodevelopmental and neuropsychiatric disorders [150,199,204].

In line with these human studies, we have demonstrated that $reln^{+/-}$ mouse males displayed a statistically significant drop of 11.89% in SYP1 compared to sex-matched normal animals, whereas no modifications were detected comparing $reln^{+/+}$ and $reln^{+/-}$ females [200]. In $reln^{+/-}$ male and female mice, reductions in SYP1 levels were particularly evident in the molecular layer, whereas in heterozygous mice of both sexes a reduction in CNTN6 occurred in all the three cortical layers of the vermis. In addition, alterations in the levels of expression of SYP1 in the molecular layer of male $reln^{+/-}$ mice ensued across all lobules except lobule VII, but they were limited to lobule II for the granular layer and lobule VII for the Purkinje cell layer.

Thus, the widespread reduction of SYP1 and of CNTN6 in the molecular layer of $reln^{+/-}$ male mice well matched with the autistic phenotype in humans [150].

In the vermis (and the whole cerebellum), there is proof for a topographic segregation of the areas controlling motion versus those connected to cognitive and affective functions, and the diverse lobules are coupled with precise zones of the brain and spinal cord [205]. The CNS areas that handle sensorimotor inputs are directly or indirectly connected with the anterior lobe (lobules I–V of the vermis), lobule VIII, and, to a lesser grade, with lobule VI; on the contrary, cortical association areas that collect non-motor responses are linked to lobules VI and VII. Existing clinical data indicate that the vermis is the chief target of the limbic system, and physiological and behavioral observations implicate the vermis in the regulation of emotions [206]. Therefore, the neurochemical modifications of the cerebellar cortex in heterozygous mice are fully in line with the possibility that the social and communication aberrations typical of autism rest on anomalies of the limbic system and its connections [207,208].

At post-mortem, a numerical reduction of the Purkinje neurons in the posterior cerebellum was long ago described in autistic subjects [184,209], but it did not appear to disturb the vermis [189]. Hypoplasia in lobules VI and VII was initially detected in vivo using MRI [145], but subsequent observations proved the existence of two distinct autistic subtypes related to vermian hypoplasia or hyperplasia [146]. A systematic review and meta-analysis of the accounts of structural MRI has then established that the reduction in size of lobules VI–X (i.e., the lobules included in the posterior cerebellum) showed a remarkable heterogeneity that associated to differences in time of life and intelligence quotient (IQ) merely in lobules VI–VII [210]. Other observations showed that the posterior/inferior vermis, i.e., lobules VII, VIIIb (left), and IX, was more prone to pathological deviations [211], with a decrease of the gray matter after quantitative MRI [190,212,213]. Therefore, it appears that the cerebellar phenotype of the heterozygous *Reeler* mouse is fully compatible with that in humans and that a deeper structural and neurochemical characterization may be useful to direct the discovery of new biomarkers of translational interest.

3.3.3. Schizophrenia and the Heterozygous *Reeler* Mouse

Schizophrenia is a ruinous psychiatric condition that affects about 1% of the population. Its main clinical symptoms are hallucinations, delusions, and cognitive disturbances. These symptoms derive from brain dysfunctions that derive from genetic and environmental factors [214]. However, schizophrenia is not strictly a genetic disease, although gene deletions, duplications, and variations may be risk factors for the disorder. At present, the gene(s) that could be involved in the pathology remain elusive for the most (see OMIM #181500), but a microdeletion in a region of chromosome 22, called 22q11, was recently established to be involved in a small percentage of cases [215].

Genetic studies have shown a link between *RELN* and schizophrenia [216] and, over the past ten years, many SNPs in the *RELN* gene loci occurred in parallel with the beginning and/or severity of the clinical signs [217], but results still are under debate and need further verification [218]. One should perhaps emphasize that observations on gene expression have converged to show that the genes implicated in schizophrenia are more highly expressed during fetal than postnatal life [219], thus making more difficult to ascertain their true role in the etiology of the condition.

Imaging

Structural MRI findings in schizophrenia have been recently reviewed [220]. There is enough information to propose that the condition is associated with a continuing development of gray matter aberrations, chiefly throughout the first stages of the disease. Reduction of the depth of the cerebral cortex in the superior temporal and inferior frontal regions was reported in individuals that later became psychotic. In patients with first episode psychosis, there was, instead, a reduction in the thickness of the superior and inferior frontal cortex, and in the volume of the thalamus. In chronic schizophrenia, the gray matter decreased further in the frontal and temporal areas, cingulate cortices, and thalamus, particularly in patients with unfortunate outcomes. Structural modifications of the white matter occurred only in a small number of longitudinal studies.

As the human phenotype is still very far from clear, it is not surprising that the few MRI observations in *Reeler* mice are still insufficient to draw any definitive consideration of translational relevance (for MRI data on Reeler see 3.3.2 Imaging).

Histopathology

Although gross structural alterations of the brain were lacking, subtle pathological changes in specific populations of neurons and in cell-to-cell communication occurred in schizophrenic patients, see [221] for a recent review. Histopathology mainly consisted in modifications of the number and density of neurons at the level of the whole brain and/or specific neuronal subpopulations, and in morphological and neurochemical alterations of these neurons.

a) Cerebral Cortex

As discussed above for autism, the most widely investigated area of the brain has been the PFC that, in general terms, displayed an increased neuronal density and an altered neuroplasticity with age-related differences between normal and schizophrenic subjects. More specifically, a statistical meta-analysis of thirty papers published between 1993 and 2012, concluded that the density of cortical neurons increased with age irrespective of the condition, but the rate of accretion was much slower in the schizophrenics [222]. However, other cortical areas, such as e.g., the dorsal ACC, displayed no changes in neuronal and glial densities after stereological analysis [223].

The above-mentioned meta-analysis [222] has also taken into consideration the density of inhibitory neurons after immunolabeling with GAD67, PV, or calbindin, and found that it was greater in schizophrenic patients compared to controls before the age of 40, but lower thereafter.

Notably, both Reln and GAD67 mRNAs were downregulated in the PFC of schizophrenic subjects with no relation to neuronal damage [224]. In keeping with these observations, it appeared that in the PFC there was a vulnerability of the inhibitory circuits, with markers of the inhibitory interneurons showing some of the more consistent alterations [225]. More precisely, these alterations consisted in a reduction in the levels of the GAD67 mRNA and protein in subsets of GABAergic basket cells containing PV [222,226,227] or cholecystokinin (CCK) [226]. Notably, these two populations of basket cells are responsible of the inhibition of the pyramidal neurons giving rise, respectively, to the cortical θ and γ oscillations altered in schizophrenia. In addition, the pyramidal neurons targeted by the PV+ basket cells expressed lower levels of the $GABA_A$ receptor α1 [226].

It is also interesting that the levels of RELN and GAD67 mRNAs in microdissected GABAergic neurons of PFC layer 1 were lower in schizophrenics, but unchanged in layer 5 of the same patients [228]. In addition, in the dorsolateral division of the PFC, the GABAergic chandelier neurons targeting the axon initial segment of the pyramidal neurons displayed remarkable neurochemical alterations. These changes were particularly evident in layers 2/3, where immunoreactivity for the GABA membrane transporter GAT1 diminished, in parallel with an increase of the GABA$_A$ receptor α2 subunit in the axons of their target pyramidal neurons [229].

Occurrence of dendritic spine pathology was another prominent feature of the schizophrenic human brain [230,231]. Spine loss mainly affected the smaller spines of the pyramidal neurons in layer 3 of the neocortex and arose during development, possibly because of altered mechanisms of generation, pruning, and/or upkeep [230].

As already mentioned in the section dedicated to autism, investigations on the cerebral cortex of the heterozygous *Reeler* reported a reduction in the levels of GAD67 [53,177], in full accordance with the human studies. A study carried out on mice whose mothers were stressed during pregnancy showed that the downregulation of Reln and GAD67 was associated with a hypermethylation of their promoters [232], this being one the mechanisms in support for the contribution of an altered epigenetic control in the down-regulation of RELN expression in schizophrenia, see [233] for review.

b) Hippocampus

The human hippocampal pathology in schizophrenia is by far less clear than in the cortex. Some initial studies have, in fact, reported a decrease in area or overall volume of the hippocampus, or in the number, size, and density of neurons, as well as a disarray of the pyramidal cells, with greatest differences affecting the pyramidal cell density in left CA4; however, several other subsequent surveys were negative, see [234] for review. In any case, hippocampal alterations in schizophrenics are not specific, as they display several common traits with those in autism.

We have previously discussed the histological changes in the hippocampus of the heterozygous *Reeler* mice in relation to autism. These modifications recall, in toto or in part, those in schizophrenia. Additional information detailed, in individual hippocampal layers, the decrease of neuronal GAD67 in CA1, CA2 and dentate gyrus, and the reduction of PV immunoreactive interneurons in CA1 and CA2, in the perspective to validate these mice as a model of schizophrenia [111]. In translational terms, the aforementioned impairment of LTP in heterozygous mice [182] is of interest, as it also occurs in schizophrenic patients [235].

c) Cerebellum

In the cerebellum of schizophrenic patients, there was a loss of distal and terminal dendritic branches and a decrease in density of the dendritic spines of the Purkinje neurons [236]. Again, these histological alterations are not specific for the condition, being evident also in autism. In addition to such changes, in the schizophrenic cerebellum there were altered levels of expression of the general presynaptic marker SYP1, of complexin II, a marker of the excitatory synapses, but not of complexin I that, instead, labels the inhibitory synapses [237]. Thus, some of the structural changes described in the heterozygous *Reeler* mouse in relation to autism also in cerebellum recollected the human schizophrenic phenotype.

4. Does the Behavior of Heterozygous *Reeler* Mice Recall the Human Conditions Related to RELN?

The recapitulation of the behavioral modifications typical of human autism, schizophrenia, or epilepsy in heterozygous *Reeler* mice still is a subject of debate. The dissimilar outcome of behavioral experiments performed in different laboratories is not surprising, because neuropsychiatric behaviors in humans primarily regard social interaction, communication, and restricted interest, and these behaviors are, obviously, very difficult to measure objectively in mice [238].

It is perhaps worth mentioning here that most of our knowledge on the effects of Reln in the cognitive or behavioral field derives from work on mouse hippocampus. This is not surprising as this part of the brain, as discussed previously, has been the primary focus of numerous investigations also in human patients affected by neuropsychiatric disturbs. Several behaviors comparable to those observed in these human disturbs also occur in *reln*$^{+/-}$ mice [239–241], as well as the deficits in reversal learning after visual discrimination tasks that were hypothesized to follow a diminished visual attention [240]. In addition, testing $reln^{+/-}$ mice for anxiety-related behavior, motor impulsivity and morphine-induced analgesia yielded a different behavioral profile from that of wild-type littermates in that they displayed, starting form adolescence, a decreased inhibition and emotionality. To these modifications, a small increase of impulsive behavior and different pain thresholds also occurred in adult mice [242]. Heterozygous mice were also tested in a complex series of PPI protocols (unimodal and cross-modal) to conclude that they exhibited a multifaceted configuration of changes in startle reactivity and sensorimotor gating, with both resemblances to and dissimilarities from schizophrenia [243]. At least partly in line with these latter observations, other studies failed, incompletely or in full, to validate the behavioral analogies between neuropsychiatric patients and $reln^{+/-}$ mice [181,244–248]. For example, Salinger and co-workers were unsuccessful to find differences between $reln^{+/-}$ and $reln^{+/+}$ mice after testing gait, emotionality, social aggression, spatial working memory, novel-object detection, fear conditioning, and sensorimotor reflex modulation [244]. In another survey [246], heterozygous *Reeler* mice were evaluated for cognitive plasticity in an instrumental reversal learning task, impulsivity in an inhibitory control task, attentional function in a three-choice serial reaction time task, and working memory in a delayed matching-to-position task to conclude that there were no differences in comparison to $reln^{+/+}$ littermates in prefrontal-related cognitive trials. However, $reln^{+/-}$ mice were deficient in two operant tasks. From these observations, the authors concluded that heterozygous *Reeler* mice were *not* a good model for the essential prefrontal-dependent cognitive shortfalls detected in schizophrenia, although they could be useful to model learning deficits in a more general sense.

In another paper it was reported that heterozygous and wild-type mice displayed comparable levels of general activity, coordination, thermal nociception, startle responses, anxiety-like behavior, shock threshold; identical cued freezing behavior, and comparable spatial learning in Morris water maze tasks, albeit a significant decrease in contextual fear conditioned learning was observed in $reln^{+/-}$ mice only [181]. These authors have then hypothesized that the pharmacological administration of Reln in heterozygous mice could restore the response to PPI. They were unable to find differences in the acoustic startle reflex among treated and untreated animals, but Reln-treated $reln^{+/-}$ mice showed a substantial increase in the percent inhibition to 78-, 86- and 90-dB pre-pulse [180].

One study has specifically focused onto the $reln^{+/-}$ mouse behavioral phenotype in young (P50–70) and fully adult (older than P75) animals to conclude that they were not useful to model schizophrenia [245]. An ample series of behavioral test was used (Irwin test; rotarod; spontaneous locomotor activity; social behavior; light-dark transition; startle response and pre-pulse inhibition; hot plate). Heterozygous mice were like their wild-type littermates at either age, though completely adult male $reln^{+/-}$ mice were involved in social exploration for a longer time. In addition, performance on the rotarod deteriorated with age.

Indeed, age appeared to be a further issue of complexity. In fact, adult $reln^{+/-}$ mice did not display discernible changes in activity, motor coordination, anxiety, or environmental perception compared to wild-type littermate controls. However, juvenile animals displayed not as much of anxiety- and risk assessment-related behaviors in the elevated plus-maze [182,241]. In addition, in one of these two studies it was demonstrated that young $reln^{+/-}$ mice had a hippocampal-dependent shortfall in associative learning and impulsivity–anxiety-related behavior [182]. Additionally, one study, starting from the clinical observations that reported the occurrence of vocal and motor anomalies in autistic patients, has described that $reln^{+/-}$ mice had a general delay in the development of their repertoire of neonatal vocal and motor behaviors [249].

Finally, one must consider that gender apparently influenced some behaviors, although very few studies have focused on this issue. Among these studies, young heterozygous female mice were described to be more active in the light/dark transition test than the heterozygous males that were, instead, more aggressive than females during social interaction [241].

5. Usefulness of the *Reeler* Mouse in Translational Studies: Concluding Remarks

The analysis of the literature discussed above requires one trying to draw some conclusions about the true usefulness of the *Reeler* mouse in translational studies.

At first, it may perhaps be useful to remember that, as discussed, *RELN* is causative of LIS2 and a small percentage of ADLTE, whereas only tentative associations up to now hold for the other conditions here considered (see Figure 1 and Table 1).

Remarkably, both LIS2 and ADLTE are rare diseases. Very few cases of LIS2 (around ten) so far come about in the literature (see OMIM #257320). Similarly, patients with lateral temporal epilepsy (LTE) are only about 10% of all temporal epilepsies, and the real prevalence of ADLTE, which has been up to now reported in Europe, USA, and Japan, is unknown, but it may account for about 19% of familial idiopathic focal epilepsies [250,251]. When one considers the human conditions related to the Reln signaling pathway, one still encounters a group of rare diseases. The actual frequency of *VLDLR*-associated cerebellar hypoplasia is unknown, but initial reports regarded not more than twenty-five affected individuals in Canada and USA [113,252], although the condition occurs worldwide, *PAFAH1B1*-associated lissencephaly is very rare as the prevalence of classic lissencephaly ranges from 11.7 to 40 per million births [120]. To date, sixty-six affected individuals and seven asymptomatic individuals with the ATTTC repeat insertion within *DAB1* have been reported in ten relatives from the south of the Iberian Peninsula, and no individuals with SCA37 from other geographic areas have been described [116]. SCA7 has a prevalence of less than 1:100,000 and accounts for about 2% of all SCAs [253].

Therefore, one must deal with the paradox of the relatively little interest for translational studies on the very conditions for which the *Reeler* mouse and/or mice with mutations of the genes of the Reln pathway fully meet the criteria for construct and face validity. Thus, the homozygous Reeler mice appear to be more interesting to the neurobiologist than to the clinician and their study will surely be still rewarding in terms of our comprehension of neurodevelopment, as the model already helped to establish that many functional and circuit features of cortical neurons are relatively independent from positional cues and cortical lamination, e.g., [179].

Very differently, the prevalence of autism in the worldwide population is around 1% [254] and that of schizophrenia is just below [221]. As the two conditions are very diffuse in the human population, there is an obvious translational interest for the heterozygous *Reeler* mouse as a model for the two disorders. However, such an interest is again paradoxical, as the validity of these mice to extract information about the human pathologies remains dubious. The first explanation for this uncertainty lies, beyond any doubt, in the substantial lack of construct validity, which is the direct consequence of the complex genetic background of autism and schizophrenia. As regarding face validity, the present survey of the literature clearly points out that there are several similarities but also dissimilarities between the human and the mouse phenotypes. Among dissimilarities, one must consider the heterogeneity of results of the behavioral experiments in mouse. Further complexity derives by the vast array of clinical symptoms in humans. Structurally, most of the imaging and post-mortem findings in humans are not specific for each of the two conditions. However, one must consider that both the human and mouse phenotype converges to indicate the cerebral cortex, hippocampus, and cerebellum as the primary foci of the pathologies and the inhibitory interneurons as major players in the context of the circuitry involved.

A serious drawback to a full validation of the heterozygous *Reeler* mouse as a model of autism and/or schizophrenia lies in the observation that the alterations so far described in mouse are very subtle in both structural, functional and neurochemical terms. The relatively low resolution of current neuroimaging procedures, and the difficulty to obtain post-mortem samples amenable for neurochemical, electrophysiological, and fine (ultra) structural analyses make it very difficult to establish whether the alterations in heterozygous *Reeler* mice have a true biological significance that goes beyond mere statistics [255,256]. In the affirmative, one could take advantage of these alterations to discover novel biomarkers that will be helpful for an earlier and more precise diagnosis in the human practice.

Author Contributions: All authors contributed to write the manuscript.

Funding: The original research work carried out at the Department of Veterinary Sciences described in this paper was funded by Local Grants of the University of Turin to LL and AM and FFABR 2017 from the Italian MIUR to CC. AG was in receipt of a Local Grant of the Catholic University of the Sacred Heart, Milano.

Conflicts of Interest: The authors declare no conflict of interest.

Abbreviations

ACC	anterior cingulate cortex
ADLTE	autosomal-dominant lateral temporal epilepsy
ApoER2	apolipoprotein E2
ARX	aristaless-related homeobox gene
ASD	autism spectrum disorders
ATXN7	ataxin 7
CCK	cholecystokinin
CNS	central nervous system
CNTN6	contactin 6
DCX	doublecortin
DTI	diffusion tractography imaging
ETL7	temporal lobe epilepsy-7
GFP	green fluorescent protein
HCN	hyperpolarization-activated cyclic nucleotide–gated
HdEEG	high-density electroencephalography
ILS	isolated lissencephaly sequence
IQ	intelligence quotient
LCH	lissencephaly with cerebellar hypoplasia
LGI1	leucine-rich, glioma inactivated 1 gene
LIS1	lissencephaly 1
LIS2	lissencephaly 2
LIS3	lissencephaly 3
LTD	long-term depression
LTE	lateral temporal epilepsy
LTP	long-term potentiation
MAP2	microtubule-associated protein 2
MDS	Miller-Dieker syndrome
MEMRI	manganese-enhanced MRI
NCAM2	neural cell adhesion molecule 2
PAFAH1B1	platelet-activating factor acetylhydrolase IB subunit α
PDD-NOS	pervasive developmental disorder-not otherwise specified
PFC	prefrontal cortex
PPI	pre-pulse inhibition
PTP	post tetanic potentiation
PV	parvalbumin
RELN	Reelin gene (human)
Reln	Reelin gene (mouse)
RELN	Reelin glycoprotein (human)
Reln	Reelin glycoprotein (mouse)
ROI	region-of-interest
SBH	subcortical band heterotopia
SCA37	spinocerebellar ataxia type 37
SCA7	spinocerebellar ataxia type 7
SNP	single nucleotide polymorphism
SYP1	synaptophysin 1
TUBA1A	α tubulin 1A
VENs	von Economo neurons
VLDLR	very low-density lipoprotein receptor

References

1. Andersen, T.E.; Finsen, B.; Goffinet, A.M.; Issinger, O.G.; Boldyreff, B. A reeler mutant mouse with a new, spontaneous mutation in the reelin gene. *Brain Res. Mol. Brain Res.* **2002**, *105*, 153–156. [CrossRef]
2. Tissir, F.; Goffinet, A.M. Reelin and brain development. *Nat. Rev. Neurosci.* **2003**, *4*, 496–505. [CrossRef] [PubMed]
3. D'Arcangelo, G.; Miao, G.G.; Chen, S.C.; Soares, H.D.; Morgan, J.I.; Curran, T. A protein related to extracellular matrix proteins deleted in the mouse mutant reeler. *Nature* **1995**, *374*, 719–723. [CrossRef] [PubMed]
4. Falconer, D.S. Two new mutants, 'trembler' and 'reeler', with neurological actions in the house mouse (*Mus musculus* L.). *J. Genet.* **1951**, *50*, 192–201. [CrossRef]
5. Caviness, V.S.; Rakic, P. Mechanisms of Cortical Development: A View from Mutations in Mice. *Annu. Rev. Neurosci.* **1978**, *1*, 297–326. [CrossRef]
6. Goffinet, A.M. Events governing organization of postmigratory neurons: Studies on brain development in normal and reeler mice. *Brain Res. Rev.* **1984**, *7*, 261–296. [CrossRef]
7. Folsom, T.D.; Fatemi, S.H. The involvement of Reelin in neurodevelopmental disorders. *Neuropharmacology* **2013**, *68*, 122–135. [CrossRef]
8. DeSilva, U.; D'Arcangelo, G.; Braden, V.V.; Chen, J.; Miao, G.G.; Curran, T.; Green, E.D. The human reelin gene: Isolation, sequencing, and mapping on chromosome 7. *Genome Res.* **1997**, *7*, 157–164. [CrossRef]
9. Hong, S.E.; Shugart, Y.Y.; Huang, D.T.; Shahwan, S.A.; Grant, P.E.; Hourihane, J.O.; Martin, N.D.; Walsh, C.A. Autosomal recessive lissencephaly with cerebellar hypoplasia is associated with human RELN mutations. *Nat. Genet.* **2000**, *26*, 93–96. [CrossRef]
10. Fatemi, S.H. Reelin glycoprotein in autism and schizophrenia. *Int. Rev. Neurobiol.* **2005**, *71*, 179–187.
11. Fatemi, S.H.; Stary, J.M.; Halt, A.R.; Realmuto, G.R. Dysregulation of Reelin and Bcl-2 proteins in autistic cerebellum. *J. Autism Dev. Disord.* **2001**, *31*, 529–535. [CrossRef] [PubMed]
12. Robertson, H.R.; Feng, G. Annual Research Review: Transgenic mouse models of childhood-onset psychiatric disorders. *J. Child Psychol. Psychiatry* **2011**, *52*, 442–475. [CrossRef] [PubMed]
13. Miles, J.H. Autism spectrum disorders—A genetics review. *Genet. Med.* **2011**, *13*, 278–294. [CrossRef] [PubMed]
14. Vorstman, J.A.S.; Parr, J.R.; Moreno-De-Luca, D.; Anney, R.J.L.; Nurnberger, J.I., Jr.; Hallmayer, J.F. Autism genetics: Opportunities and challenges for clinical translation. *Nat. Rev. Genet.* **2017**, *18*, 362–376. [CrossRef]
15. Geyer, M.A. Developing translational animal models for symptoms of schizophrenia or bipolar mania. *Neurotox. Res.* **2008**, *14*, 71–78. [CrossRef]
16. Chadman, K.K. Animal models for autism in 2017 and the consequential implications to drug discovery. *Exp. Opin. Drug Discov.* **2017**, *12*, 1187–1194. [CrossRef]
17. Zaki, M.; Shehab, M.; El-Aleem, A.A.; Abdel-Salam, G.; Koeller, H.B.; Ilkin, Y.; Ross, M.E.; Dobyns, W.B.; Gleeson, J.G. Identification of a novel recessive RELN mutation using a homozygous balanced reciprocal translocation. *Am. J. Med. Genet. A* **2007**, *143*, 939–944. [CrossRef]
18. Hirotsune, S.; Takahara, T.; Sasaki, N.; Hirose, K.; Yoshiki, A.; Ohashi, T.; Kusakabe, M.; Murakami, Y.; Muramatsu, M.; Watanabe, S. The reeler gene encodes a protein with an EGF-like motif expressed by pioneer neurons. *Nat. Genet.* **1995**, *10*, 77–83. [CrossRef]
19. Ogawa, M.; Miyata, T.; Nakajima, K.; Yagyu, K.; Seike, M.; Ikenaka, K.; Yamamoto, H.; Mikoshiba, K. The reeler gene-associated antigen on Cajal-Retzius neurons is a crucial molecule for laminar organization of cortical neurons. *Neuron* **1995**, *14*, 899–912. [CrossRef]
20. D'Arcangelo, G. Reelin in the years: Controlling neuronal migration and maturation in the mammalian brain. *Adv. Neurosci.* **2014**, *2014*, 597395. [CrossRef]
21. Hiesberger, T.; Trommsdorff, M.; Howell, B.W.; Goffinet, A.; Mumby, M.C.; Cooper, J.A.; Herz, J. Direct binding of Reelin to VLDL receptor and ApoE receptor 2 induces tyrosine phosphorylation of disabled-1 and modulates tau phosphorylation. *Neuron* **1999**, *24*, 481–489. [CrossRef]
22. Assadi, A.H.; Zhang, G.; Beffert, U.; McNeil, R.S.; Renfro, A.L.; Niu, S.; Quattrocchi, C.C.; Antalffy, B.A.; Sheldon, M.; Armstrong, D.D.; et al. Interaction of reelin signaling and Lis1 in brain development. *Nat. Genet.* **2003**, *35*, 270–276. [CrossRef] [PubMed]

23. Bahi-Buisson, N.; Cavallin, M. Tubulinopathies overview. In *GeneReviews®*; Adam, M.P., Ardinger, H.H., Pagon, R.A., Wallace, S.E., Eds.; University of Washington: Seattle, WA, USA, 2016.
24. Lo, N.C.; Chong, C.S.; Smith, A.C.; Dobyns, W.B.; Carrozzo, R.; Ledbetter, D.H. Point mutations and an intragenic deletion in LIS1, the lissencephaly causative gene in isolated lissencephaly sequence and Miller-Dieker syndrome. *Hum. Mol. Genet.* **1997**, *6*, 157–164.
25. Kato, M.; Dobyns, W.B. Lissencephaly and the molecular basis of neuronal migration. *Hum. Mol. Genet.* **2003**, *12*, R89–R96. [CrossRef]
26. Lecourtois, M.; Poirier, K.; Friocourt, G.; Jaglin, X.; Goldenberg, A.; Saugier-Veber, P.; Chelly, J.; Laquerriere, A. Human lissencephaly with cerebellar hypoplasia due to mutations in TUBA1A: Expansion of the foetal neuropathological phenotype. *Acta Neuropathol.* **2010**, *119*, 779–789. [CrossRef]
27. Ross, M.E.; Swanson, K.; Dobyns, W.B. Lissencephaly with cerebellar hypoplasia (LCH): A heterogeneous group of cortical malformations. *Neuropediatrics* **2001**, *32*, 256–263. [CrossRef]
28. Sergi, C.; Zoubaa, S.; Schiesser, M. Norman-Roberts syndrome: Prenatal diagnosis and autopsy findings. *Prenat. Diagn.* **2000**, *20*, 505–509. [CrossRef]
29. Badea, A.; Nicholls, P.J.; Johnson, G.A.; Wetsel, W.C. Neuroanatomical phenotypes in the reeler mouse. *Neuroimage* **2007**, *34*, 1363–1374. [CrossRef]
30. Silva, A.C.; Lee, J.H.; Wu, C.W.H.; Tucciarone, J.; Pelled, G.; Aoki, I.; Koretsky, A.P. Detection of cortical laminar architecture using manganese-enhanced MRI. *J. Neurosci. Meth.* **2008**, *167*, 246–257. [CrossRef]
31. Harsan, L.A.; David, C.; Reisert, M.; Schnell, S.; Hennig, J.; von Elverfeld, D.; Staiger, J.F. Mapping remodeling of thalamocortical projections in the living reeler mouse brain by diffusion tractography. *Proc. Natl. Acad. Sci. USA* **2013**, *110*, E1797–E1806. [CrossRef]
32. Pappas, G.D.; Kriho, V.; Liu, W.S.; Tremolizzo, L.; Lugli, G.; Larson, J. Immunocytochemical localization of reelin in the olfactory bulb of the heterozygous reeler mouse: an animal model for schizophrenia. *Neurol. Res.* **2003**, *25*, 819–830. [CrossRef] [PubMed]
33. Katsuyama, Y.; Terashima, T. Developmental anatomy of reeler mutant mouse. *Dev. Growth Differ.* **2009**, *51*, 271–286. [CrossRef] [PubMed]
34. Wyss, J.M.; Stanfield, B.B.; Cowan, W.M. Structural abnormalities in the olfactory bulb of the Reeler mouse. *Brain Res.* **1980**, *188*, 566–571. [CrossRef]
35. Marrone, M.C.; Marinelli, S.; Biamonte, F.; Keller, F.; Sgobio, C.A.; Ammassari-Teule, M.; Bernardi, G.; Mercuri, N.B. Altered cortico-striatal synaptic plasticity and related behavioural impairments in reeler mice. *Eur. J. Neurosci.* **2006**, *24*, 2061–2070. [CrossRef]
36. Cariboni, A.; Rakic, S.; Liapi, A.; Maggi, R.; Goffinet, A.; Parnavelas, J.G. Reelin provides an inhibitory signal in the migration of gonadotropin-releasing hormone neurons. *Development* **2005**, *132*, 4709–4718. [CrossRef]
37. Stanfield, B.B.; Wyss, J.M.; Cowan, W.M. The projection of the supramammillary region upon the dentate gyrus in normal and reeler mice. *Brain Res.* **1980**, *198*, 196–203. [CrossRef]
38. Baba, K.; Sakakibara, S.; Setsu, T.; Terashima, T. The superficial layers of the superior colliculus are cytoarchitectually and myeloarchitectually disorganized in the reelin-deficient mouse, reeler. *Brain Res.* **2007**, *1140*, 205–215. [CrossRef]
39. Terashima, T. Distribution of mesencephalic trigeminal nucleus neurons in the reeler mutant mouse. *Anat. Rec.* **1996**, *244*, 563–571. [CrossRef]
40. Nishikawa, S.; Goto, S.; Yamada, K.; Hamasaki, T.; Ushio, Y. Lack of Reelin causes malpositioning of nigral dopaminergic neurons: Evidence from comparison of normal and Reln (rl) mutant mice. *J. Comp. Neurol.* **2003**, *461*, 166–173. [CrossRef]
41. Takaoka, Y.; Setsu, T.; Misaki, K.; Yamauchi, T.; Terashima, T. Expression of reelin in the dorsal cochlear nucleus of the mouse. *Brain Res. Dev. Brain Res.* **2005**, *159*, 127–134. [CrossRef]
42. Goffinet, A.M. The embryonic development of the inferior olivary complex in normal and reeler (rlORL) mutant mice. *J. Comp. Neurol.* **1983**, *219*, 10–24. [CrossRef] [PubMed]
43. Terashima, T.; Inoue, K.; Inoue, Y.; Mikoshiba, K.; Tsukada, Y. Observations on the brainstem-spinal descending systems of normal and reeler mutant mice by the retrograde HRP method. *J. Comp. Neurol.* **1984**, *225*, 95–104. [CrossRef] [PubMed]
44. Tanaka, Y.; Okado, H.; Terashima, T. Retrograde infection of precerebellar nuclei neurons by injection of a recombinant adenovirus into the cerebellar cortex of normal and reeler mice. *Arch. Histol. Cytol.* **2007**, *70*, 51–62. [CrossRef] [PubMed]

45. Villeda, S.A.; Akopians, A.L.; Babayan, A.H.; Basbaum, A.I.; Phelps, P.E. Absence of Reelin results in altered nociception and aberrant neuronal positioning in the dorsal spinal cord. *Neuroscience* **2006**, *139*, 1385–1396. [CrossRef] [PubMed]
46. Yip, J.W.; Yip, Y.P.; Nakajima, K.; Capriotti, C. Reelin controls position of autonomic neurons in the spinal cord. *Proc. Natl. Acad. Sci. USA* **2000**, *97*, 8612–8616. [CrossRef]
47. Phelps, P.E.; Rich, R.; Dupuy-Davies, S.; Rios, Y.; Wong, T. Evidence for a cell-specific action of Reelin in the spinal cord. *Dev. Biol.* **2002**, *244*, 180–198. [CrossRef]
48. Stanfield, B.B.; Cowan, W.M. The morphology of the hippocampus and dentate gyrus in normal and reeler mice. *J. Comp. Neurol.* **1979**, *185*, 393–422. [CrossRef]
49. Pinto Lord, M.C.; Caviness, V.S., Jr. Determinants of cell shape and orientation: A comparative Golgi analysis of cell-axon interrelationships in the developing neocortex of normal and reeler mice. *J. Comp. Neurol.* **1979**, *187*, 49–69. [CrossRef]
50. Niu, S.; Yabut, O.; D'Arcangelo, G. The Reelin signaling pathway promotes dendritic spine development in hippocampal neurons. *J. Neurosci.* **2008**, *28*, 10339–10348. [CrossRef]
51. Olson, E.C.; Kim, S.; Walsh, C.A. Impaired neuronal positioning and dendritogenesis in the neocortex after cell-autonomous Dab1 suppression. *J. Neurosci.* **2006**, *26*, 1767–1775. [CrossRef]
52. Niu, S.; Renfro, A.; Quattrocchi, C.C.; Sheldon, M.; D'Arcangelo, G. Reelin promotes hippocampal dendrite development through the VLDLR/ApoER2-Dab1 pathway. *Neuron* **2004**, *41*, 71–84. [CrossRef]
53. Liu, W.S.; Pesold, C.; Rodriguez, M.A.; Carboni, G.; Auta, J.; Lacor, P.; Larson, J.; Condie, B.G.; Guidotti, A.; Costa, E. Down-regulation of dendritic spine and glutamic acid decarboxylase 67 expressions in the reelin haploinsufficient heterozygous reeler mouse. *Proc. Natl. Acad. Sci. USA* **2001**, *98*, 3477–3482. [CrossRef] [PubMed]
54. Chameau, P.; Inta, D.; Vitalis, T.; Monyer, H.; Wadman, W.J.; van Hooft, J.A. The N-terminal region of reelin regulates postnatal dendritic maturation of cortical pyramidal neurons. *Proc. Natl. Acad. Sci. USA* **2009**, *106*, 7227–7232. [CrossRef] [PubMed]
55. Manita, S.; Suzuki, T.; Homma, C.; Matsumoto, T.; Odagawa, M.; Yamada, K.; Ota, K.; Matsubara, C.; Inutsuka, A.; Sato, M.; et al. Top-Down Cortical Circuit for Accurate Sensory Perception. *Neuron* **2015**, *86*, 1304–1316. [CrossRef] [PubMed]
56. Larkum, M.E.; Petro, L.S.; Sachdev RN, S.; Muckli, L. A Perspective on cortical layering and layer-spanning neuronal elements. *Front. Neuroanat.* **2018**, *12*, 56. [CrossRef]
57. Lörincz, A.; Notomi, T.; Tamás, G.; Shigemoto, R.; Nusser, Z. Polarized and compartment-dependent distribution of HCN1 in pyramidal cell dendrites. *Nat. Neurosci.* **2002**, *5*, 1185–1193. [CrossRef]
58. Kupferman, J.V.; Basu, J.; Russo, M.J.; Guevarra, J.; Cheung, S.K.; Siegelbaum, S.A. Reelin signaling specifies the molecular identity of the pyramidal neuron distal dendritic compartment. *Cell* **2014**, *158*, 1335–1347. [CrossRef]
59. Meseke, M.; Neumuller, F.; Brunne, B.; Li, X.; Anstotz, M.; Pohlkamp, T.; Rogalla, M.M.; Herz, J.; Rune, G.M.; Bender, R.A. distal dendritic enrichment of HCN1 channels in hippocampal CA1 is promoted by estrogen, but does not require Reelin. *eNeuro* **2018**, *5*. [CrossRef]
60. Bliss, T.V.; Chung, S.H. An electrophysiological study of the hippocampus of the 'reeler' mutant mouse. *Nature* **1974**, *252*, 153–155. [CrossRef]
61. Silva, L.R.; Gutnick, M.J.; Connors, B.W. Laminar distribution of neuronal membrane properties in neocortex of normal and reeler mouse. *J. Neurophysiol.* **1991**, *66*, 2034–2040. [CrossRef]
62. Shah, M.M.; Hammond, R.S.; Hoffman, D.A. Dendritic ion channel trafficking and plasticity. *Trends Neurosci.* **2010**, *33*, 307–316. [CrossRef] [PubMed]
63. Chen, Y.; Beffert, U.; Ertunc, M.; Tang, T.S.; Kavalali, E.T.; Bezprozvanny, I.; Herz, J. Reelin modulates NMDA receptor activity in cortical neurons. *J. Neurosci.* **2005**, *25*, 8209–8216. [CrossRef] [PubMed]
64. Beffert, U.; Weeber, E.J.; Durudas, A.; Qiu, S.; Masiulis, I.; Sweatt, J.D.; Li, W.P.; Adelmann, G.; Frotscher, M.; Hammer, R.E.; et al. Modulation of synaptic plasticity and memory by Reelin involves differential splicing of the lipoprotein receptor Apoer2. *Neuron* **2005**, *47*, 567–579. [CrossRef] [PubMed]
65. Ishida, A.; Shimazaki, K.; Terashima, T.; Kawai, N. An electrophysiological and immunohistochemical study of the hippocampus of the reeler mutant mouse. *Brain Res.* **1994**, *662*, 60–68. [CrossRef]

66. Pujadas, L.; Gruart, A.; Bosch, C.; Delgado, L.; Teixeira, C.M.; Rossi, D.; De Lecea, L.; Martinez, A.; Delgado-Garcia, J.M.; Soriano, E. Reelin regulates postnatal neurogenesis and enhances spine hypertrophy and long-term potentiation. *J. Neurosci.* **2010**, *30*, 4636–4649. [CrossRef]
67. Rogers, J.T.; Rusiana, I.; Trotter, J.; Zhao, L.; Donaldson, E.; Pak, D.T.; Babus, L.W.; Peters, M.; Banko, J.L.; Chavis, P.; et al. Reelin supplementation enhances cognitive ability, synaptic plasticity, and dendritic spine density. *Learn. Mem.* **2011**, *18*, 558–564. [CrossRef]
68. Weeber, E.J.; Beffert, U.; Jones, C.; Christian, J.M.; Forster, E.; Sweatt, J.D.; Herz, J. Reelin and ApoE receptors cooperate to enhance hippocampal synaptic plasticity and learning. *J. Biol. Chem.* **2002**, *277*, 39944–39952. [CrossRef]
69. Parnavelas, J.G. The origin and migration of cortical neurones: New vistas. *Trends Neurosci.* **2000**, *23*, 126–131. [CrossRef]
70. D'Arcangelo, G. Reelin mouse mutants as models of cortical development disorders. *Epilepsy Behav.* **2006**, *8*, 81–90. [CrossRef]
71. Caviness, V.S., Jr. Patterns of cell and fiber distribution in the neocortex of the reeler mutant mouse. *J. Comp. Neurol* **1976**, *170*, 435–447. [CrossRef]
72. Terashima, T.; Takayama, C.; Ichikawa, R.; Inoue, Y. Dendritic arbolization of large pyramidal neurons in the motor cortex of normal and reeler mutant mouse. *Okajimas Folia Anat. Jpn.* **1992**, *68*, 351–363. [CrossRef] [PubMed]
73. Landrieu, P.; Goffinet, A. Inverted pyramidal neurons and their axons in the neocortex of reeler mutant mice. *Cell Tissue Res.* **1981**, *218*, 293–301. [CrossRef] [PubMed]
74. Terashima, T.; Inoue, K.; Inoue, Y.; Mikoshiba, K.; Tsukada, Y. Distribution and morphology of corticospinal tract neurons in reeler mouse cortex by the retrograde HRP method. *J. Comp. Neurol.* **1983**, *218*, 314–326. [CrossRef] [PubMed]
75. Markram, H.; Toledo-Rodriguez, M.; Wang, Y.; Gupta, A.; Silberberg, G.; Wu, C. Interneurons of the neocortical inhibitory system. *Nat. Rev. Neurosci.* **2004**, *5*, 793–807. [CrossRef] [PubMed]
76. Yabut, O.; Renfro, A.; Niu, S.; Swann, J.W.; Marin, O.; D'Arcangelo, G. Abnormal laminar position and dendrite development of interneurons in the reeler forebrain. *Brain Res.* **2007**, *1140*, 75–83. [CrossRef]
77. Hevner, R.F.; Daza, R.A.; Englund, C.; Kohtz, J.; Fink, A. Postnatal shifts of interneuron position in the neocortex of normal and reeler mice: Evidence for inward radial migration. *Neuroscience* **2004**, *124*, 605–618. [CrossRef]
78. Pla, R.; Borrell, V.; Flames, N.; Marin, O. Layer acquisition by cortical GABAergic interneurons is independent of Reelin signaling. *J. Neurosci.* **2006**, *26*, 6924–6934. [CrossRef]
79. Hammond, V.; So, E.; Gunnersen, J.; Valcanis, H.; Kalloniatis, M.; Tan, S.S. Layer positioning of late-born cortical interneurons is dependent on Reelin but not p35 signaling. *J. Neurosci.* **2006**, *26*, 1646–1655. [CrossRef]
80. Lakoma, J.; Garcia-Alonso, L.; Luque, J.M. Reelin sets the pace of neocortical neurogenesis. *Development* **2011**, *138*, 5223–5234. [CrossRef]
81. Nishikawa, S.; Goto, S.; Hamasaki, T.; Yamada, K.; Ushio, Y. Involvement of reelin and Cajal-Retzius cells in the developmental formation of vertical columnar structures in the cerebral cortex: Evidence from the study of mouse presubicular cortex. *Cereb. Cortex* **2002**, *12*, 1024–1030. [CrossRef]
82. Nishibe, M.; Katsuyama, Y.; Yamashita, T. Developmental abnormality contributes to cortex-dependent motor impairments and higher intracortical current requirement in the reeler homozygous mutants. *Brain Struct. Funct.* **2018**, *223*, 2575–2587. [CrossRef] [PubMed]
83. Simmons, P.A.; Lemmon, V.; Pearlman, A.L. Afferent and efferent connections of the striate and extrastriate visual cortex of the normal and reeler mouse. *J. Comp. Neurol.* **1982**, *211*, 295–308. [CrossRef] [PubMed]
84. Wagener, R.J.; David, C.; Zhao, S.; Haas, C.A.; Staiger, J.F. The somatosensory cortex of reeler mutant mice shows absent layering but intact formation and behavioral activation of columnar somatotopic maps. *J. Neurosci.* **2010**, *30*, 15700–15709. [CrossRef] [PubMed]
85. Pielecka-Fortuna, J.; Wagener, R.J.; Martens, A.K.; Goetze, B.; Schmidt, K.F.; Staiger, J.F.; Lowel, S. The disorganized visual cortex in reelin-deficient mice is functional and allows for enhanced plasticity. *Brain Struct. Funct.* **2015**, *220*, 3449–3467. [CrossRef]
86. Guy, J.; Wagener, R.J.; Mock, M.; Staiger, J.F. persistence of functional sensory maps in the absence of cortical layers in the somsatosensory cortex of Reeler mice. *Cereb. Cortex* **2015**, *25*, 2517–2528. [CrossRef]

87. Prume, M.; Rollenhagen, A.; Lubke, J.H.R. Structural and synaptic organization of the adult reeler mouse somatosensory neocortex: A comparative fine-scale electron microscopic study of Reeler with wild type mice. *Front. Neuroanat.* **2018**, *12*, 80. [CrossRef]
88. Grossberg, S. Towards a unified theory of neocortex: Laminar cortical circuits for vision and cognition. *Prog. Brain Res.* **2007**, *165*, 79–104.
89. D'Souza, R.D.; Burkhalter, A.A. Laminar Organization for Selective Cortico-Cortical Communication. *Front. Neuroanat.* **2017**, *11*, 71. [CrossRef]
90. Guy, J.; Staiger, J.F. The Functioning of a Cortex without Layers. *Front. Neuroanat.* **2017**, *11*, 54. [CrossRef]
91. Mikoshiba, K.; Nagaike, K.; Kohsaka, S.; Takamatsu, K.; Aoki, E.; Tsukada, Y. Developmental studies on the cerebellum from reeler mutant mouse in vivo and in vitro. *Dev. Biol.* **1980**, *79*, 64–80. [CrossRef]
92. Altman, J.; Bayer, S.A. *Development of the Cerebellar System in Relation to Its Evolution, Structure and Functions*; CRC Press: Boca Raton, FL, USA, 1997.
93. Cocito, C.; Merighi, A.; Giacobini, M.; Lossi, L. alterations of cell proliferation and apoptosis in the hypoplastic Reeler cerebellum. *Front. Cell. Neurosci.* **2016**, *10*, 141. [CrossRef] [PubMed]
94. Castagna, C.; Merighi, A.; Lossi, L. Cell death and neurodegeneration in the postnatal development of cerebellar vermis in normal and Reeler mice. *Ann. Anat.* **2016**, *207*, 76–90. [CrossRef] [PubMed]
95. Mariani, J.; Crepel, F.; Mikoshiba, K.; Changeux, J.P.; Sotelo, C. Anatomical, physiological and biochemical studies of the cerebellum from Reeler mutant mouse. *Philos. Trans. R. Soc. B* **1977**, *281*, 1–28. [CrossRef] [PubMed]
96. Heckroth, J.A.; Goldowitz, D.; Eisenman, L.M. Purkinje cell reduction in the reeler mutant mouse: A quantitative immunohistochemical study. *J. Comp. Neurol.* **1989**, *279*, 546–555. [CrossRef]
97. Yuasa, S.; Kitoh, J.; Oda, S.; Kawamura, K. Obstructed migration of Purkinje cells in the developing cerebellum of the reeler mutant mouse. *Anat. Embryol.* **1993**, *188*, 317–329. [CrossRef]
98. Castagna, C.; Aimar, P.; Alasia, S.; Lossi, L. Post-natal development of the Reeler mouse cerebellum: An ultrastructural study. *Ann. Anat.* **2014**, *196*, 224–235. [CrossRef]
99. Mariani, J. Extent of multiple innervation of Purkinje cells by climbing fibers in the olivocerebellar system of weaver, reeler, and staggerer mutant mice. *J. Neurobiol.* **1982**, *13*, 119–126. [CrossRef]
100. Terashima, T.; Inoue, K.; Inoue, Y.; Mikoshiba, K.; Tsukada, Y. Observations on Golgi epithelial cells and granule cells in the cerebellum of the reeler mutant mouse. *Brain Res.* **1985**, *350*, 103–112. [CrossRef]
101. Keays, D.A.; Tian, G.; Poirier, K.; Huang, G.J.; Siebold, C.; Cleak, J.; Oliver, P.L.; Fray, M.; Harvey, R.J.; Molnár, Z.; et al. Mutations in αtubulin cause abnormal neuronal migration in mice and lissencephaly in humans. *Cell* **2007**, *128*, 45–57. [CrossRef]
102. Bahi-Buisson, N.; Poirier, K.; Fourniol, F.; Saillour, Y.; Valence, S.; Lebrun, N.; Hully, M.; Bianco, C.F.; Boddaert, N.; Elie, C.; et al. The wide spectrum of tubulinopathies: What are the key features for the diagnosis? *Brain* **2014**, *137*, 1676–1700. [CrossRef]
103. Aiken, J.; Buscaglia, G.; Bates, E.A.; Moore, J.K. The α-tubulin gene TUBA1A in brain development: A key ingredient in the neuronal isotype blend. *J. Dev. Biol.* **2017**, *5*, 8. [CrossRef] [PubMed]
104. Goncalves, F.G.; Freddi, T.A.L.; Taranath, A.; Lakshmanan, R.; Goetti, R.; Feltrin, F.S.; Mankad, K.; Teixeira, S.R.; Hanagandi, P.B.; Arrigoni, F. Tubulinopathies. *Top. Magn. Reson. Imaging* **2018**, *27*, 395–408. [CrossRef] [PubMed]
105. Romaniello, R.; Arrigoni, F.; Fry, A.E.; Bassi, M.T.; Rees, M.I.; Borgatti, R.; Pilz, D.T.; Cushion, T.D. Tubulin genes and malformations of cortical development. *Eur. J. Med. Genet.* **2018**, *61*, 744–754. [CrossRef] [PubMed]
106. Dazzo, E.; Fanciulli, M.; Serioli, E.; Minervini, G.; Pulitano, P.; Binelli, S.; Di, B.C.; Luisi, C.; Pasini, E.; Striano, S.; et al. Heterozygous reelin mutations cause autosomal-dominant lateral temporal epilepsy. *Am. J. Hum. Genet.* **2015**, *96*, 992–1000. [CrossRef]
107. Michelucci, R.; Pulitano, P.; Di Bonaventura, C.; Binelli, S.; Luisi, C.; Pasini, E.; Striano, S.; Striano, P.; Coppola, G.; La Neve, A.; et al. The clinical phenotype of autosomal dominant lateral temporal lobe epilepsy related to reelin mutations. *Epilepsy Behav.* **2017**, *68*, 103–107. [CrossRef]
108. Ceská, K.; Aulická, Š.; Horák, O.; Danhofer, P.; Ríha, P.; Marecek, R.; Šenkyrík, J.; Rektor, I.; Brázdil, M.; Oslejsková, H. Autosomal dominant temporal lobe epilepsy associated with heterozygous reelin mutation: 3 T brain MRI study with advanced neuroimaging methods. *Epilepsy Behav. Case Rep.* **2019**, *11*, 39–42. [CrossRef]

109. Hwang, E.; Brown, R.E.; Kocsis, B.; Kim, T.; McKenna, J.T.; McNally, J.M.; Han, H.B.; Choi, J.H. Optogenetic stimulation of basal forebrain parvalbumin neurons modulates the cortical topography of auditory steady-state responses. *Brain Struct. Funct.* **2019**, *224*, 1505–1518. [CrossRef]
110. Ammassari-Teule, M.; Sgobio, C.; Biamonte, F.; Marrone, C.; Mercuri, N.B.; Keller, F. Reelin haploinsufficiency reduces the density of PV+neurons in circumscribed regions of the striatum and selectively alters striatal-based behaviors. *Psychopharmacology* **2009**, *204*, 511–521. [CrossRef]
111. Nullmeier, S.; Panther, P.; Dobrowolny, H.; Frotscher, M.; Zhao, S.; Schwegler, H.; Wolf, R. Region-specific alteration of GABAergic markers in the brain of heterozygous reeler mice. *Eur. J. Neurosci.* **2011**, *33*, 689–698. [CrossRef]
112. Ding, L.; Satish, S.; Zhou, C.; Gallagher, M.J. Cortical activation in generalized seizures. *Epilepsia* **2019**, *60*, 1932–1941. [CrossRef]
113. Boycott, K.M.; Bonnemann, C.; Herz, J.; Neuert, S.; Beaulieu, C.; Scott, J.N.; Venkatasubramanian, A.; Parboosingh, J.S. Mutations in VLDLR as a cause for autosomal recessive cerebellar ataxia with mental retardation (dysequilibrium syndrome). *J. Child Neurol.* **2009**, *24*, 1310–1315. [CrossRef] [PubMed]
114. Trommsdorff, M.; Gotthardt, M.; Hiesberger, T.; Shelton, J.; Stockinger, W.; Nimpf, J.; Hammer, R.E.; Richardson, J.A.; Herz, J. Reeler/Disabled-like disruption of neuronal migration in knockout mice lacking the VLDL receptor and ApoE receptor 2. *Cell* **1999**, *97*, 689–701. [CrossRef]
115. Korwek, K.M.; Trotter, J.H.; LaDu, M.J.; Sullivan, P.M.; Weeber, E.J. ApoE isoform-dependent changes in hippocampal synaptic function. *Mol. Neurodegener.* **2009**, *4*, 21. [CrossRef] [PubMed]
116. Matilla-Dueñas, A.; Volpini, V. Spinocerebellar ataxia type 37. In *GeneReviews®*; Adam, M.P., Ardinger, H.H., Pagon, R.A., Wallace, S.E., Eds.; University of Washington: Seattle, WA, USA, 2019.
117. Serrano-Munuera, C.; Corral-Juan, M.; Stevanin, G.; San Nicolás, H.; Roig, C.; Corral, J.; Campos, B.; De Jorge, L.; Morcillo-Suárez, C.; Navarro, A.; et al. New subtype of spinocerebellar ataxia with altered vertical eye movements mapping to chromosome 1p32 subtype of SCA with altered vertical eye movements. *JAMA Neurol.* **2013**, *70*, 764–771. [CrossRef] [PubMed]
118. Seixas, A.I.; Loureiro, J.R.; Costa, C.; Ordóñez-Ugalde, A.S.; Marcelino, H.; Oliveira, C.L.; Loureiro, J.L.; Dhingra, A.; Brandão, E.; Cruz, V.T.; et al. A Pentanucleotide ATTTC Repeat Insertion in the Non-coding Region of DAB1, Mapping to SCA37, Causes Spinocerebellar Ataxia. *Am. J. Hum. Genet.* **2017**, *101*, 87–103. [CrossRef] [PubMed]
119. Ware, M.L.; Fox, J.W.; González, J.L.; Davis, N.M.; De Rouvroit, C.L.; Russo, C.J.; Chua, S.C.; Goffinet, A.M.; Walsh, C.A. Aberrant splicing of a mouse disabled homolog, mdab1, in the scrambler Mouse. *Neuron* **1997**, *19*, 239–249. [CrossRef]
120. Dobyns, W.B.; Das, S. PAFAH1B1-Associated Lissencephaly/Subcortical Band Heterotopia. In *GeneReviews®*; Adam, M.P., Ardinger, H.H., Pagon, R.A., Wallace, S.E., Eds.; University of Washington: Seattle, WA, USA, 2014.
121. Katayama, K.I.; Hayashi, K.; Inoue, S.; Sakaguchi, K.; Nakajima, K. Enhanced expression of Pafah1b1 causes over-migration of cerebral cortical neurons into the marginal zone. *Brain Struct. Funct.* **2017**, *222*, 4283–4291. [CrossRef]
122. Hunt, R.F.; Dinday, M.T.; Hindle-Katel, W.; Baraban, S.C. LIS1 Deficiency Promotes Dysfunctional synaptic integration of granule cells generated in the developing and adult dentate gyrus. *J. Neurosci.* **2012**, *32*, 12862–12875. [CrossRef]
123. Zhang, G.; Assadi, A.H.; McNeil, R.S.; Beffert, U.; Wynshaw-Boris, A.; Herz, J.; Clark, G.D.; D'Arcangelo, G. The Pafah1b complex interacts with the Reelin receptor VLDLR. *PLoS ONE* **2007**, *2*, e252. [CrossRef]
124. Enevoldson, T.P.; Sanders, M.D.; Harding, A.E. Autosomal dominant cerebellar ataxia with pigmentary macular dystrophy. A clinical and genetic study of eight families. *Brain* **1994**, *117*, 445–460. [CrossRef]
125. McCullough, S.D.; Xu, X.; Dent, S.Y.; Bekiranov, S.; Roeder, R.G.; Grant, P.A. Reelin is a target of polyglutamine expanded ataxin-7 in human spinocerebellar ataxia type 7 (SCA7) astrocytes. *Proc. Natl. Acad. Sci. USA* **2012**, *109*, 21319–21324. [CrossRef] [PubMed]
126. Lammert, D.B.; Howell, B.W. RELN Mutations in Autism Spectrum Disorder. *Front. Cell Neurosci.* **2016**, *10*, 84. [CrossRef] [PubMed]
127. Persico, A.M.; D'Agruma, L.; Maiorano, N.; Totaro, A.; Militerni, R.; Bravaccio, C.; Wassink, T.H.; Schneider, C.; Melmed, R.; Trillo, S.; et al. Reelin gene alleles and haplotypes as a factor predisposing to autistic disorder. *Mol. Psychiatry* **2001**, *6*, 150–159. [CrossRef] [PubMed]

128. Zhang, H.; Liu, X.; Zhang, C.; Mundo, E.; Macciardi, F.; Grayson, D.R.; Guidotti, A.R.; Holden, J.J.A. Reelin gene alleles and susceptibility to autism spectrum disorders. *Mol. Psychiatry* **2002**, *7*, 1012–1017. [CrossRef] [PubMed]
129. Holt, R.; Barnby, G.; Maestrini, E.; Bacchelli, E.; Brocklebank, D.; Sousa, I.S.; Mulder, E.J.; Kantojärvi, K.; Järvelä, I.; Klauck, S.M.; et al. Linkage and candidate gene studies of autism spectrum disorders in European populations. *Eur. J. Hum. Genet.* **2010**, *18*, 1013–1019. [CrossRef] [PubMed]
130. Devlin, B.; Bennett, P.; Dawson, G.; Figlewicz, D.A.; Grigorenko, E.L.; McMahon, W.; Minshew, N.; Pauls, D.; Smith, M.; Spence, M.A.; et al. Alleles of a reelin CGG repeat do not convey liability to autism in a sample from the CPEA network. *Am. J. Med. Genet.* **2004**, *126*, 46–50. [CrossRef]
131. Bonora, E.; Beyer, K.S.; Lamb, J.A.; Parr, J.R.; Klauck, S.M.; Benner, A.; Paolucci, M.; Abbott, A.; Ragoussis, I.; Poustka, A.; et al. Analysis of reelin as a candidate gene for autism. *Mol. Psychiatry* **2003**, *8*, 885–892. [CrossRef]
132. Wang, Z.; Hong, Y.; Zou, L.; Zhong, R.; Zhu, B.; Shen, N.; Chen, W.; Lou, J.; Ke, J.; Zhang, T.; et al. Reelin gene variants and risk of autism spectrum disorders: An integrated meta-analysis. *Am. J. Med. Genet.* **2014**, *165*, 192–200. [CrossRef]
133. Parihar, R.; Ganesh, S. Autism genes: The continuum that connects us all. *J. Genet.* **2016**, *95*, 481–483. [CrossRef]
134. De Rubeis, S.; He, X.; Goldberg, A.P.; Poultney, C.S.; Samocha, K.; Ercument Cicek, A.; Kou, Y.; Liu, L.; Fromer, M.; Walker, S.; et al. Synaptic, transcriptional and chromatin genes disrupted in autism. *Nature* **2014**, *515*, 209–215. [CrossRef]
135. Neale, B.M.; Kou, Y.; Liu, L.; Ma'ayan, A.; Samocha, K.E.; Sabo, A.; Lin, C.F.; Stevens, C.; Wang, L.S.; Makarov, V.; et al. Patterns and rates of exonic de novo mutations in autism spectrum disorders. *Nature* **2012**, *485*, 242–245. [CrossRef] [PubMed]
136. Iossifov, I.; O'Roak, B.J.; Sanders, S.J.; Ronemus, M.; Krumm, N.; Levy, D.; Stessman, H.A.; Witherspoon, K.T.; Vives, L.; Patterson, K.E.; et al. The contribution of de novo coding mutations to autism spectrum disorder. *Nature* **2014**, *515*, 216–221. [CrossRef] [PubMed]
137. Gaugler, T.; Klei, L.; Sanders, S.J.; Bodea, C.A.; Goldberg, A.P.; Lee, A.B.; Mahajan, M.; Manaa, D.; Pawitan, Y.; Reichert, J.; et al. Most genetic risk for autism resides with common variation. *Nat. Genet.* **2014**, *46*, 881–885. [CrossRef] [PubMed]
138. Fatemi, S.H. Reelin mutations in mouse and man: From reeler mouse to schizophrenia, mood disorders, autism and lissencephaly. *Mol. Psychiatry* **2001**, *6*, 129–133. [CrossRef]
139. Ecker, C. The neuroanatomy of autism spectrum disorder: An overview of structural neuroimaging findings and their translatability to the clinical setting. *Autism* **2017**, *21*, 18–28. [CrossRef]
140. Lange, N.; Travers, B.G.; Bigler, E.D.; Prigge, M.B.; Froehlich, A.L.; Nielsen, J.A.; Cariello, A.N.; Zielinski, B.A.; Anderson, J.S.; Fletcher, P.T.; et al. Longitudinal volumetric brain changes in autism spectrum disorder ages 6–35 years. *Autism Res.* **2015**, *8*, 82–93. [CrossRef]
141. Shen, M.D.; Nordahl, C.W.; Young, G.S.; Wootton-Gorges, S.L.; Lee, A.; Liston, S.E.; Harrington, K.R.; Ozonoff, S.; Amaral, D.G. Early brain enlargement and elevated extra-axial fluid in infants who develop autism spectrum disorder. *Brain* **2013**, *136*, 2825–2835. [CrossRef]
142. Schumann, C.M.; Bloss, C.S.; Barnes, C.C.; Wideman, G.M.; Carper, R.A.; Akshoomoff, N.; Pierce, K.; Hagler, D.; Schork, N.; Lord, C.; et al. Longitudinal magnetic resonance imaging study of cortical development through early childhood in autism. *J. Neurosci.* **2010**, *30*, 4419–4427. [CrossRef]
143. Hazlett, H.C.; Poe, M.D.; Gerig, G.; Styner, M.; Chappell, C.; Smith, R.G.; Vachet, C.; Piven, J. Early brain overgrowth in autism associated with an increase in cortical surface area before age 2 years. *Arch. Gen. Psychiatry* **2011**, *68*, 467–476. [CrossRef]
144. Minshew, N.J.; Sweeney, J.A.; Bauman, M.L.; Webb, S.J. Neurologic aspects of autism. In *Handbook of Autism and Pervasive Developmental Disorders*; Volkmar, F.R., Paul, R., Klin, A., Cohen, D., Eds.; John Wiley & Sons, Inc.: Hoboken, NJ, USA, 2005; pp. 473–514. [CrossRef]
145. Courchesne, E.; Yeung-Courchesne, R.; Hesselink, J.R.; Jernigan, T.L. Hypoplasia of cerebellar vermal lobules VI and VII in autism. *N. Engl. J. Med.* **1988**, *318*, 1349–1354. [CrossRef]
146. Courchesne, E.; Saitoh, O.; Townsend, J.; Yeung-Courchesne, R.; Press, G.; Lincoln, A.; Haas, R.; Schreibman, L. Cerebellar hypoplasia and hyperplasia in infantile autism. *Lancet* **1994**, *343*, 63–64. [CrossRef]

147. Scott, J.A.; Schumann, C.M.; Goodlin-Jones, B.L.; Amaral, D.G. A comprehensive volumetric analysis of the cerebellum in children and adolescents with autism spectrum disorder. *Autism Res.* **2009**, *2*, 246–257. [CrossRef] [PubMed]
148. Piven, J.; Saliba, K.; Bailey, J.; Arndt, S. An MRI study of autism: The cerebellum revisited. *Neurology* **1997**, *49*, 546–551. [CrossRef] [PubMed]
149. Lucibello, S.; Verdolotti, T.; Giordano, F.M.; Lapenta, L.; Infante, A.; Piludu, F.; Tartaglione, T.; Chieffo, D.; Colosimo, C.; Mercuri, E.; et al. Brain morphometry of preschool age children affected by autism spectrum disorder: Correlation with clinical findings. *Clin. Anat.* **2019**, *32*, 143–150. [CrossRef] [PubMed]
150. Oguro-Ando, A.; Zuko, A.; Kleijer, K.T.E.; Burbach, J.P.H. A current view on contactin-4,-5, and-6: Implications in neurodevelopmental disorders. *Mol. Cell. Neurosci.* **2017**, *81*, 72–83. [CrossRef] [PubMed]
151. Kemper, T.L.; Bauman, M.L. The contribution of neuropathologic studies to the understanding of autism. *Neurol. Clin.* **1993**, *11*, 175–187. [CrossRef]
152. Amaral, D.G.; Schumann, C.M.; Nordahl, C.W. Neuroanatomy of autism. *Trends Neurosci.* **2008**, *31*, 137–145. [CrossRef]
153. Varghese, M.; Keshav, N.; Jacot-Descombes, S.; Warda, T.; Wicinski, B.; Dickstein, D.L.; Harony-Nicolas, H.; De Rubeis, S.; Drapeau, E.; Buxbaum, J.D.; et al. Autism spectrum disorder: Neuropathology and animal models. *Acta Neuropathol.* **2017**, *134*, 537–566. [CrossRef]
154. Wegiel, J.; Kuchna, I.; Nowicki, K.; Imaki, H.; Wegiel, J.; Marchi, E.; Ma, S.Y.; Chauhan, A.; Chauhan, V.; Bobrowicz, T.W.; et al. The neuropathology of autism: Defects of neurogenesis and neuronal migration, and dysplastic changes. *Acta Neuropathol.* **2010**, *119*, 755–770. [CrossRef]
155. Wegiel, J.; Flory, M.; Kuchna, I.; Nowicki, K.; Ma, S.Y.; Imaki, H.; Wegiel, J.; Frackowiak, J.; Kolecka, B.M.; Wierzba-Bobrowicz, T.; et al. Neuronal nucleus and cytoplasm volume deficit in children with autism and volume increase in adolescents and adults. *Acta Neuropathol. Commun.* **2015**, *3*, 2. [CrossRef]
156. Casanova, M.F. Neuropathological and genetic findings in autism: The significance of a putative minicolumnopathy. *Neuroscientist* **2006**, *12*, 435–441. [CrossRef] [PubMed]
157. Mukaetova-Ladinska, E.B.; Arnold, H.; Jaros, E.; Perry, R.; Perry, E. Depletion of MAP2 expression and laminar cytoarchitectonic changes in dorsolateral prefrontal cortex in adult autistic individuals. *Neuropathol. Appl. Neurobiol.* **2004**, *30*, 615–623. [CrossRef] [PubMed]
158. Raymond, G.V.; Bauman, M.L.; Kemper, T.L. Hippocampus in autism: A Golgi analysis. *Acta Neuropathol.* **1996**, *91*, 117–119. [CrossRef] [PubMed]
159. Hutsler, J.J.; Zhang, H. Increased dendritic spine densities on cortical projection neurons in autism spectrum disorders. *Brain Res.* **2010**, *1309*, 83–94. [CrossRef] [PubMed]
160. Camacho, J.; Ejaz, E.; Ariza, J.; Noctor, S.C.; Martínez-Cerdeño, V.N. RELN-expressing neuron density in layer I of the superior temporal lobe is similar in human brains with autism and in age-matched controls. *Neurosci. Lett.* **2014**, *579*, 163–167. [CrossRef]
161. Courchesne, E.; Mouton, P.R.; Calhoun, M.E.; Semendeferi, K.; Ahrens-Barbeau, C.; Hallet, M.J.; Barnes, C.C.; Pierce, K. Neuron number and size in prefrontal cortex of children with autism. *JAMA* **2011**, *306*, 2001–2010. [CrossRef]
162. Hashemi, E.; Ariza, J.; Rogers, H.; Noctor, S.C.; Martínez-Cerdeño, V.N. The number of parvalbumin-expressing interneurons is decreased in the prefrontal cortex in autism. *Cereb. Cortex* **2017**, *27*, 1931–1943.
163. Jacot-Descombes, S.; Uppal, N.; Wicinski, B.; Santos, M.; Schmeidler, J.; Giannakopoulos, P.; Heinsein, H.; Schmitz, C.; Hof, P.R. Decreased pyramidal neuron size in Brodmann areas 44 and 45 in patients with autism. *Acta Neuropathol.* **2012**, *124*, 67–79. [CrossRef]
164. Zhubi, A.; Chen, Y.; Guidotti, A.; Grayson, D.R. Epigenetic regulation of RELN and GAD1 in the frontal cortex (FC) of autism spectrum disorder (ASD) subjects. *Int. J. Dev. Neurosci.* **2017**, *62*, 63–72. [CrossRef]
165. Van Kooten, I.A.J.; Palmen, S.J.M.C.; Von Cappeln, P.; Steinbusch, H.W.M.; Korr, H.; Heinsen, H.; Hof, P.R.; Van Engeland, H.; Schmitz, C. Neurons in the fusiform gyrus are fewer and smaller in autism. *Brain* **2008**, *131*, 987–999. [CrossRef]
166. Oblak, A.L.; Rosene, D.L.; Kemper, T.L.; Bauman, M.L.; Blatt, G.J. Altered posterior cingulate cortical cyctoarchitecture, but normal density of neurons and interneurons in the posterior cingulate cortex and fusiform gyrus in autism. *Autism Res.* **2011**, *4*, 200–211. [CrossRef] [PubMed]

167. Kennedy, D.P.; Semendeferi, K.; Courchesne, E. No reduction of spindle neuron number in frontoinsular cortex in autism. *Brain Cogn.* **2007**, *64*, 124–129. [CrossRef] [PubMed]
168. Allman, J.M.; Watson, K.K.; Tetreault, N.A.; Hakeem, A.Y. Intuition and autism: A possible role for Von Economo neurons. *Trends Cogn. Sci.* **2005**, *9*, 367–373. [CrossRef] [PubMed]
169. Santos, M.; Uppal, N.; Butti, C.; Wicinski, B.; Schmeidler, J.; Giannakopoulos, P.; Heinsen, H.; Schmitz, C.; Hof, P.R. Von Economo neurons in autism: A stereologic study of the frontoinsular cortex in children. *Brain Res.* **2011**, *1380*, 206–217. [CrossRef] [PubMed]
170. Simms, M.L.; Kemper, T.L.; Timbie, C.M.; Bauman, M.L.; Blatt, G.J. The anterior cingulate cortex in autism: Heterogeneity of qualitative and quantitative cytoarchitectonic features suggests possible subgroups. *Acta Neuropathol.* **2009**, *118*, 673–684. [CrossRef] [PubMed]
171. Uppal, N.; Wicinski, B.; Buxbaum, J.D.; Heinsen, H.; Schmitz, C.; Hof, P.R. Neuropathology of the Anterior Midcingulate Cortex in Young Children with Autism. *J. Neuropathol. Exp. Neurol.* **2014**, *73*, 891–902. [CrossRef] [PubMed]
172. Weidenheim, K.M.; Goodman, L.; Dickson, D.W.; Gillberg, C.; Råstam, M.; Rapin, I. Etiology and Pathophysiology of Autistic Behavior: Clues from Two Cases with an Unusual Variant of Neuroaxonal Dystrophy. *J. Child Neurol.* **2001**, *16*, 809–819. [CrossRef]
173. Hussman, J.P.; Chung, R.H.; Griswold, A.J.; Jaworski, J.M.; Salyakina, D.; Ma, D.; Konidari, I.; Whitehead, P.L.; Vance, J.M.; Martin, E.R.; et al. A noise-reduction GWAS analysis implicates altered regulation of neurite outgrowth and guidance in autism. *Mol. Autism* **2011**, *2*, 1. [CrossRef]
174. Ichinohe, N.; Knight, A.; Ogawa, M.; Ohshima, T.; Mikoshiba, K.; Yoshihara, Y.; Terashima, T.; Rockland, K.S. Unusual Patch–Matrix Organization in the Retrosplenial Cortex of the Reeler Mouse and *Shaking Rat Kawasaki*. *Cereb. Cortex* **2007**, *18*, 1125–1138. [CrossRef]
175. Ichinohe, N. Small-Scale Module of the Rat Granular retrosplenial cortex: An example of the minicolumn-like structure of the cerebral cortex. *Front. Neuroanat.* **2012**, *5*, 69. [CrossRef]
176. Lui, J.; Hansen, D.; Kriegstein, A. Development and Evolution of the Human Neocortex. *Cell* **2011**, *146*, 18–36. [CrossRef] [PubMed]
177. Romano, E.; Fuso, A.; Laviola, G. Nicotine restores Wt-like levels of reelin and GAD67 gene expression in brain of heterozygous reeler mice. *Neurotox. Res.* **2013**, *24*, 205–215. [CrossRef] [PubMed]
178. Bailey, A.; Luthert, P.; Dean, A.; Harding, B.; Janota, I.; Montgomery, M.; Rutter, M.; Lantos, P. A clinicopathological study of autism. *Brain* **1998**, *121*, 889–905. [CrossRef] [PubMed]
179. Lawrence, Y.A.; Kemper, T.L.; Bauman, M.L.; Blatt, G.J. Parvalbumin-, calbindin-, and calretinin-immunoreactive hippocampal interneuron density in autism. *Acta Neurol. Scand.* **2010**, *121*, 99–108. [CrossRef] [PubMed]
180. Rogers, J.T.; Zhao, L.; Trotter, J.H.; Rusiana, I.; Peters, M.M.; Li, Q.; Donaldson, E.; Banko, J.L.; Keenoy, K.E.; Rebeck, G.W.; et al. Reelin supplementation recovers sensorimotor gating, synaptic plasticity and associative learning deficits in the heterozygous reeler mouse. *J. Psychopharmacol.* **2013**, *27*, 386–395. [CrossRef]
181. Qiu, S.; Zhao, L.F.; Korwek, K.M.; Weeber, E.J. Differential Reelin-Induced Enhancement of NMDA and AMPA Receptor Activity in the Adult Hippocampus. *J. Neurosci.* **2006**, *26*, 12943. [CrossRef]
182. Qiu, S.; Korwek, K.M.; Pratt-Davis, A.R.; Peters, M.; Bergman, M.Y.; Weeber, E.J. Cognitive disruption and altered hippocampus synaptic function in Reelin haploinsufficient mice. *Neurobiol. Learn. Mem.* **2006**, *85*, 228–242. [CrossRef]
183. Hellwig, S.; Hack, I.; Kowalski, J.; Brunne, B.; Jarowyj, J.; Unger, A.; Bock, H.H.; Junghans, D.; Frotscher, M. Role for Reelin in neurotransmitter release. *J. Neurosci.* **2011**, *31*, 2352–2360. [CrossRef]
184. Bauman, M.; Kemper, T.L. Histoanatomic observations of the brain in early infantile autism. *Neurology* **1985**, *35*, 866–874. [CrossRef]
185. Schumann, C.M.; Amaral, D.G. Stereological Analysis of Amygdala Neuron Number in Autism. *J. Neurosci.* **2006**, *26*, 7674–7679. [CrossRef]
186. Wegiel, J.; Flory, M.; Kuchna, I.; Nowicki, K.; Ma, S.Y.; Imaki, H.; Wegiel, J.; Cohen, I.L.; London, E.; Wisniewski, T.; et al. Stereological study of the neuronal number and volume of 38 brain subdivisions of subjects diagnosed with autism reveals significant alterations restricted to the striatum, amygdala and cerebellum. *Acta Neuropathol. Commun.* **2014**, *2*, 141. [CrossRef] [PubMed]
187. Morgan, J.T.; Barger, N.; Amaral, D.G.; Schumann, C.M. Stereological study of amygdala glial populations in adolescents and adults with autism spectrum disorder. *PLoS ONE* **2014**, *9*, e110356. [CrossRef] [PubMed]

188. Boyle, M.P.; Bernard, A.; Thompson, C.L.; Ng, L.; Boe, A.; Mortrud, M.; Hawrylycz, M.J.; Jones, A.R.; Hevner, R.F.; Lein, E.S. Cell-type-specific consequences of reelin deficiency in the mouse neocortex, hippocampus, and amygdala. *J. Comp. Neurol.* **2011**, *519*, 2061–2089. [CrossRef] [PubMed]
189. Fatemi, S.H.; Aldinger, K.A.; Ashwood, P.; Bauman, M.L.; Blaha, C.D.; Blatt, G.J.; Chauhan, A.; Chauhan, V.; Dager, S.R.; Dickson, P.E.; et al. Consensus paper: Pathological role of the cerebellum in autism. *Cerebellum* **2012**, *11*, 777–807. [CrossRef] [PubMed]
190. D'Mello, A.M.; Crocetti, D.; Mostofsky, S.H.; Stoodley, C.J. Cerebellar gray matter and lobular volumes correlate with core autism symptoms. *Neuroimage Clin.* **2015**, *7*, 631–639. [CrossRef]
191. Hampson, D.R.; Blatt, G.J. Autism spectrum disorders and neuropathology of the cerebellum. *Front. Neurosci.* **2015**, *9*, 420. [CrossRef] [PubMed]
192. Skefos, J.; Cummings, C.; Enzer, K.; Holiday, J.; Weed, K.; Levy, E.; Yuce, T.; Kemper, T.; Bauman, M. Regional alterations in purkinje cell density in patients with autism. *PLoS ONE* **2014**, *9*, e81255. [CrossRef]
193. Fatemi, S.H.; Halt, A.R.; Realmuto, G.; Earle, J.; Kist, D.A.; Thuras, P.; Merz, A. Purkinje cell size is reduced in cerebellum of patients with autism. *Cell. Mol. Neurobiol.* **2002**, *22*, 171–175. [CrossRef]
194. Wegiel, J.; Kuchna, I.; Nowicki, K.; Imaki, H.; Wegiel, J.; Ma, S.Y.; Azmitia, E.C.; Banerjee, P.; Flory, M.; Cohen, I.L.; et al. Contribution of olivofloccular circuitry developmental defects to atypical gaze in autism. *Brain Res.* **2013**, *1512*, 106–122. [CrossRef]
195. Whitney, E.R.; Kemper, T.L.; Rosene, D.L.; Bauman, M.L.; Blatt, G.J. Density of cerebellar basket and stellate cells in autism: Evidence for a late developmental loss of Purkinje cells. *J. Neurosci. Res.* **2009**, *87*, 2245–2254. [CrossRef]
196. Maloku, E.; Covelo, I.R.; Hanbauer, I.; Guidotti, A.; Kadriu, B.; Hu, Q.; Davis, J.M.; Costa, E. Lower number of cerebellar Purkinje neurons in psychosis is associated with reduced reelin expression. *Proc. Natl. Acad. Sci. USA* **2010**, *107*, 4407–4411. [CrossRef] [PubMed]
197. Magliaro, C.; Cocito, C.; Bagatella, S.; Merighi, A.; Ahluwalia, A.; Lossi, L. The number of Purkinje neurons and their topology in the cerebellar vermis of normal and reln haplodeficient mouse. *Ann. Anat.* **2016**, *207*, 68–75. [CrossRef] [PubMed]
198. Keller, R.; Basta, R.; Salerno, L.; Elia, M. Autism, epilepsy, and synaptopathies: A not rare association. *Neurol. Sci.* **2017**, *38*, 1353–1361. [CrossRef] [PubMed]
199. Mercati, O.; Huguet, G.; Danckaert, A.; André-Leroux, G.; Maruani, A.; Bellinzoni, M.; Rolland, T.; Gouder, L.; Mathieu, A.; Buratti, J.; et al. CNTN6 mutations are risk factors for abnormal auditory sensory perception in autism spectrum disorders. *Mol. Psychiatry* **2016**, *22*, 625–633. [CrossRef] [PubMed]
200. Castagna, C.; Merighi, A.; Lossi, L. Decreased expression of synaptophysin 1 (SYP1 major synaptic vesicle protein p38) and contactin 6 (CNTN6/NB3) in the cerebellar vermis of reln haplodeficient mice. *Cell. Mol. Neurobiol.* **2019**, *39*, 833–856. [CrossRef] [PubMed]
201. Sundberg, M.; Tochitsky, I.; Buchholz, D.E.; Winden, K.; Kujala, V.; Kapur, K.; Cataltepe, D.; Turner, D.; Han, M.J.; Woolf, C.J.; et al. Purkinje cells derived from TSC patients display hypoexcitability and synaptic deficits associated with reduced FMRP levels and reversed by rapamycin. *Mol. Psychiatry* **2018**, *23*, 2167–2183. [CrossRef]
202. Tassano, E.; Uccella, S.; Giacomini, T.; Severino, M.; Fiorio, P.; Gimelli, G.; Ronchetto, P. Clinical and molecular characterization of two patients with CNTN6 copy number variations. *Cytogenet. Genome Res.* **2018**, *156*, 144–149. [CrossRef]
203. Garcia-Ortiz, J.E.; Zarazúa-Niño, A.I.; Hernández-Orozco, A.A.; Reyes-Oliva, E.A.; Pérez-Ávila, C.E.; Becerra-Solano, L.E.; Galán-Huerta, K.A.; Rivas-Estilla, A.M.; Córdova-Fletes, C. Case Report: Whole exome sequencing unveils an inherited truncating variant in CNTN6 (p. Ser189Ter) in a mexican child with autism spectrum disorder. *J. Autism Dev. Disord.* **2019**. [CrossRef]
204. Hu, J.; Liao, J.; Sathanoori, M.; Kochmar, S.; Sebastian, J.; Yatsenko, S.A.; Surti, U. CNTN6 copy number variations in 14 patients: A possible candidate gene for neurodevelopmental and neuropsychiatric disorders. *J. Neurodev. Disord.* **2015**, *7*, 26. [CrossRef]
205. Stoodley, C.J.; Schmahmann, J.D. Evidence for topographic organization in the cerebellum of motor control versus cognitive and affective processing. *Cortex* **2010**, *46*, 831–844. [CrossRef]
206. Schmahmann, J.D.; Weilburg, J.B.; Sherman, J.C. The neuropsychiatry of the cerebellum—insights from the clinic. *Cerebellum* **2007**, *6*, 254–267. [CrossRef] [PubMed]

207. Catani, M.; Jones, D.K.; Daly, E.; Embiricos, N.; Deeley, Q.; Pugliese, L.; Curran, S.; Robertson, D.; Murphy, D.G. Altered cerebellar feedback projections in Asperger syndrome. *Neuroimage* **2008**, *41*, 1184–1191. [CrossRef] [PubMed]
208. Catani, M.; Dell'Acqua, F.; de Schotten, M.T. A revised limbic system model for memory, emotion and behaviour. *Neurosci. Biobehav. Rev.* **2013**, *37*, 1724–1737. [CrossRef] [PubMed]
209. Bauman, M.L. Microscopic neuroanatomic abnormalities in autism. *Pediatrics* **1991**, *87*, 791–796.
210. Stanfield, A.C.; McIntosh, A.M.; Spencer, M.D.; Philip, R.; Gaur, S.; Lawrie, S.M. Towards a neuroanatomy of autism: A systematic review and meta-analysis of structural magnetic resonance imaging studies. *Eur. Psychiatry* **2008**, *23*, 289–299. [CrossRef]
211. Limperopoulos, C.; Bassan, H.; Gauvreau, K.; Robertson, R.L., Jr.; Sullivan, N.R.; Benson, C.B.; Avery, L.; Stewart, J.; Soul, J.S.; Ringer, S.A.; et al. Does cerebellar injury in premature infants contribute to the high prevalence of long-term cognitive, learning, and behavioral disability in survivors? *Pediatrics* **2007**, *120*, 584–593. [CrossRef]
212. D'Mello, A.M.; Stoodley, C.J. Cerebro-cerebellar circuits in autism spectrum disorder. *Front. Neurosci.* **2015**, *9*, 408. [CrossRef]
213. Stoodley, C.J. Distinct regions of the cerebellum show gray matter decreases in autism, ADHD, and developmental dyslexia. *Front. Syst. Neurosci.* **2014**, *8*, 92. [CrossRef]
214. Insel, T.R. Rethinking schizophrenia. *Nature* **2010**, *468*, 187–193. [CrossRef]
215. Van, L.; Boot, E.; Bassett, A.S. Update on the 22q11.2 deletion syndrome and its relevance to schizophrenia. *Curr. Opin. Psychiatry* **2017**, *30*, 191–196. [CrossRef]
216. Ishii, K.; Kubo, K.I.; Nakajima, K. Reelin and Neuropsychiatric Disorders. *Front. Cell. Neurosci.* **2016**, *10*, 229. [CrossRef] [PubMed]
217. Luo, X.; Chen, S.; Xue, L.; Chen, J.H.; Shi, Y.W.; Zhao, H. SNP variation of RELN gene and schizophrenia in a chinese population: A hospital-based case-control study. *Front. Genet.* **2019**, *10*, 175. [CrossRef] [PubMed]
218. Tost, H.; Weinberger, D.R. RELN rs7341475 and schizophrenia risk: Confusing, yet somehow intriguing. *Biol. Psychiatry* **2011**, *69*, e19. [CrossRef] [PubMed]
219. Weinberger, D.R. Future of Days Past: Neurodevelopment and Schizophrenia. *Schizophr. Bull.* **2017**, *43*, 1164–1168. [CrossRef]
220. Dietsche, B.; Kircher, T.; Falkenberg, I. Structural brain changes in schizophrenia at different stages of the illness: A selective review of longitudinal magnetic resonance imaging studies. *Aust. N. Z. J. Psychiatry* **2017**, *51*, 500–508. [CrossRef]
221. Kahn, R.S.; Sommer, I.E.; Murray, R.M.; Meyer-Lindenberg, A.; Weinberger, D.R.; Cannon, T.D.; O'Donovan, M.; Correll, C.U.; Kane, J.M.; Van Os, J.; et al. Schizophrenia. *Nat. Rev. Dis. Primers* **2015**, *1*, 15067. [CrossRef]
222. Bakhshi, K.; Chance, S.A. The neuropathology of schizophrenia: A selective review of past studies and emerging themes in brain structure and cytoarchitecture. *Neuroscience* **2015**, *303*, 82–102. [CrossRef]
223. Hoistad, M.; Heinsen, H.; Wicinski, B.; Schmitz, C.; Hof, P.R. Stereological assessment of the dorsal anterior cingulate cortex in schizophrenia: Absence of changes in neuronal and glial densities. *Neuropathol. Appl. Neurobiol.* **2013**, *39*, 348–361. [CrossRef]
224. Guidotti, A.; Auta, J.; Davis, J.M.; Di-Giorgi-Gerevini, V.; Dwivedi, Y.; Grayson, D.R.; Impagnatiello, F.; Pandey, G.; Pesold, C.; Sharma, R.; et al. Decrease in reelin and glutamic acid decarboxylase67 (GAD67) expression in schizophrenia and bipolar disorder: A postmortem brain study. *Arch. Gen. Psychiatry* **2000**, *57*, 1061–1069. [CrossRef]
225. Dienel, S.J.; Lewis, D.A. Alterations in cortical interneurons and cognitive function in schizophrenia. *Neurobiol. Dis.* **2019**, *131*, 104208. [CrossRef]
226. Curley, A.A.; Lewis, D.A. Cortical basket cell dysfunction in schizophrenia. *J. Physiol.* **2012**, *590*, 715–724. [CrossRef] [PubMed]
227. Lewis, D.A.; Curley, A.A.; Glausier, J.R.; Volk, D.W. Cortical parvalbumin interneurons and cognitive dysfunction in schizophrenia. *Trends Neurosci.* **2012**, *35*, 57–67. [CrossRef] [PubMed]
228. Ruzicka, W.B.; Zhubi, A.; Veldic, M.; Grayson, D.R.; Costa, E.; Guidotti, A. Selective epigenetic alteration of layer I GABAergic neurons isolated from prefrontal cortex of schizophrenia patients using laser-assisted microdissection. *Mol. Psychiatry* **2007**, *12*, 385–397. [CrossRef] [PubMed]
229. Lewis, D.A. The chandelier neuron in schizophrenia. *Dev. Neurobiol.* **2011**, *71*, 118–127. [CrossRef] [PubMed]

230. Glausier, J.R.; Lewis, D.A. Dendritic spine pathology in schizophrenia. *Neuroscience* **2013**, *251*, 90–107. [CrossRef]
231. MacDonald, M.L.; Alhassan, J.; Newman, J.T.; Richard, M.; Gu, H.; Kelly, R.M.; Sampson, A.R.; Fish, K.N.; Penzes, P.; Wills, Z.P.; et al. Selective loss of smaller spines in schizophrenia. *AJP* **2017**, *174*, 586–594. [CrossRef]
232. Matrisciano, F.; Tueting, P.; Dalal, I.; Kadriu, B.; Grayson, D.R.; Davis, J.M.; Nicoletti, F.; Guidotti, A. Epigenetic modifications of GABAergic interneurons are associated with the schizophrenia-like phenotype induced by prenatal stress in mice. *Neuropharmacology* **2013**, *68*, 184–194. [CrossRef]
233. Guidotti, A.; Grayson, D.R.; Caruncho, H.J. Epigenetic RELN dysfunction in schizophrenia and related neuropsychiatric disorders. *Front. Cell. Neurosci.* **2016**, *10*, 89. [CrossRef]
234. Gothelf, D.; Soreni, N.; Nachman, R.P.; Tyano, S.; Hiss, Y.; Reiner, O.; Weizman, A. Evidence for the involvement of the hippocampus in the pathophysiology of schizophrenia. *Eur. Neuropsychopharmacol.* **2000**, *10*, 389–395. [CrossRef]
235. Konradi, C.; Yang, C.K.; Zimmerman, E.I.; Lohmann, K.M.; Gresch, P.; Pantazopoulos, H.; Berretta, S.; Heckers, S. Hippocampal interneurons are abnormal in schizophrenia. *Schizophr. Res.* **2011**, *131*, 165–173. [CrossRef]
236. Mavroudis, I.A.; Petrides, F.; Manani, M.; Chatzinikolaou, F.; Ciobica, A.S.; Padurariu, M.; Kazis, D.; Njau, S.N.; Costa, V.G.; Baloyannis, S.J. Purkinje cells pathology in schizophrenia. A morphometric approach. *Rom. J. Morphol. Embryol.* **2017**, *58*, 419–424. [PubMed]
237. Eastwood, S.L.; Cotter, D.; Harrison, P.J. Cerebellar synaptic protein expression in schizophrenia. *Neuroscience* **2001**, *105*, 219–229. [CrossRef]
238. Bey, A.L.; Jiang, Y.H. Overview of mouse models of autism spectrum disorders. *Curr. Protoc. Pharmacol.* **2014**, *66*, 5–26. [PubMed]
239. Tueting, P.; Costa, E.; Dwivedi, Y.; Guidotti, A.; Impagnatiello, F.; Manev, R.; Pesold, C. The phenotypic characteristics of heterozygous reeler mouse. *Neuroreport* **1999**, *10*, 1329–1334. [CrossRef]
240. Brigman, J.L.; Padukiewicz, K.E.; Sutherland, M.L.; Rothblat, L.A. Executive functions in the heterozygous reeler mouse model of schizophrenia. *Behav. Neurosci.* **2006**, *120*, 984–988. [CrossRef]
241. Ognibene, E.; Adriani, W.; Macri, S.; Laviola, G. Neurobehavioural disorders in the infant reeler mouse model: Interaction of genetic vulnerability and consequences of maternal separation. *Behav. Brain Res.* **2007**, *177*, 142–149. [CrossRef]
242. Ognibene, E.; Adriani, W.; Granstrem, O.; Pieretti, S.; Laviola, G. Impulsivity–anxiety-related behavior and profiles of morphine-induced analgesia in heterozygous reeler mice. *Brain Res.* **2007**, *1131*, 173–180. [CrossRef]
243. Barr, A.M.; Fish, K.N.; Markou, A.; Honer, W.G. Heterozygous reeler mice exhibit alterations in sensorimotor gating but not presynaptic proteins. *Eur. J. Neurosci.* **2008**, *27*, 2568–2574. [CrossRef]
244. Salinger, W.L.; Ladrow, P.; Wheeler, C. Behavioral phenotype of the reeler mutant mouse: Effects of RELN gene dosage and social isolation. *Behav. Neurosci.* **2003**, *117*, 1257–1275. [CrossRef]
245. Podhorna, J.; Didriksen, M. The heterozygous reeler mouse: Behavioural phenotype. *Behav. Brain Res.* **2004**, *153*, 43–54. [CrossRef]
246. Krueger, D.D.; Howell, J.L.; Hebert, B.F.; Olausson, P.; Taylor, J.R.; Nairn, A.C. Assessment of cognitive function in the heterozygous reeler mouse. *Psychopharmacology* **2006**, *189*, 95–104. [CrossRef] [PubMed]
247. Michetti, C.; Romano, E.; Altabella, L.; Caruso, A.; Castelluccio, P.; Bedse, G.; Gaetani, S.; Canese, R.; Laviola, G.; Scattoni, M.L. Mapping pathological phenotypes in reelin mutant mice. *Front. Pediatr.* **2014**, *2*, 95. [CrossRef] [PubMed]
248. Teixeira, C.M.; Martín, E.D.; Sahún, I.; Masachs, N.; Pujadas, L.; Corvelo, A.; Bosch, C.; Rossi, D.; Martinez, A.; Maldonado, R.; et al. Overexpression of Reelin Prevents the Manifestation of Behavioral Phenotypes Related to Schizophrenia and Bipolar Disorder. *Neuropsychopharmacology* **2011**, *36*, 2395–2405. [CrossRef] [PubMed]
249. Romano, E.; Michetti, C.; Caruso, A.; Laviola, G.; Scattoni, M.L. Characterization of neonatal vocal and motor repertoire of reelin mutant mice. *PLoS ONE* **2013**, *8*, e64407. [CrossRef] [PubMed]
250. Ottman, R.; Risch, N.; Hauser, W.A.; Pedley, T.A.; Lee, J.H.; Barker-Cummings, C.; Lustenberger, A.; Nagle, K.J.; Lee, K.S.; Scheuer, M.L.; et al. Localization of a gene for partial epilepsy to chromosome 10q. *Nat. Genet.* **1995**, *10*, 56–60. [CrossRef] [PubMed]

251. Michelucci, R.; Pasini, E.; Nobile, C. Lateral temporal lobe epilepsies: Clinical and genetic features. *Epilepsia* **2009**, *50*, 52–54. [CrossRef] [PubMed]
252. Boycott, K.M.; Flavelle, S.; Bureau, A.; Glass, H.C.; Fujiwara, T.M.; Wirrell, E.; Davey, K.; Chudley, A.E.; Scott, J.N.; McLeod, D.R.; et al. Homozygous deletion of the very low density lipoprotein receptor gene causes autosomal recessive cerebellar hypoplasia with cerebral gyral simplification. *Am. J. Hum. Genet.* **2005**, *77*, 477–483. [CrossRef]
253. Garden, G. Spinocerebellar Ataxia Type 7. In *GeneReviews®*; Adam, M.P., Ardinger, H.H., Pagon, R.A., Wallace, S.E., Eds.; University of Washington: Seattle, WA, USA, 1993.
254. Lai, M.C.; Lombardo, M.V.; Baron-Cohen, S. Autism. *Lancet* **2014**, *383*, 896–910. [CrossRef]
255. Marino, M.J. The use and misuse of statistical methodologies in pharmacology research. *Biochem. Pharmacol.* **2014**, *87*, 78–92. [CrossRef]
256. Motulsky, H.J. Common misconceptions about data analysis and statistics. *Br. J. Pharmacol.* **2015**, *172*, 2126–2132. [CrossRef]

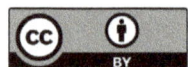

© 2019 by the authors. Licensee MDPI, Basel, Switzerland. This article is an open access article distributed under the terms and conditions of the Creative Commons Attribution (CC BY) license (http://creativecommons.org/licenses/by/4.0/).

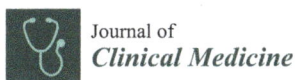

Review

Bioengineered Skin Substitutes: The Role of Extracellular Matrix and Vascularization in the Healing of Deep Wounds

Francesco Urciuolo [1,2,*], **Costantino Casale** [1], **Giorgia Imparato** [3] **and Paolo A. Netti** [1,2,3]

[1] Department of Chemical, Materials and Industrial Production Engineering (DICMAPI) University of Naples Federico II, P.le Tecchio 80, 80125 Naples, Italy; costantino.casale@unina.it (C.C.); nettipa@unina.it (P.A.N.)
[2] Interdisciplinary Research Centre on Biomaterials (CRIB), University of Naples Federico II P.le Tecchio 80, 80125 Naples, Italy
[3] Center for Advanced Biomaterials for HealthCare@CRIB, Istituto Italiano di Tecnologia, Largo Barsanti e Matteucci 53, 80125 Naples, Italy; giorgia.imparato@iit.it
* Correspondence: urciuolo@unina.it

Received: 15 October 2019; Accepted: 26 November 2019; Published: 1 December 2019

Abstract: The formation of severe scars still represents the result of the closure process of extended and deep skin wounds. To address this issue, different bioengineered skin substitutes have been developed but a general consensus regarding their effectiveness has not been achieved yet. It will be shown that bioengineered skin substitutes, although representing a valid alternative to autografting, induce skin cells in repairing the wound rather than guiding a regeneration process. Repaired skin differs from regenerated skin, showing high contracture, loss of sensitivity, impaired pigmentation and absence of cutaneous adnexa (i.e., hair follicles and sweat glands). This leads to significant mobility and aesthetic concerns, making the development of more effective bioengineered skin models a current need. The objective of this review is to determine the limitations of either commercially available or investigational bioengineered skin substitutes and how advanced skin tissue engineering strategies can be improved in order to completely restore skin functions after severe wounds.

Keywords: skin substitutes; tissue engineering; wound healing; extracellular matrix; bottom-up tissue engineering; vascularization; bioreactors; dermal substitutes; scar tissue

1. Introduction

The skin is the largest organ of the body, accounting for about 15% of the total adult body weight. It is made up of three layers: the epidermis, dermis, and the hypodermis (Figure 1, [1]). Bioengineered skin substitutes, in the form of either cellularized engineered skin grafts or acellular dermal regeneration templates (DRT), have been developed to address two main issues still affecting the repair of extended deep wounds [2–10]: firstly, limiting the amount of healthy skin removed from the patient needed for closure; and secondly, acting as promoter for the restoration of the physiologic conditions of the skin avoiding the formation of severe scars. Skin acts not only as a barrier between the organism and the environment preventing invasion of pathogens and fending off chemical and physical assaults [11], it also plays a crucial role in the regulation of body temperature, moisture, and trafficking of water and solutes [12]. In addition, the sensory system of the skin allows the sensing of pain, temperature, light touch, discriminative touch, vibration and pressure. Finally, other important adnexal structures, such as sweat glands and hair follicles, contribute to the functionality of the healthy skin. In addition to the epidermis, severe damage due to burns, chronic ulcers and reconstructive surgeries, induce the destruction of the dermis. Unlike the epidermis, the dermis is characterized by an impaired healing process in which the final assembly of the extracellular matrix (ECM) is far from physiologic conditions.

This mismatch compromises the reestablishment of the aforementioned regulatory functions of the whole organ [13–15]. The components of the ECM of the dermis (collagen elastin, hyaluronic acid, fibronectin, perlacan, water and other molecules), possess specific three-dimensional arrangements of sequences orchestrating the cross-talk among the different cell populations comprising the skin. Ultimately, such cross-talk affects the attachment, migration, differentiation and morphogenetic phenomena. For instance, the ECM promotes 'appropriate' communications between keratinocytes and the fibroblasts, and it is responsible for the formation and maintenance of the adnexal structures such as hair follicles, sweat glands and innervations [16–18]. Furthermore, when such adnexal structures become compromised, the self-regeneration of the epidermis cannot occur, and the wound becomes hard to heal. The repair of a deep wound can be divided into four subsequent phases [19,20]: (i) the coagulation and homeostasis phase (immediately after injury); (ii) the inflammatory phase (shortly after injury to tissue), during which swelling takes place; (iii) the proliferation period, where new tissues and blood vessels are formed; and (iv) the maturation phase, in which remodeling of new tissues takes place. How the maturation phase takes place determines the difference between repair and regeneration. The former is a "mere" closure process where fibroblasts bridge the wound gap by organizing their ECM differently from the healthy status. The latter restores the organization of the ECM that will appear indistinguishable from the healthy status [21]. The impaired ECM organization featuring the repair process depresses the regulatory and repository role of the extracellular space that ultimately forms an extended scar characterized by the loss of biological functionalities, inducing the insurgence of severe aesthetics and mobility-associated concerns. A classical approach to skin grafting and repairing is depicted in Figure 2. After debridement of the wound bed, a DRT is applied. Fibroblasts and endothelial cells from the recipient take at least one month to invade the DRT. After this time, it is possible to apply a split thickness skin graft (STSG): an epidermis with a layer of dermis removed from healthy sites of the patient. Both vascularization and fibroblast-secreted ECM molecules affect the take of the STSG that serves to trigger the regeneration of the epidermis due to the lack of adnexa and basal lamina [22–26]. As shown in Figure 2, with a period of two years, the remodeling of the neodermis occurs. To date, even though progress in biomaterials science and tissue engineering has led to the realization of different classes of skin substitutes (either cellularized or not), their healing potential is still limited in triggering a repair process instead of regeneration. In addition to economics, safety and regulatory (in case of allogenic or xenogeneic materials) concerns, in this work the currently available skin substitutes will be reviewed in the light of the composition of the dermis compartment and how this can affect the regeneration process. DRT can be fabricated starting from connective tissues of either allogenic or xenogeneic origin after removal of the cellular component [27,28]. The decellularization processes remove the associated risk of transmission of pathogens, preserving the composition of the ECM. On the other hand, the functionality of molecules of the ECM resulting from the decellularization processes compromise the correct signal presentation to the cells [16–18]. Pre-cellularization with endothelial cells, fibroblasts and keratinocytes seems to improve the biological performance of reconstructed three-dimensional matrices of both natural or synthetic origins [2,27,29–31], by speeding up the vascularization, the synthesis of neodermis, the take of the STSG and the closure of the wounds [32–34]. Nevertheless, the reconstructed three-dimensional matrices used to accommodate living cells prior to the implant are composed of exogenous biomatrices that possess composition, stiffness and three-dimensional arrangements that are quite different from the native dermis. For this reason, some doubts on their effectiveness in triggering a regeneration process have been raised [17]. Finally, a tissue engineering strategy that use patients' own cells to build up in vitro a human-like vascularized ECM featured by the absence of any exogenous material, is presented as an alternative to guide the wound toward a physiological regeneration process [35–37].

2. Tissue Engineering Strategies for Skin Regeneration

Tissue engineering aims at developing strategies to allow tissue and organ regeneration [32] by two approaches: (i) In in vitro tissue engineering the patient's human skin is re-built in a laboratory using either endogenous or allogenic cell lines (keratinocytes and fibroblasts); after a period of cultivation in three-dimensional matrices [24] and bioreactors [10,38], the engineered skin is then implanted [32]; (ii) in in vivo tissue engineering a three-dimensional matrix is introduced in the wound bed; such matrices are bio-functionalized in order to attract both cells and growth factors supporting skin regeneration [38]. The use of de novo fabricated skin becomes necessary when skin self-regeneration is hindered by adverse conditions [10]; in particular, when severe burns (second-, third-, and fourth-degree burns), chronic ulcers, surgery or trauma lead to the destruction of the dermis and underlying tissues (fat, muscle or bone) are exposed [39,40]. Bioengineered skin substitutes can be classified according to the following categories.

- Cellularized epithelial tissues: used for superficial wounds, when the dermis is not (or is partially) damaged; autologous, allogenic or xenogeneic epithelial tissues are cultured in vitro and then implanted. In this case, the application of an STSG is not required. Engineered epithelial tissues are in general formed by cell sheets two or three cell layers thick [41,42].
- Cellularized dermis: when the dermis is damaged, autologous or allogenic fibroblasts are embedded in a three-dimensional matrix and then implanted in the wound bed. This procedure implies a second surgical step for the application of an epithelial layer using an STSG as shown in Figure 2 [41,42].
- Cellularized composite skin (or full thickness): engineered tissues containing both epithelial and dermal tissues. They are composed of epithelial tissue grown on a dermis surrogate composed of fibroblasts entrapped in a biomaterial [4,41–43]. Due to the presence of an epidermis layer, the application of an STSG can be avoided.
- Acellular dermal substitutes: or derma regeneration templates (DRT) that are porous 3D biomaterials (non-containing cells) applied in the missing dermis after wound debridement. This procedure implies a second surgical step for the application of an epithelial layer coming from an STSG, as shown in Figure 2 [4,41–43].

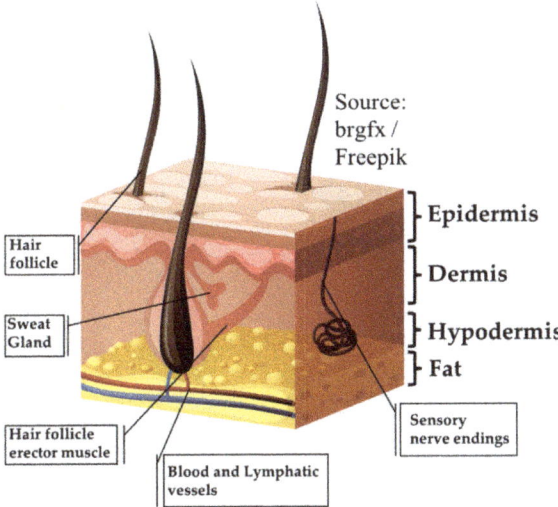

Figure 1. Main components of the human skin. (Image source: brgfx/Freepik).

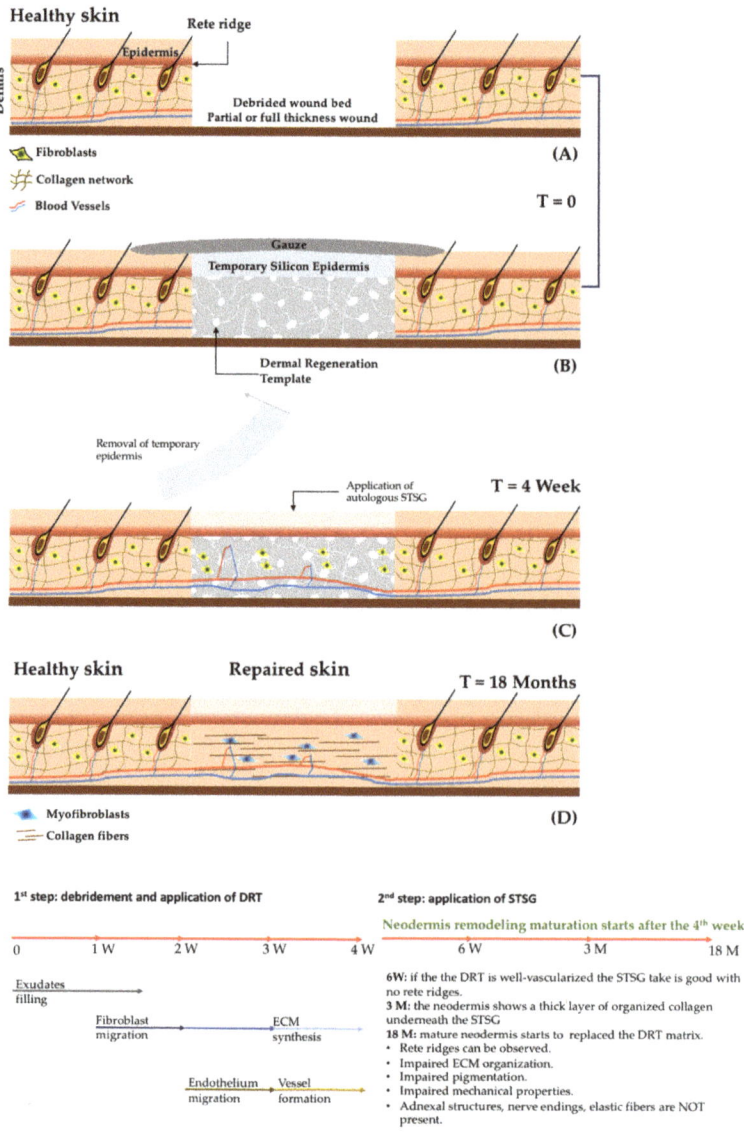

Figure 2. The main steps of a two-step procedure to treat deep and partial wounds with the application of a DRT. (**A**) Healthy skin and wound bed after debridement. (**B**) Application of a DRT possessing an artificial silicone epidermis and covered with gauze. (**C**) Removal of the silicone epidermis and application of the STSG. (**D**) Long-term appearance of the repaired dermis. (**E**) Cellular end extracellular dynamics occurring during the wound healing process after the application of a DRT. W = week; M = month. DRT, dermal regeneration templates; STSG, split thickness skin graft; ECM, extracellular matrix.

2.1. Dermal Regeneration Templates (DRT): Materials and Fabrication Techniques

Porous and fibrous materials. Regardless of the tissue engineering strategy used (in vitro vs. in vivo approaches), a 3D scaffold supporting cell growth is required [42]. Scaffolds are biomaterials acting as temporary porous structures mimicking the 3D architecture of human tissue. In the case of skin tissue engineering, the tissue that one would like to mimic is the dermis. The scaffolds mimicking the dermis can be made by either natural or synthetic polymers (or a combination of both) and, regardless of their origin, they must have different characteristics: non-immunogenic; biocompatible; be able to resist the activity of proteolytic enzymes; stiff and flexible in order to withstand surgical procedures; be able to control the wound contracture; and to possess a degradation rate synchronous with the neo-dermis ingrowth and assembling. Furthermore, the scaffold should support epidermis attachment, maintenance and stratification, and it should promote the blood vessels' influx when implanted [23,34,42]. Three-dimensional porous structures can be obtained by different fabrication techniques allowing the production of different 3D architectures. Starting from melt polymers or polymer solutions, the use of porogen agents, or phase separation techniques, allows the production of sponge-like structures with interconnected pores and porosity ranging from 50 to 500 μm [44]. When porogens are used, the final mechanical properties of the scaffold can be modulated by varying the polymer concentration, the volume fraction and the dimension of the porogens. Phase separation technique exploits the thermodynamic instability of either polymeric solutions or blends [42]. The instability can be induced physically (i.e., temperature) or chemically (i.e., introduction of a solvent/non-solvent agent). The thermodynamic instability induces a segregation process with the formation of a dispersed and a continuum phase. The dispersed phase forms globular structures and after its removal porosity is created. The parameters affecting the final properties of the scaffold (mechanical properties, porosity, pore diameter and pore interconnection) are the initial composition of the polymer solution and, in the case of thermally induced phase separation, the cooling/heating rate is used to induce the thermodynamic instability. Woven and non-woven assembly of nano-fibers using electrospinning allows the production of porous structures categorized as fibrillar scaffolds [30,45,46]. Nanofibrous materials can be also produced by means of different techniques such as self-assembly, phase separation, fiber bonding and electrospinning. This kind of structure is able to mimic better the fibrous nature of the natural extracellular matrix. In in vitro tissue engineering, such preformed structures (either porous or fibrous) are colonized by the cells after the preparation, since their fabrication techniques represent severe conditions for cell viability. This could represent a limitation because a homogenous cell seeding through the thickness of the scaffolds is difficult to achieve and sophisticated bioreactors need to be used [38,47–49]. Hydrogels represent another class of fibrous scaffolds. These are highly hydrated 3D structures obtained by physical, ionic or covalent cross-linking of different polymers of both natural or synthetic origins [49–52]. Three-dimensional hydrogels can be obtained by the assembly and crosslinking of a liquid monomeric phase. This represents an advantage because the monomeric solution can be mixed with the cell suspension. At the end of the gelling process, cells remain entrapped in the 3D structures obtaining a homogenous cellularization of the final 3D scaffold. Although the final properties can be modulated by different parameters (monomer concentration, temperature, pH, UV radiation, ionic strength) the presence of cells poses the same constraints on the control of the final mechanical properties. For instance, UV radiation, pH, temperature and other methods used to induce cross-link of polymeric networks may affect cell viability. Hydrogel are, in general, considered soft materials. Hydrogels composed of gelatin–chitosan hydrogels [53], fibronectin–hyaluronan, or dextran-based hydrogels, in combination with nano-fibrous poly lactic-co-glycolic acid (PLGA) scaffolds have been extensively used for wound healing and regeneration applications [54–56]. In particular, dextran-based hydrogels demonstrated efficient vascularization. Composite hydrogels formed by glycosaminoglycan (GAG)–collagen showed good wound healing in rabbit models [56]. Self-assembling peptide-based hydrogel scaffolds have been reported to reduce burn wound healing time and skin cell proliferation [56].

Protein-based naturals biomaterials. Biomaterials of protein nature can be realized using (but not limited to) collagen, gelatin, silk and fibrinogen. Collagen is the most abundant structural protein of the human dermis secreted by fibroblasts, and is responsible for tensile stiffness. Collagen in skin tissue engineering is used as both acellular scaffold or cell-populated scaffold [56]. Collagen for tissue engineering application is extracted from animals: bovine, ovine and avian are the mostly exploited sources. Examples of acellular/porous scaffolds are the commercially available dermis substitutes Alloderm® or Integra®, while examples of cell-populated collagen hydrogels are represented by Apligraft® and Transcyte®. In addition, collagen-based biomaterials have been processed in the form of membranes, sponges, composite sponges and electrospun biomaterials with nanometric features [56]. Gelatin is a protein obtained by collagen denaturation possessing higher advantages in terms of cell adhesion and inducing a reduced immunogenic response. In the treatment of wounds and burns, gelatin has been used as electrospun nanofibers [57], membranes [58] and gelatin sponges loaded with growth factors [59]. Silk fibroin in the form of sponges, nanofibers and porous films have shown decreased inflammatory response, and promising results in wound healing and skin regeneration has been reported [60].

Polysaccharide-based biomaterials. Polysaccharide-based biomaterials are mainly used in the form of hydrogels. Those mostly used in skin regeneration and wound healing are dextran [54], cellulose [26], chitosan [61], alginate [62] and hyaluronic acid (HA) [63–65]. Among these, HA has been extensively used in skin regeneration leading to the commercialization of different skin substitutes, such as Hyaff®, Laserskin® and Hyalograft®.

Synthetic and composite biomaterials. Synthetic biomaterials comprise [30] the class of aliphatic polyesters, such as polylactic acid (PLA), polyglycolic (PGA) and polycaprolactone (PCL). They possess controllable mechanical stiffness and high process flexibility and are biocompatible and nontoxic. Moreover, PLA, PGA, PCL, and their blends and copolymers are FDA approved. An example of a commercially available skin substitute made using such materials is Dermagraft®.

Decellularized matrices. To date, no biomaterials yet exist that are able to mimic the composition of the native extracellular matrix as a whole [16–18]. Decellularized matrices of allogenic or xenogeneic origin should bridge such a gap. This is very important in skin regeneration because the lack of a functional extracellular matrix is the main cause affecting the impaired wound healing process. Currently available decellularized biomaterials comprise decellularized mesothelium, intestine, amniotic membrane, dermis and skin flaps [9]. Allogenic dermis can be obtained by treating fresh dermis from a cadaver with Dispase–Triton X-100 or NaCl–sodium dodecyl sulfate (SDS). In this way, collagen bundles and basement membranes retain their structure. The abstained biomaterial is further lyophilized. An FDA-approved decellularized dermis obtained with such a technique is Alloderm® [9]. Its use in combination with split-thickness autologous skin grafts allows complete cellularization of skin defects after 12 weeks post application when applied to full-thickness or partial-thickness burn wounds, thereby reducing subsequent scarring [65]. Other acellular dermal matrices are of porcine origin (e.g., Permacol®) and the decellularization process is similar to that of Alloderm®. Different techniques use a foaming process in order to destroy the cellular component, as well as any immunogenic agent. On the other hand, foaming compromises extracellular matrix structure and functions. In general, this kind of decellularized dermis is similar to porous scaffolds and is used for hemostatic applications. Other kinds of decellularized matrices are derived from the mesothelium, including peritoneum, pleura and pericardium [27,66,67]. Decellularized peritoneum is obtained using detergent agents and the processes are designed to maximize the preservation of the extracellular matrix architecture and composition. Because growth factors have a limited shelf life, such biomaterials are often combined with fibroblast growth factor (FGF) and epidermal growth factor (EGF) to promote wound repair. Decellularized mesothelium of porcine origin is used, for instance, in breast reconstruction. Bovine sources are another font of decellularized mesothelium showing a faster healing process than that observed for other decellularized dermis substitutes such as Alloderm® [27]. The intestine is another source to obtain decellularized extracellular matrices.

Interestingly, many cytokines and growth factors (FGF and TGF-β families) are retained after the decellularization process. Different applications have been reported comprising the reconstruction of cornea, urethra, vagina, and lung. In the case of dermis reconstruction, decellularized intestine and, in particular, the decellularized small intestine submucosa, is a very promising scaffold due to its capability in promoting angiogenesis. OaSIS® and SurgySIS® (Cook Surgical, Bloomington, IN, USA) are two decellularized matrices from small intestine submucosa [9,68]. The human amniotic membrane is rich in basement membrane and avascular stromal matrix. Decellularization can be obtained using ethylenediaminetetraacetic acid (EDTA) and aprotinin, SDS, DNAase and RNAase. Nevertheless, such a process induces the reduction of anti-inflammatory and anti-scarring components by reducing their superiority compared to other matrices. Clinical applications can be found in the reconstruction of the ocular surface, while different studies have been performed on skin reconstruction in nude mice models [27].

2.2. Tissue Engineering Strategies

2.2.1. Traditional Tissue Engineering

Tissue engineering aims at producing functional and living human tissue in vitro that can be implanted to restore and to replace damaged tissues and organs [32], or can be used in vitro as living testing platforms [68]. The classical approach involves the extraction of cells from humans (primary cells or stem cells), their expansion and seeding in a biomaterial [32], followed by a dynamic culture to promote the neo tissue growth [10,38,47,49]. After cell expansion, the skin tissue engineering process involves at least three steps. (i) Fibroblasts are seeded in a biomaterial; this cellular construct acts as a dermis surrogate where the scaffold represents the temporary extracellular matrix of the fibroblast. (ii) After a variable culture period (two weeks–one month), to allow fibroblast attachment and production of endogenous extracellular matrix components, keratinocytes are seeded on the top of the engineered dermis and kept in submerged culture. (iii) After approximately two weeks, the culture conditions are switched from submerged to air liquid interface (ALI) in order to promote the stratification of the epidermis with the formation of the stratum corneum [2,69]. Such full-thickness engineered skin can be eventually implanted, but different requirements need to be satisfied [70]. The engineered skin must be safe for the patient because any cultured cell material possesses an associated risk of contamination, and viral or bacterial infection. Moreover, in the case of allogenic or xenogeneic cells and materials, there is also an associated risk of rejection. The tissue engineered skin should be effective in providing real benefit for the patient: it should attach correctly to the wound area, it should undergo normal healing limiting or discouraging the formation of a scar, and it should restore the correct pigmentation and barrier functions. Then, it should support the vascular network ingrowth [2,24] with subsequent development of other structures useful for the normal life of the patient: innervation should be promoted in order to restore the sensing properties [71] and the growth of both hair follicles and sweat glands [72]. Finally, tissue engineered skin should be cost-effective in order to achieve a concrete clinical uptake. One of the strengths of the tissue engineering approach is the possibility to have fine control over the properties of the final tissue. Indeed, by modulating the initial properties of the scaffold used to accommodate human fibroblasts and optimizing the culture conditions (culture media composition, mechanical stimulation, hydrodynamic stimulation) it is possible to obtain engineered skin with desired properties [10,38,47–49,70]. It has been demonstrated that uniaxial and biaxial stretch can induce the alignment of the de novo synthesized collagen network [73]. Furthermore, by engineering either the stiffness or the porosity of the scaffold, it is possible to control the assembly of the de novo synthesized extracellular matrix [74]. This allows, for instance, to match the final properties of the engineered skin with the properties of the patient's skin in order to lower the structural and functional differences between the restored zone and the surrounding skin [13,21,43,75–78].

2.2.2. Modular Tissue Engineering: Building a Tissue from the Bottom Up

Modular tissue engineering strategy applies the concept of tissue engineering but at a sub-millimeter scale. Cells are arranged in 3D architectures in the form of micromodules or micro tissues, or building blocks having at least one dimension ranging from 50 to 200 µm. Such micrometric tissues can be either scaffold-free or scaffold-based, and they act as building blocks for the fabrication of larger structures [78]. Scaffold-free microtissues can be obtained by organizing cells in sheets [79] (with a thickness ranging from 50 to 100 µm) or spheres [80,81] (diameters up to 200 µm). Scaffold-based microtissues are obtained by entrapping cells in micrometric scaffolds, such as porous microspheres [81], non-porous microspheres [82–85], non-spherical microparticles [78] or wires of hydrogels [84]. Sheets of human fibroblast are obtained by culturing fibroblasts in flat dishes and promoting the synthesis of the extracellular matrix. When the sheets achieve confluency, they are detached from the culture dishes and, by stacking different sheets of cells, a thicker tissue can be obtained [85]. When placed in close proximity, cell–cell contacts and extracellular matrix–extracellular matrix contacts lead to the formation of continuum structures made by fibroblasts embedded in their own extracellular matrix. One of the limitations of this technique is represented by the high cell density. This induces the formation of a dermis equivalent featuring a cell: ECM ratio higher than that found in the human dermis. The presence of high traction forces exerted by fibroblasts on the immature collagen fibers induces the formation of a highly packed ECM. Moreover, the over-expressed cell density increases the metabolic request. For these reasons, the cell-sheets are often characterized by a very low thickness and by the presence of a necrotic core. The detachment of the cell sheets from the culture plate and the subsequent stacking procedures represent other issues [86–88]. The fabrication of centimeter-sized tissues can be obtained by casting spherical microtissues in molds having any shape and dimensions [83]. Fibroblasts can be entrapped in both spherical and non-spherical hydrogels under continuous conditions using microfluidic devices [89,90]. Dermal microtissues obtained using this approach have been successfully used to build up large pieces of living dermis in vitro. In this direction, fibroblasts laden hydrogel has been used as a building block to fabricate a doll-shaped dermis equivalent [83]. In this study, the possibility of building up a centimeter-sized piece of dermis was demonstrated, but the final tissue underwent sever contracture. Since fibroblasts were imbedded in collagen hydrogel, the lack of a mature cell-synthesized extracellular matrix capable of withstanding the traction force of fibroblasts caused the shrinking of the final tissue. Finally, the presence of an exogenous collagen did not guarantee the complete replication of the native extracellular microenvironment [83]. To reduce the presence of exogenous matrices and promote the synthesis and the assembly of an endogenous dermal microenvironment, human fibroblasts have been seeded in porous gelatin microspheres kept in suspension cultures [89]. Under optimized culture conditions, fibroblasts were able to produce and assemble their extracellular matrix in the inner pores of the microspheres. The microspheres were designed in order to degrade during the extracellular matrix assembly process so the final microtissue was a sort of a sub-millimeter-sized "ball of human dermis", named Dermal-µTissue (Figure 3), composed of fibroblasts and fibroblast-assembled-collagen, elastin and hyaluronic acid [83,91,92]. Dermal-µTissues, having an average diameter of about 200 µm, have been cast in centimeter-sized molds in order to promote biological sintering. The molds containing the Dermal-µTissues have been inserted in bioreactors working under engineered fluid dynamic regimes, which have been developed to improve mass transport during the assembly of the Dermal-µTissue [91,92]. In these works, shear stress and optimized fluid velocity fields were used to guide the correct assembly of the de novo synthetized ECM [92,93]. Moreover, the final dermis equivalent was completely formed by a fibroblast assembled extracellular matrix, leading to the fabrication of skin substitutes with superior functionalities compared to the engineered skin composed of exogenous ECM. For instance, when cultured in vitro in the presence of human keratinocytes and dorsal root ganglion cells, the first spontaneous formation of follicle-like structures in vitro [72] and functional innervation [35] were observed. Finally, tissue wire technology can be used to produce living fibers treated as textile and woven fibers [84]. These modular approaches lead to several advantages, such as fine control over the final architecture, control over the final shape, and control over the spatial organization of engineered biologic structures [79–87,92,93].

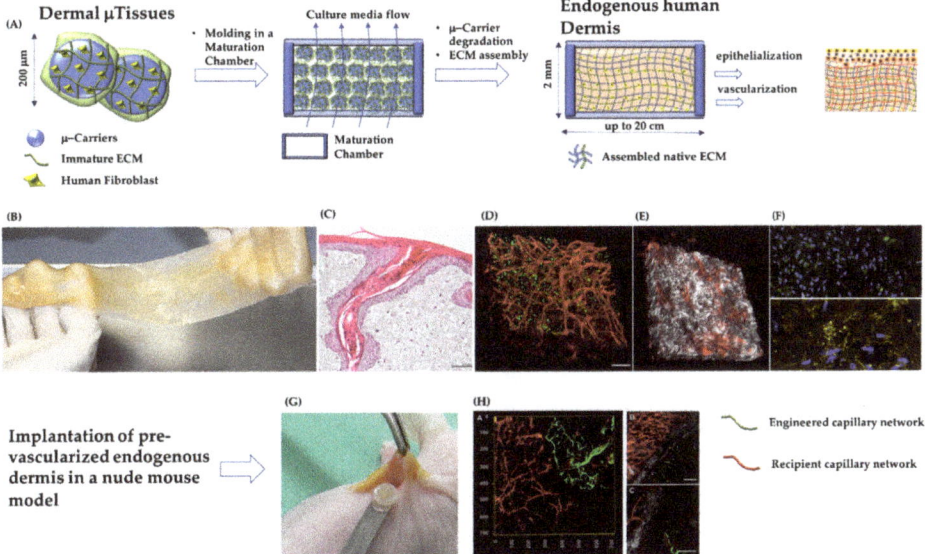

Figure 3. The main steps for the production of a DRT composed of fibroblast-assembled/pre-vascularized human dermis substitutes, and its morphological features before and after implantation in a nude mice model. (**A**) From left to right: production of Dermal-µTissues; their molding and assembly in a maturation chamber that is kept under dynamic culture conditions; formation of a continuum of fibroblasts embedded in their own dermal extracellular matrix; epithelization and vascularization of the endogenous human dermis. (**B**) Fabrication of large pieces of endogenous human dermis (major dimension 20 cm). (**C**) Histology of the endogenous human dermis supporting the differentiation of epidermis with the formation of spontaneous rete ridge profile. (**D**) Vascularized endogenous human dermis: cell nuclei in green and capillary network in red. (**E**) Vascularized endogenous human dermis: fibroblast-assembled collagen bundles observed under label-free multiphoton microscopy in gray; capillary network in red. (**F**) Top: fibroblast-assembled hyaluronic acid in green, cell nuclei in blue; Bottom: fibroblast-assembled elastin network in yellow, cell nuclei in blue. (**G**) Implantation of a piece of the pre-vascularized endogenous human dermis. (**H**) Connection between engineered capillary network (green) and recipient capillary network (red); fibroblast-assembled collagen in gray. Figure 3B, 3D, 3E, 3G, and 3H are from reference [34] "Mazio, C. et al. Pre-vascularized dermis model for fast and functional anastomosis with host vasculature. Biomat. 192, 159–170 (2019)". Authors obtained permision from Elsevier: License Number 4681910194044.

Three-Dimensional Bio-Printing

Three-dimensional bio-printing [94] techniques are used to achieve correct positioning of different cell types. The aim is the fabrication of intricate biologic architectures with high spatial resolution in a standardized manner [82,95–97]. Moreover, the obtainment of a full-thickness human skin equivalent takes at least four weeks, representing an issue in the case of production of autologous skin engineering grafts that should be implanted in a shorter time frame. The positioning of different cell strata in their final configuration could reduce the time required for the development of the full-thickness graft. Other advantages of 3D printing techniques are represented by the possibility of printing a vascular network and its insertion in its final configuration in important adnexal structures such as the hair follicle precursors [97–100]. This should represent a plus in the case of deep skin damage where neither innervation nor hair follicle development during the healing process has been observed [20]. Finally, the use of 3D printing techniques aims at reducing the batch-to-batch variability by providing a standardized and controlled process. By precisely locating different matrix materials, growth factors, and different cells in a layer-by-layer assembly, functional living skin tissues would be fabricated possessing designed and personalized structures with neither size nor shape limitations, in a high throughput, and in a highly reproducible manner. In general, the equipment used to print skin tissues consists of independently controlled cell-dispensing channels. Electromechanical valves operate the dispenser, which is positioned on a three-axis robotic stage possessing high spatial resolution (below 50 µm). The dispenser can deliver pre-hydrogel solutions containing cells. Once delivered, the hydrogel solution solidifies via chemical or physical routes. According to this strategy, fibroblasts embedded in rat tail collagen have been printed layer-by-layer, forming a dermis surrogate upon which keratinocytes have been deposited in order to form the epidermal layer [101]. In this study, it was demonstrated that a 3D dermis can be formed in an automated and controlled fashion by printing nanoliter droplets of collagen containing living cells [95,99]. A printed skin equivalent can be obtained using fibrin hydrogels as bio-ink containing cells [95,100]. It was demonstrated that a dermis equivalent as large as 100 cm^2 could be obtained in less than 35 minutes. After this time, a layer of keratinocytes was printed on the top of the dermis equivalent and, after confluency was obtained (24 h), the bilayer engineered skin was implanted in immunodeficient mouse. After implantation, the dermis was able to integrate with the recipient tissue and the epidermis was able to differentiate until forming the stratum corneum. Nevertheless, the dermal–epidermal interface did not present the physiological rete ridge profile. Finally, techniques for the printing of a microvasculature network have been assessed. Endothelial cells can be inserted in fibrinogen solution and printed in a gelling bath according to a prescribed 3D architecture. Together with the vascular network, a hydrogel solution containing fibroblasts can be printed by means of an independent dispenser in order to obtain a more complex dermis formed by a connective tissue equivalent containing a 3D designed microvasculature [102].

3. Commercially Available Skin Substitutes

3.1. Acellular Dermal Substitutes

The most used commercially available acellular dermal substitutes (Table 1) are composed of natural extracellular matrix components and can be divided in two categories: decellularized extracellular matrices and reconstructed extracellular matrices. The first category is formed by natural connective tissues (dermis, mesothelium, intestine) deprived of any cellular components and allergenic/immunogenic agents.

The most used commercially available decellularized matrices (Table 1) for the treatment of deep wounds after burns and trauma, or for reconstruction and treatment of diabetic/venous/pressure ulcers are (but not limited to): Alloderm®, Dermacell®, Dermamatrix®, SureDerm®, OASIS®, Permacoll® and EZ-DERM®. Alloderm®, Dermacell®, Dermamatrix® and SureDerm®, are decellularized cadaveric dermis, non-cross-linked, that can be incorporated into the wound bed [4,6–9,40,42,103,104]. In general, such systems retain the basement membrane after the decellularization process but lack an epidermal layer. The acellular matrix provides a good natural 3D environment for fibroblasts and endothelial cells influx in order to promote the formation of a new extracellular matrix and vascular network. OASIS®, Permacoll® and EZ-DERM® are decellularized matrices of porcine origins. OASIS® is obtained using similar processing methods to those of human derived matrices but start from porcine small intestine submucosa. Permacoll® and EZ-DERM® are decellularized porcine dermis that are further cross-linked. Alloderm® was approved and considered as banked human tissue by the FDA; it has been used to treat burns since 1992 and has also been used to treat severe soft tissue defects [105]. This product has been shown to have good graft take rates and to reduce subsequent scarring of full-thickness wounds, even though the graft take of split-skin grafts in a one-step procedure is low. Alloderm® is considered medically necessary in post-mastectomy breast reconstructive surgery for at least one of the following indications: there is insufficient tissue expander or implant coverage by the pectoralis major muscle and additional coverage is required; there are thin post-mastectomy skin flaps that are at risk of dehiscence or necrosis; or the infra-mammary fold and lateral mammary folds have been undermined during mastectomy and re-establishment of these landmarks is needed [39]. By retrieving information form the websites of Dermacell® and Dermamatrix®, it is possible to note that they are intended for soft tissue reconstruction (face defects, nasal reconstruction, abdomen, etc.) and for breast reconstruction. Moreover, different clinical trials involving Dermacell® and Dermamatrix® can be retrieved by consulting the database of clinicaltrials.gov. SureDerm® is indicated by the manufacturer as suitable for gingival and root reconstruction. EZ-DERM® is a porcine-derived xenograft in which the collagen has been chemically cross-linked with aldehyde in order to provide strength and durability [106]; it has FDA 510(k) approval for the treatment of partial-thickness burns and venous, diabetic, and pressure ulcers. In a randomized study involving 157 patients affected by partial-thickness burns, it was found to have satisfactory results: non-correct positioning = 1.5%, infection = 3.0%, incomplete epithelialization at time of separation = 2.2%, need for additional excision and grafting = 4.5%, and hypertrophic scaring = 3.3% [106]. OASIS® Wound Matrix and OASIS® Ultra Tri-Layer Matrix are considered medically necessary for treatment of chronic, noninfected, partial- or full-thickness lower-extremity vascular ulcers, which have not adequately responded following a one-month period of conventional ulcer therapy. They are regulated by the FDA as a Class II (moderate risk) device and received FDA 510(k) approval (K061711), on 19 July, 2006 [39]. OASIS® Wound Matrix was subjected to a randomized controlled study in 120 patients with chronic venous leg ulcers. Significantly more wounds (55% vs. 34%) were observed to be healed in comparison with conventional therapy [67].

Using other routes, the production of acellular dermis is obtained in vitro using the main constituents of the connective tissues (collagen, elastin, glycosaminoglycan, etc.) which are extracted from animals and then reconstructed. Once extracted and purified, the extracellular matrix components can be eventually combined together and processed to form 3D porous structures according to the techniques discussed in Section 2.1 (e.g., cross-linking, lyophilization and electrospinning). In the class of reconstructed extracellular matrices (Table 1), we find: Integra®, Biobrane®, Matriderm® and Hyalomatrix®. Integra® Dermal Regeneration Template consists of a bi-layered extracellular matrix of fibers of cross-linked bovine collagen and chondroitin-6-sulfate (a component of cartilage) with a silicone membrane as transient epithelium. Once the neodermis is formed, the disposable silicone sheet is removed, and an ultrathin autograft is placed over the neodermis [9,20,26]. Integra® Dermal Regeneration Template is considered medically necessary in the post-excisional treatment of severe burns when autografting is not feasible. It has an FDA PMA for treatment of life-threatening, full-thickness or deep partial-thickness thermal injuries where sufficient autograft is not available at the time of excision or not desirable due to the physiologic condition of the individual [39]. This product also has an FDA PMA for repair scar contractures. An issue affecting this kind of skin substitute is the time required for neovascularization. Indeed, when the dermis bed is not well vascularized, or it takes a long time to achieve vascularization, the take of the STSG is compromised. Matriderm® becomes vascularized faster than Integra®, supporting the take of a split-skin graft in a one-step procedure. This is due to the presence of elastin in the Matriderm® model, which is able to attract more vascular cells than the chondroitin-6-sulphate present in Integra®. Biobrane® is an acellular dermal matrix composed of bovine type 1 collagen, silicone and nylon, and mechanically bonded to a flexible knitted nylon fabric. The semipermeable membrane is comparable to human epidermis and controls the loss of water vapor, allows for drainage of exudates, and provides permeability to topical antibiotics. The nylon/silicone membrane provides a flexible adherent covering for the wound surface [2,6,9,10,31,39,41,57,61,67,76,99,107,108]. Biobrane® holds an FDA 510(k) approval for the treatment of clean partial-thickness burn wounds and donor site wounds. It is considered medically necessary [39] for the treatment of burn wounds when all of the following criteria are met: the treatment is specific to non-infected partial-thickness burn wounds and donor site wounds;

excision of the burn wound is complete (e.g., nonviable tissue are removed) and homeostasis achieved; sufficient autograft tissue is not available at the time of excision; and autograft is not desirable due to the individual's physiologic condition (e.g., individual has multisystem injuries such that creating new wounds may cause undue stress). It has been shown to be as effective as frozen human allografts. Furthermore, when used on excised full-thickness burns, it reduces hospitalization time in the case of pediatric patients with second-degree burn injuries. Nylon present in Biobrane® is not incorporated, making such an acellular matrix a wound dressing rather than a skin substitute. Hyalomatrix® [2,6,9,42,107,109–111] is a bilayer, esterified hyaluronic acid (HYAFF®) matrix with an outer silicone membrane. The connective-mimicking layer HYAFF® is a long-acting derivative of hyaluronic acid providing a microenvironment suitable for optimal tissue repair and accelerated wound healing. Specifically intended for the treatment of deep burns and full-thickness wounds, it also provides a wound preparation support for the implantation of autologous skin grafts.

3.2. Cellularized Dermal Substitutes

Cellularized skin substitutes can be divided into three categories: (1) Epithelial sheets: formed by epithelial cells embedded in or seeded on polymeric membranes. Such engineered epithelial tissues will not be discussed in this review because the scope of the survey is to elucidate the role of dermis regeneration during the closure of deep wounds. (2) Dermis equivalents: composed of 3D porous matrices or hydrogels containing fibroblasts. (3) Full-thickness (or composite) skin equivalents: composed of a dermis equivalent and epidermis.

In the class of cellularized dermis (Table 2) we find (but are not limited to): Dermagraft®, TransCyte®, and Hyalograft3D®. Dermagraft® is classified by the FDA as an interactive wound and burn dressing approved under the PMA process as a class III, high-risk device, and requires clinical data to support their claims for use: treatment of full-thickness diabetic foot ulcers of greater than six weeks duration that extend through the dermis, but without tendon, muscle, joint capsule, or bone exposure. It is a living dermal replacement composed of a bio-absorbable PLGA mesh seeded with cryopreserved neonatal allogeneic foreskin fibroblasts. Dermagraft® is considered medically necessary when used for at least one of the following indications: the treatment of full-thickness diabetic foot ulcers of greater than six weeks duration that have not adequately responded to standard therapy, that extend through the dermis, but without tendon, muscle, joint capsule or bone exposure; or when used on wounds with dystrophic epidermolysis bullosa. It is advised that this material should be used in patients that have adequate blood supply [39]. This dermal substitute appears to produce results as good as allografts with regard to wound infection, wound exudate, wound-healing time, wound closure and graft take, and is more readily removed than allograft, with significantly higher levels of patient satisfaction [111]. The advantages of this skin substitute include good resistance to tearing, ease of handling and lack of rejection [112]. TransCyte® is a nylon mesh coated with bovine collagen and seeded with allogenic neonatal human foreskin fibroblasts which proliferate and synthesize growth factors and extracellular matrix components. It was shown that the presence of a cell-assembled ECM was able to hasten the re-epithelialization process of partial-thickness burns [113]. Furthermore, a multicenter randomized clinical study showed it to be even superior to frozen human cadaver allograft for the temporary closure of excised burn wounds [114].

TransCyte® received an FDA PMA as a temporary wound covering for surgically excised full-thickness and deep partial-thickness burn wounds (detailed reports can be retrieved on the web site of the FDA). It is considered medically necessary for the following uses: temporary wound covering to treat surgically excised full-thickness (third-degree) and deep partial-thickness (second-degree) thermal burn wounds in persons who require such a covering before autograft placement; and the treatment of mid-dermal to indeterminate depth burn wounds that typically require debridement, and that may be expected to heal without autografting [39].

Hyalograft3D (FDA 510(k) approval) comprises esterified hyaluronic acid fibers seeded with autologous fibroblasts and covered by a silicone membrane. Its use in diabetic ulcer therapy has been reported, showing significant improvement of the wound closure compared to other devices [115]. Apligraft® consists of neonatal fibroblasts seeded onto a bovine type I collagen gel and neonatal keratinocytes cultured on top of this dermal layer [116–118]. It gained an FDA PMA based on its efficacy with venous ulcers. Apligraf® also has an FDA PMA for use in the treatment of diabetic foot ulcers.

In the case of venous insufficiency, it is considered medically necessary for at least one of the following indications: chronic, non-infected, partial- or full-thickness ulcers due to venous insufficiency; standard therapeutic compression also in use; and at least one month of conventional ulcer therapy (such as standard dressing changes, and standard therapeutic compression) has been ineffective [39]. In the case of diabetic foot ulcers, it is considered medically necessary for at least one of the following indications: full-thickness neuropathic diabetic foot ulcers that extend through the dermis but without tendon, muscle, joint capsule, or bone exposure; and at least four weeks of conventional ulcer therapy (such as surgical debridement, complete off-loading and standard dressing changes) has been ineffective. It has been reported that adding Apligraf® to compression therapy for chronic venous ulcers doubled the number of healed wounds at six months. Furthermore, in chronic diabetic foot ulcers, 56% of patients in the Apligraf® group had reached complete healing by 12 weeks compared with only 38% in the control group with moist gauze dressing treatment [118]. Use of Apligraft® in other skin defects, such as donor-site wounds and epidermolysis bullosa [119], has been reported. Disadvantages are its uneven pigmentation and contracture, short shelf life of five days, fragility, the risk of disease transfer due to its allogeneic constituents, and the high cost [4]. Tissuetech® is composed of hyaluronic acid-based matrix seeded with fibroblasts with autologous keratinocytes on top. It was shown to be effective in the treatment of the lower limbs. Furthermore, in 401 diabetic ulcers, 70.3% treated with Tissuetech® healed within less than one year [2,42,107]. OrCel® is a bi-layered skin substitute formed by human derma fibroblasts entrapped in a bovine collagen sponge, with human keratinocytes on top.

OrCel® has received an FDA PMA for the treatment of fresh, clean split-thickness donor sites associated with mitten-hand deformities in individuals who have recessive dystrophic epidermolysis bullosa. It is considered medically necessary for the following indications: epidermolysis bullosa in children after reconstructive surgery; and full-thickness (third-degree) or partial-thickness (second-degree burns) [3,39,41,116,120,121]. Once placed in the defect, OrCel® dissolves and is replaced by the patient's own skin.

Table 1. Acellular dermal substitutes.

Product	Composition	Indications	FDA Status
ALLODERM®	Acellular human dermis– non crosslinked	Repair or replacement of damaged or inadequate integument tissue	HCT/P
DERMACELL®	Acellular human dermis– non crosslinked	Chronic non-healing wounds	HCT/P
DERMAMATRIX®	Acellular human dermis– non crosslinked	Soft tissue replacement Breast Reconstruction	Available through the Musculoskeletal Transplant Foundation which meets and exceeds the standards and regulations of the American Association of Tissue Banks (AATB) and the Food and Drug Administration (FDA)
SUREDERM®	Acellular human dermis– non crosslinked	Soft tissue replacement	HCT/P
OASIS®	Porcine acellular lyophilized small intestine submucosa– non crosslinked	Acute, chronic and burns wounds. It delivers growth factors to stimulate and cell migration angiogenesis	510(k)
PERMACOLL®	Porcine acellular diisocyanite -crosslinked	Full-thickness defects such as burns and for soft tissue reconstruction such as hernia repair	510(k)

Table 1. Cont.

Product	Composition	Indications	FDA Status
EZ-DERM®	Porcine aldehyde cross-linked reconstituted dermal collagen	Partial-thickness burns	510(k)
INTEGRA®	Acellular Bovine type I collagen and chondroitin-6-sulfate copolymer coated with a thin silicone elastomer-crosslinked	Deep partial thickness and full thickness burns	PMA (1996) 510(k) (2002)
BIOBRANE®	Ultrathin silicone as epidermal analog film and 3D nylon filament as dermal analog with type I collagen peptides	Partial-thickness burns in children; toxic epidermal necrolysis, paraneoplastic pemphigus and chronic wounds	510(k)
MATRIDERM®	Bovine non-crosslinked lyophilized dermis, coated with α-elastin hydrolysate	Full-thickness burns	510(k)
HYALOMATRIX®	Acellular non-woven pad of benzyl ester of hyaluronic acid and a silicone membrane–non crosslinked	Burns, chronic wounds.	510(k)

Adapted from [9,29,39,40]. FDA status (retrieved from FDA website): A preamendment device is one that was in commercial distribution before May 28, 1976, the date the Medical Device Amendments were signed into law. After the Medical Device Amendments became law, the classification of devices was determined by FDA classification panels. Eventually all Class III devices will require a PMA. However, preamendment Class III devices require a PMA only after FDA publishes a regulation calling for PMA submissions. The preamendment devices must have a PMA filed for the device by the effective date published in the regulation in order to continue marketing the device. The CFR will state the date that a PMA is required. Prior to the PMA effective date, the devices must have a cleared Premarket Notification 510(k) prior to marketing. Class III Preamendment devices that require a 510(k) are identified in the CFR as Class III and include the statement "Date premarket approval application (PMA) or notice of completion of product development protocol (PDP) is required. No effective date has been established of the requirement for premarket approval.".

Table 2. Cellularized skin substitutes.

Product	Composition	Indications	Status
DERMAGRAFT® (d)	Human cultured neonatal fibroblasts seeded on polyglactin scaffold	Treatment of diabetic foot ulcers, epidermolysisbullosa	PMA (2001)
TRANSCYTE® (d)	Nylon mesh coated with bovine collagen and seeded with allogenic neonatal human foreskin fibroblasts	Full and partial thickness burns	PMA (1998)
ICX-SKN® (d)	A fibrin matrix seeded with neonatal human fibroblasts	Deep dermal wounds	-
DENOVODERM® (d)	Autologous fibroblasts in collagen hydrogel	Deep defect of the skin	In development, under clinical trials
HYALOGRAFT3D® (d)	Based on estherified hyaluronic acid derivate with cultured fibroblasts and covered by a silicone membrane	Use in diabetic ulcer therapy has been reported	510(k)
APLIGRAFT® (ft)	Bovine collagen matrix seeded with neonatal foreskin fibroblasts and keratinocytes	Treatment of various forms of epidermolysisbullosa Diabetic and venous ulcers	PMA Commercially available in the USA
TISSUETECH® (ft)	Hyaluronic acid with cultured autologous keratinocytes and fibroblasts (Hyalograft 3D® + Laserskin®)	Ulcers	-
PERMADERM® (ft)	Autologous fibroblasts and keratinocytes in culture with bovine collagen and GAG substrates	Sever Burns	-
ORCEL® (ft)	Type I bovine collagen matrix seeded with allogeneic neonatal foreskin fibroblasts and keratinocyte	Donor sites in Epidermolysis Bullosa Fresh, clean split thickness donor site wounds in burn patients	PMA (2001)
DENOVOSKIN® (ft)	Autologous fibroblasts in collagen hydrogel and autologous keratinocytes	Deep defect of the skin	In development, under clinical trials

D = composed of one layer (engineered dermis); FT = full-thickness, composed of engineered dermis and engineered epidermis. Adapted from [9,29,39,40]. FDA status: see caption in Table 1.

3.3. Clinical Effectiveness of Skin Substitutes

3.3.1. Effectiveness of Acellular Dermal Regeneration Templates

Dermal substitutes must guarantee correct regeneration of the dermis compartment [13]. After implantation, a dermal substitute has to allow a fast recruitment of endothelial cells in order to guarantee the correct take of a thin STSG. As a long-term aim, the skin substitute should guide a correct regeneration avoiding the formation of scar tissue. It has been recognized that an ideal dermal substitute must satisfy the following requirements [38]:

- avoid the immune response, inflammation and any kind of rejection;
- protect the wounds from infection and loss of fluid;
- easy to handle and flexible, but stiff enough to withstand surgical procedures;
- enable the influx of cells (fibroblasts and endothelial cells) that will build the neodermis;
- stable enough to guarantee the correct neo-synthesis and assembly of immature extracellular matrix; on the other hand, its rate of degradation should be synchronous with the rate of formation of the neo-tissue;
- enable a correct vascularization in less than 14 days post implantation in order to increase the probability of the take of the STSG;
- be able to guide the regeneration avoiding the formation of scar tissue.

To date it is difficult to make a comparison between the efficacy of the different commercially available dermal substitutes because of the lack of long-term follow-up studies in which different dermal substitutes have been studied in parallel. Even where different clinical studies exist for each of the skin substitutes, it is difficult to make an objective comparison due to different factors. Notably, different studies use different methods for the evaluation of the success of the healing. Indeed, different scales exist to evaluate the features of the scar after implantation: Vancouver Scar Scale, Hamilton Burn Scar Rating, Patient and Observer Scar Assessment Scale, Manchester Scar Scale and Visual Analog Scale [121–124]. Moreover, the studies are conducted starting from different type of wounds (burns, ulcers, trauma, etc.). Finally, the experience of the surgeon plays a crucial role in the success of the take of both dermal regeneration template and STSG. This is highlighted by analyzing the results on the take of grafts coming from multicenter and single center studies: the former possesses higher degrees of uncertainty than the latter [124].

Nevertheless, it is possible to extrapolate some general indications showing the benefits and downsides of the different dermal substitutes. By focusing attention on partial- to full-thickness wounds, the gold standard treatment is the application of a partial- or full-thickness STSG. The application of an STSG is an autografting procedure and possesses two main issues: (i) the use of an STSG is an invasive technique because after the removal of large parts of healthy tissues, other damage is induced; and (ii) if the total burn surface is higher than 25% of the total body area, the donor site cannot provide enough tissue to cover the wounded area. For this reason, the majority of the clinical trials have been conducted by comparing the efficacy of a dermis substitute to the efficacy of the gold standard treatment. Among the acellular dermal substitutes, Integra®, Matriderm® and Alloderm® have been subjected to a systematic review [38] thanks to the availability of long-term follow-up studies starting from similar wounds (partial- or full-thickness wounds due to thermal burns). The comparison between the dermal substitutes and the control groups has been performed by analyzing primary outcomes (graft take, wound infection, scar quality) and secondary outcomes (donor site morbidity, convalescence of the patient, need to re-graft). Compared with an STSG, only Integra® showed a significantly lower take ($p < 0.001$). Concerning the infection rate, a value of 85% of infection in patients having a total burn surface of 45% and treated with Integra® has been reported [125,126]. However, other studies reported no difference in infection percentage between Integra® and the control group [26,126,127]. A 6% rate of infection has been detected in a study where Alloderm® was used [127]. Matriderm® did not reveal any difference of infection rate compared with the controls [128]. Concerning scar quality, data only showed better scar quality for Integra® compared to that of an STSG. For all other models, no significant differences were detected in scar quality compared with the control groups. A relevant increase in donor site healing (lower donor site morbidity) has been detected in all studies [38]. This is because by using a dermal substitute to fill the wound bed, the thickness of the STSG can be reduced to 0.006 of an inch, compared to 0.01 of an inch for gold standard treatments.

With the exception of Integra®, few data concerning the mortality and length of stay of patients have been found [38]. No significant differences in rates of re-graft were reported between the dermal substitutes and control groups. Other studies have compared five dermal substitutes (involving Integra®, Matriderm® and Hyalomatrix®) in a preclinical pig model [110]. No difference was found at the end of the survey (six months after implantation) in terms of scar quality and healing properties. A difference was found in the evolution of the healing process. Integra® took more time for fibroblast and blood vessel influx and was still present, as a fragmented matrix, at the end of the survey. Hyalomatrix® showed a lower degradation rate than Matriderm®, but both had completely disappeared at the end of the survey. The quality of the scar assessed with the Vancouver Scar Scale was similar. A long-term follow-up revealed both histological and clinical outcomes in a randomized study using Integra® and Nevelia® [103]. Nevelia® is a porous degradable matrix of about 2 mm thickness made of stabilized native collagen type 1 from calf hides and a silicone sheet of about 200 µm thickness mechanically reinforced with a polyester fabric, and does not contain any chondroitin-6-sulphate GAG. Collagen is purified from calf hides from animals younger than nine months sourced from safe countries. Collagen is then cross-linked with a very low percentage of glutaraldehyde. Clinical results were evaluated through the healing time, Manchester Scar Scale (MSS) and Visual Analog Scale (VAS) up to three years. The differences in healing time between groups, pain and self-estimation was not statistically significant up to a one-year follow-up. Nevelia® showed early regenerative properties in terms of epidermal proliferation and dermal renewal at three weeks, compared with Integra®. Furthermore, Nevelia® showed a more evident angiogenesis vs. Integra®, evaluated as α-SMA immunohistochemistry. Differences in the MSS score were statistically significant at three years follow up in favor of Nevelia® group ($p = 0.001$), together with clinical outcomes. Histological and immunohistochemistry data showed that Nevelia® allows faster neo-angiogenesis and tissue regeneration with neo-formed tissue architecture closer to the physiology of the skin. This data confirms the importance of both vascularization and neodermis influx within the dermal substitute. Indeed, it is well accepted that the faster the vascularization, the higher the take of the STSG. Integra® contains a fraction of chondroitin-6-sulphate GAG that had two side effects: firstly, such a kind of GAG slows the influx of endothelial cells; secondly, the presence of such a high hydrophilic component may retain lesion inflammatory exudates. Furthermore, the high degree of cross-linking in Integra® masks both the adhesion site for fibroblasts and the proteolytic degradation sites, hampering the recipient cells' influx and the degradation of such exogenous ECM. Finally, it seems that rapid vascularization and presence of endogenous dermal cells (fibroblast and vascular network) may play a crucial role in the effectiveness of the dermal substitute.

3.3.2. Effectiveness of Cellularized Skin Substitutes

The introduction of cellularized skin substitutes in the treatment of full-thickness wounds has been necessary in order to overcome some limitations of the acellular dermis. In particular, the presence of dermic cell lines (fibroblast or endothelial cells) serves to reduce the time for neodermis influx after implant. By using acellular dermal substitutes, surgeons have to wait at least four weeks for the implantation of the STSG in order to allow fibroblast and endothelial cells' influx. Without such cellular components, the take of the STSG is not possible. Moreover, the larger the delay before the STSG is implanted, the higher the probability of infection. Thus, the success of the regeneration process is strictly related to both "colonization" time and the quality of the neodermis formed in the porosity of the acellular dermis. A cell populated scaffold introduced in the wound bed aims at reducing such colonization time as a primary task. We can highlight additional requirements that engineered skin substitutes have to possess compared with acellular substitutes:

- Safety concerns: any cultured cell material carries the risk of transmitting viral or bacterial infection, and some support materials (such as bovine collagen and murine feeder cells) may also have a disease risk.
- Clinical efficacy: since the biological risk is higher, the benefits in terms of quality of the healed tissue must be significantly superior, and not only equal, to conventional therapies.
- Convenience: in general, the cost of tissue engineered products is at least ten-fold higher compared to that of non-cellularized materials; in order to achieve clinical uptake, the benefits must include the reduction of hospitalization time, surgical operations after the implants, pain and the associated cost of the treatment.

To date, the use of tissue engineered products for the treatment of burns, although it has received broad scientific success, seems to be not convenient in terms of commercial outcomes. For this reason, many companies have focused their attention on the commercialization of engineered tissues for the treatment of chronic diseases: venous valve insufficiency, arterial diseases, diabetes, vasculitis, skin malignancies and blistering diseases. Regardless of the origin of the wound, the major aim is to reestablish the physiological conditions of the dermis layer. The cells that act to maintain the dermis are the fibroblasts [108], which synthesize and assemble collagen, elastin, and proteoglycans. When inflammation occurs, fibroblasts migrate to the wound site, attracted by bFGF and TGF-β secreted by inflammatory cells and platelets, where the fibroblasts are stimulated to replicate, migrate into the wound, and secrete IGF-1, bFGF, TGF-β, platelet-derived growth factor, and KGF, enabling fibroblast–keratinocyte interaction. When the wound is chronic, the continuous inflammation state induces a premature and stress-induced cellular senescence of the fibroblasts. Moreover, a decreased proliferative potential, impaired capacity to react to growth factors and abnormal protein production is observed. When the percentage of senescent cells in the defect is greater than 15%, wounds are described as hard to heal [14,15,129,130]. The use of Dermagraft® for the treatment of non-healing ulcers has been demonstrated in different clinical studies [130–132]. Summarizing the results, it is possible to establish that the percentage of healing using Dermagraft® ranged from 50% to 71.4%. The complete closure of the wound can be obtained only for ulcers with 12 months of duration or less.

The most popular bi-layered skin substitute (containing fibroblasts and keratinocytes) is Apligraf®, which has been studied since 1999. It has been demonstrated that use of such a bi-layered engineered skin is an effective treatment for ulcers of greater than one-year duration, with a percentage of wound closure of about 50%. Moreover, the number of osteomyelitis and lower-limb amputations were less frequent in the Apligraf® group. The advantage of dermal–epidermal substitutes is the presence of the living epidermal layer that avoids the use of gauzes and two-step procedures. This reduces the risk of infections and improves the healing process due to the presence of fibroblast–keratinocyte cross-talk, which plays a crucial role in the healing process of deep wounds. One of the limitations of the aforementioned categories of skin grafts is the presence of allogenic cell lines, which contain an associated biological risk. This limitation is being overcame by developing models containing autologous cell lines. Two models that use autologous fibroblasts and keratinocytes are denovoDerm® and denovoSkin®, which are under clinical trials at University Children's Hospital of Zurich [71,133–135]. Finally, to deeply investigate on both FDA status and the effectiveness of current skin substitutes the reader can refer to "FDA" and "clinicaltrial" databases by searching for the desired skin model [136,137].

4. Advanced Bioengineered Skin Equivalents: A Future Perspective

4.1. Pre–Vascularization of Dermis Substitutes

The treatment and the evolution of deep wounds due to thermal burns is schematized in Figure 2A-D. After the debridement of the wound, the bed is filled with a DRT supporting an artificial layer of silicone-based epidermis. After a period of four weeks, the epidermal layer is detached and an autologous STSG is applied. In a clinical study that used Integra® as the DRT, 20 patients presenting deep wounds were treated using the procedure described in Figure 2A-D. The evolution of the wound was analyzed by means of histology, immunocytochemistry and the Vancouver Scar Scale [20]. It was observed that the vascularization of the DRT played a crucial role in the take of the STSG. For instance, if the STSG was applied after two or three weeks, the take rate was very low. On the contrary, if the STSG was applied after the fourth week, the take increased up to 95%. Histological and immunostaining analyses demonstrated that at two weeks the vascularization of DRT was poor but increased four weeks after implantation. These data suggest that vascularization of the DRT and the take of the STSG are strictly related [20].

Other relevant findings concern the evolution of the dermis compartment over the time. Weekly histological investigation revealed that influx of exudates and host fibroblasts occurred during weeks one–two. At three weeks, the influx of endothelial cells and the synthesis of immature extracellular matrix components by fibroblasts began. During week four, the formation of a capillary network (Figure 2E) was observed. After the application of the STSG, the wound continued its evolution: at week six a well-organized capillary network was observed, but the dermis–epidermis interface presented no rete ridge profile; at month three, a layer of endogenous collagen network was observed underneath the STSG; after two months, the wound was completely repaired but the neo-tissue was different from the healthy skin. Finally, the complete substitution of the initial DRT with the neodermis occurred at two years post implantation. Even though the patients recovered partial mobility of the damaged parts, it was observed that the repaired zone showed an impaired pigmentation, the mechanical properties between healthy and repaired sites were different, and the organization of the collagen network of the neodermis was different than that of the collagen in the healthy dermis. Finally, neither elastin nor adnexa were present, and differentiation of fibroblasts in myofibroblasts was observed. On the basis of such findings two main issues affecting the DRT emerge: (i) the lack of vascularization [22,23]; and (ii) the limited capability in inducing regeneration instead of repairing processes [135]. The take of the STSG has huge implications related to the repairing process, patient mortality, and morbidity and healthcare costs. Indeed, a low take percentage increases the number of re-grafts and the risk of infection by causing either the death of the patient or an increase of hospitalization time in case of morbidity. To increase the take of STSGs, new emerging strategies involve the use of pre-vascularized DRTs [22,23,33,34,36]. By seeding a DRT with adipose tissue-derived microvasculature fragments, a faster vascularization after implants was observed [138]. Complete reperfusion of the DRT occurred at day six. The percentage of the take was high if the STSG was applied just after day six, indicating that reperfusion rather than simple vascularization played a crucial role in the take. These data suggest that pre-vascularization of the DRT can contribute to shortening the timeframe needed for the application of an STSG. On the other hand, a one-step surgery, which may decrease the number of surgical operations, cannot be performed yet. To do this, not only vascularization, but also fast reperfusion should be promoted.

4.2. Engineered Skin Composed of Fibroblast-Assembled Extracellular Matrix

The lack of vascularization at the moment of implantation has been recognized as the main issue affecting the take of the STSG. No studies have been performed yet on the role that the extracellular matrix comprising the DRT may play on both vascularization and longtime dermal remodeling [17]. The dermis compartment of the totality of the skin substitutes (either cellularized or acellular) are composed by exogenous extracellular materials, i.e., not assembled by the fibroblasts of the patient. This should represent the limitation of the currently available tissue engineering skins. Indeed, exogenous matrices, even though of natural origins, cannot fully replicate the complexity of the living dermis. This may ultimately compromise the repository and regulatory role that the native cell-assembled extracellular matrix plays [16–18]. Such a mismatch between an exogenous material and the living dermis may be responsible for the impaired repair process at both cellular and extracellular levels. Firstly, because the repository and regulatory role of the native ECM is depressed, the growth factors secreted by fibroblasts are not correctly presented to other cell types (e.g., keratinocytes and endothelial cells) neither in space nor time, generating a possible "mistake" in cell–cell signaling [16,17]. This could explain both the delay in the vascularization time and the delayed formation of the rete ridge profile at dermal epidermal interfaces [20,26,72]. As confirmation of this, in vitro tissue engineered skin made by exogenous natural hydrogels (i.e., collagen, fibrin, etc.) presents a flat dermal–epidermal interface. On the contrary, if epithelial cells are grown on a fibroblast-assembled ECM, it is possible to observe a rete ridge profile with spontaneous formation of epithelial invagination and follicular-like structures (Figure 3C) [72], which are typical of the physiologic dermal–epidermal cross-talk mediated by the extracellular matrix [72]. The lack of endogenous ECM-mediated signaling may also explain the absence of both cutaneous adnexa and nerve endings in repaired deep wounds [20,26,129]. Secondly, when fibroblasts colonize the inner porosity of the DRT, they produce an immature extracellular matrix with a degree of assembly much lower than the degree of assembly of the surrounding healthy dermis. Such an immature protein network is not able to withstand the traction forces of the fibroblasts [74,110], generating a different architecture of the collagen fibers in the wound compared to the healthy dermis [15,19,21,77]. Macroscopically, these phenomena generate a portion of the cutis possessing different mechanical properties, different pigmentation, absence of sensing properties and high contracture, provoking both severe functional and aesthetic concerns.

To overcome such limitations, a tissue engineering strategy to produce a human dermis substitute composed of a fibroblast-assembled extracellular matrix has been developed [73,75]. The innovative idea of such strategy is to let human fibroblasts producing their own ECM in vitro. This process provides the possibility of modulating the properties of the cell-synthesized ECM, in order to obtain a final dermis having both composition and assembly degree of the collagen network relatively similar to those present in vivo. Moreover, no exogenous materials are present. This bottom-up tissue engineering strategy starts with the fabrication of dermal building blocks obtained [81] by seeding human fibroblasts in porous gelatin microspheres (Figure 3A). It has been demonstrated that by optimizing the culture conditions, the fibroblasts can produce their own extracellular matrix. Such building blocks, named Dermal-µTissues, were subsequently molded and packed in maturation chambers where both cell–cell and ECM–ECM interactions took place, leading to the formation of a continuum, up to 2 mm thick, made of an endogenous dermis containing fibroblasts and gelatin microspheres. By modulating the stiffness and the degradation rate of the gelatin microspheres and by engineering the dynamic culture conditions (Figure 3), it was possible to obtain fine control over the maturation status and assembly of both collagen and elastin networks [74,91]. During the duration of the process (approximately five weeks), gelatin microspheres were degraded by protease digestion and the final tissue, named EndoDermis, was completely made up of fibroblasts embedded in their own extracellular matrix (Figure 3A). Interestingly, the collagen network was characterized by a stiffness and degree of assembly similar to that featuring the human skin. In the ECM elastin, hyaluronic acid, fibronectin and elastin were also present (Figure 3B-F). In order to produce a pre-vascularized endogenous human dermis model, human umbilical vein endothelial cells (HUVECs) were seeded on the EndoDermis and it was allowed to form an interconnected capillary network [34] that occurred within three weeks (Figure 3D, E). At the best of our knowledge, other than a capillary network, such an engineered DRT is the first model completely formed by a fibroblast-assembled extracellular matrix [34]. After subcutaneous implant in a nude mouse model, fibroblasts and their own ECM (the neodermis) were already present and well-assembled. Thus, no additional time is required for fibroblast influx and neodermis formation. The only phenomenon required is the anastomosis and perfusion of the engineered capillary network. This was shown to occur within seven days of implantation (Figure 3H). Although further investigations are currently being conducted of a more representative wound model, such data are encouraging. In addition to vascularization, which has been recognized as a critical issue [22,23,25,33,34] affecting the effectiveness of a DRT, the described tissue engineered strategy allows the fabrication of a DRT composed of a native extracellular matrix starting from a small number of fibroblasts derived from the patient. In this way, the risks associated with the allogenic nature of the cells and the impaired ECM assembly during wound closure, can be drastically reduced. According to this idea, the formation of severe scars can be reduced.

5. Discussion and Conclusions

Dermal regeneration templates and tissue engineered skin [40] has been reviewed in the light of their effectiveness in guiding the closure of deep wounds toward a regeneration process rather than a repair process [38]. By analyzing the literature, no strategies are currently available that are able to completely restore the whole functionality of the reconstructed part, including pigmentation, mechanical properties, adnexal structures and sensing properties. In other words, the formation of severe scarring still represents a concern in the field of skin reconstruction. Many advances have been made to limit the use of thick STSGs. Indeed, using a last generation DRT, the thickness of STSGs can be reduced to 0.006 of an inch, compared to 0.01 of an inch for gold standard treatments. Furthermore, the take of STSGs has been improved by promoting the vascularization of the DRT [22,23,25]. It has been observed that a DRT composed of non-cross-linked matrices promotes the invasion of fibroblasts and endothelial cells, increasing the take of the STSG compared to the case of cross-linked matrices [9]. On the other hand, cross-linked matrices are able to better withstand contracture during the neodermis remodeling process, due to their superior stiffness. To hasten neodermis growth after implantation, tissue engineering strategies aim at cellularizing the dermis compartment prior to implantation with either fibroblasts or endothelial cells. Pre-vascularization has been shown to improve the take of the STSG and the reperfusion of the dermal bed. This aids the oxygenation of the zone and the removal of waste. The presence of fibroblasts serves to shorten the migration time of fibroblasts from the recipient and to also promote the synthesis of the neo-ECM in the wound bed [26]. Nevertheless, once assembled, the final ECM is still far from its physiologic condition. By analyzing the composition of the bioengineered skin models, it is possible to highlight that they are characterized by a common denominator: cells are always embedded in exogenous matrices (i.e., not synthesized by fibroblasts). This can represent an issue, since native ECMs possess a specific arrangement of moieties, which regulates the cross-talk between fibroblasts and keratinocytes that ultimately leads to the formation of skin adnexa and skin appendages [16–18]. The in vitro fabrication of human bioengineered dermis composed of a fibroblast-assembled ECM incorporating a vascularized network may provide a means of overcoming the scarring process. In this regard, it has been shown that a tissue engineering strategy allows the control of the assembly of the ECM produced by fibroblasts. By modulating the process variables, it is possible to produce an engineered dermis possessing composition, organization, and signal presentation capabilities relatively similar to the native dermis [19,34,35,72,74,81]. This may led to different benefits in the scenario of skin regeneration: (i) To date, the neodermis takes at least two years to form; by introducing the reconstructed patients' dermis in the wound bed, possessing the final architecture and composition at the moment of the implant, no further time will be required for neodermis formation; (ii) by controlling in vitro the degree of assembly of the ECM, it will possible to decrease the differences between repaired and healthy tissues; and (iii) the spatial organization and the functionality of ECM components is not compromised by external factors (e.g., chemicals or physical treatments) and communications among all cell types (e.g., fibroblasts, keratinocytes, nerve endings and macrophages) are correctly orchestrated.

Author Contributions: F.U. collected the majority of the data from the literature, performed a critical analysis of data retrieved from both literature and FDA-CRINICAL TRIAL database, then it wrote the manuscript with inputs from all authors (C.C., G.I. and P.A.N.). C.C. collected data from bottom up tissue engineering skin models and produced histological images and bioengineered skin samples described in the in the Figure 3. He participated to critical discussions during the editing phase. G.I. worked on the arrangement of paragraphs toghether with F.U. and contributed to the development of figures and participated to critical discussions. P.A.N. was the supervisor of the project; he gave inputs about the organization of the manuscript, he gave a crucial contribution concerning the arrangement of discussion in the scientific framework.

Acknowledgments: The authors would like to acknowledge Alessia Larocca, for her contribution in the preparation of the Graphical Abstract.

Conflicts of Interest: The authors declare no conflict of interest.

References

1. Kanitakis, J. Anatomy, histology and immunohistochemistry of normal human skin. *Eur. J. Dermatol.* **2002**, *12*, 390–401.
2. Vig, K.; Atul, C.; Shweta, T.; Saurabh, D.; Rajnish, S.; Shreekumar, P.; Vida, A.D.; Shree, R.S. Advances in Skin Regeneration Using Tissue Engineering. *Int. J. Mol. Sci.* **2017**, *18*, 789. [CrossRef] [PubMed]
3. Zhang, Z.; Michniak-kohn, B.B. Tissue Engineered Human Skin Equivalents. *Pharmaceutics* **2012**, *4*, 26–41. [CrossRef] [PubMed]
4. Matrices, D.; Skin, B. Dermal Matrices and Bioengineered Skin Substitutes: A Critical Review of Current Options. *Plast. Reconstr. Surg. Glob. Open* **2015**, *3*, e284.
5. Heimbach, D.; Luterman, A.; Burke, J.; Cram, A.; Herndon, D.; Hunt, J.; Jordan, M.; McManus, W.; Solem, L.; Warden, G.L. Artificial Dermis for Major Burns. *Ann. Surg.* **1988**, *208*, 313–320. [CrossRef] [PubMed]
6. Shahrokhi, S.; Arno, A.; Jeschke, M.G. The use of dermal substitutes in burn surgery: Acute phase. *Wound Repair Regen.* **2014**, *22*, 14–22. [CrossRef]
7. Sun, B.K.; Siprashvili, Z.; Khavari, P.A. Advances in skin grafting and treatment of cutaneous wounds. *Science* **2014**, *346*, 941–946. [CrossRef]
8. Dhivya, S.; Vijaya, V.; Santhini, E. Review article Wound dressings—A review. *BioMedicine* **2015**, *5*, 24–28. [CrossRef]
9. Van der Veen, V.C.; van der Wal, M.B.; van Leeuwen, M.C.; Ulrich, M.M.; Middelkoop, E. Biological background of dermal substitutes. *Burns* **2010**, *36*, 305–321. [CrossRef]
10. Bloemen, M.C.; van Leeuwen, M.C.; van Vucht, N.E.; van Zuijlen, P.P.; Middelkoop, E. Dermal Substitution in Acute Burns and Reconstructive Surgery: A 12-Year Follow-Up. *Plast. Reconstr. Surg.* **2010**, *125*, 1450–1459. [CrossRef]
11. Proksch, E.; Brandner, J.M.; Jensen, J. The skin: An indispensable barrier. *Exp. Dermatol.* **2008**, *17*, 1063–1072. [CrossRef] [PubMed]
12. Schlader, Z.J.; Vargas, N.T. Regulation of Body Temperature by Autonomic and Behavioral Thermoeffectors. *Exerc. Sport Sci. Rev.* **2019**, *47*, 116–126. [CrossRef] [PubMed]
13. Enoch, S.; Leaper, D.J. Basic science of wound healing. *Surgery* **2008**, *26*, 31–37.
14. Tarnuzzer, R.W.; Gregory, S. Biochemical analysis of acute and chronic wound environments. *Wound Repair Regen.* **1996**, *4*, 321–325. [CrossRef]
15. Velnar, T.; Bailey, T.; Smrkolj, V. The wound healing process: An overview of the cellular and molecular mechanisms. *J. Int. Med. Res.* **2009**, *37*, 1528–1542. [CrossRef]
16. Bowers, S.L.; Banerjee, I.; Baudino, T.A. The extracellular matrix: At the center of it all. *J. Mol. Cell Cardiol.* **2010**, *48*, 474–482. [CrossRef]
17. Rozario, T.; DeSimone, D.W. The extracellular matrix in development and morphogenesis: A dynamic view. *Dev. Biol.* **2010**, *341*, 126. [CrossRef]
18. Watt, F.M.; Fujiwara, H. Cell-Extracellular Matrix Interactions in Normal and Diseased Skin. *Cold Spring Harb. Perspect. Biol.* **2011**, *3*, a005124. [CrossRef]
19. Lombardi, B.; Casale, C.; Imparato, G.; Urciuolo, F.; Netti, P.A. Spatiotemporal Evolution of the Wound Repairing Process in a 3D Human Dermis Equivalent. *Adv. Healthc. Mater.* **2017**, *6*, 1–11. [CrossRef]
20. Moiemen, N.S.; Vlachou, E.; Staiano, J.J.; Thawy, Y.; Frame, J.D. Reconstructive Surgery with Integra Dermal Regeneration Template: Histologic Study, Clinical Evaluation, and Current Practice. *Plast. Reconstr. Surg.* **2006**, *117*, 160S–174S. [CrossRef]
21. Clark, J.A.; Leung, K.S. Mechanical properties of normal skin and hypetrophic scars. *Burns* **1996**, *22*, 443–446. [CrossRef]
22. Frueh, F.S.; Sanchez-Macedo, N.; Calcagni, M.; Giovanoli, P.; Lindenblatt, N. The crucial role of vascularization and lymphangiogenesis in skin reconstruction. *Eur. Surg. Res.* **2018**, *59*, 242–254. [CrossRef] [PubMed]
23. Laschke, M.W.; Menger, M.D. Vascularization in tissue engineering: Angiogenesis versus inosculation. *Eur. Surg. Res.* **2012**, *48*, 85–92. [CrossRef] [PubMed]

24. Chaudhari, A.A.; Vig, K.; Baganizi, D.R.; Sahu, R.; Dixit, S.; Dennis, V.; Singh, S.R.; Pillai, S.R. Future Prospects for Scaffolding Methods and Biomaterials in Skin Tissue Engineering: A Review. *Int. J. Mol. Sci.* **2016**, *17*, 1974. [CrossRef]
25. Hendrickx, B.; Verdonck, K.; Van den Berge, S.; Dickens, S.; Eriksson, E.; Vranckx, J.J.; Luttun, A. Integration of blood outgrowth endothelial cells in dermal fibroblast sheets promotes full thickness wound healing. *Stem Cells* **2010**, *28*, 1165–1177. [CrossRef]
26. Lagus, H.; Sarlomo-Rikala, M.; Böhling, T.; Vuola, J. Prospective study on burns treated with Integra®, a cellulose sponge and split thickness skin graft: Comparative clinical and histological study—Randomized controlled trial. *Burns* **2013**, *39*, 1577–1587. [CrossRef]
27. Cui, H.; Chai, Y.; Yu, Y. Review Article Progress in developing decellularized bioscaffolds for enhancing skin construction. *J. Biomed. Mater. Res. Part A* **2019**, *107*, 1849–1859.
28. Moore, M.A.; Samsell, B.; Wallis, G.; Triplett, S.; Chen, S.; Jones, A.L.; Qin, X. Decellularization of human dermis using non-denaturing anionic detergent and endonuclease: A review. *Cell Tissue Bank.* **2015**, *16*, 249–259. [CrossRef]
29. Macneil, S. Progress and opportunities for tissue-engineered skin. *Nature* **2007**, *445*, 874–880. [CrossRef]
30. Cheung, H.; Lau, K.; Lu, T.; Hui, D. A critical review on polymer-based bio-engineered materials for scaffold development. *Compos. Part B* **2007**, *38*, 291–300. [CrossRef]
31. Zhong, S.P.; Zhang, Y.Z.; Lim, C.T. Tissue scaffolds for skin wound healing and dermal reconstruction. *Nanomed. Nanobiotechnol.* **2010**, *2*, 510–525. [CrossRef] [PubMed]
32. Vacanti, C.A. The history of tissue engineering. *J. Cell. Mol. Med.* **2006**, *10*, 569–576. [CrossRef] [PubMed]
33. Domaszewska-Szostek, A.; Krzyżanowska, M.; Siemionow, M. Cell-Based Therapies for Chronic Wounds Tested in Clinical Studies. *Ann. Plast. Surg.* **2019**, *83*, e96–e109. [CrossRef] [PubMed]
34. Mazio, C.; Casale, C.; Imparato, G.; Urciuolo, F.; Attanasio, C.; De Gregorio, M.; Rescigno, F.; Netti, P.A. Pre-vascularized dermis model for fast and functional anastomosis with host vasculature. *Biomaterials* **2019**, *192*, 159–170. [CrossRef] [PubMed]
35. Martorina, F.; Casale, C.; Urciuolo, F.; Netti, P.A.; Imparato, G. In vitro activation of the neuro-transduction mechanism in sensitive organotypic human skin model. *Biomaterials* **2017**, *113*, 217–229. [CrossRef]
36. Martin, I.; Wendt, D.; Heberer, M. The role of bioreactors in tissue engineering. *TRENDS Biotechnol.* **2004**, *22*, 80–86. [CrossRef]
37. Ratcliffe, A.; Niklason, L.E.E. Bioreactors and Bioprocessing for Tiosue Engineering. *Ann. N. Y. Acad. Sci.* **2002**, *961*, 210–215. [CrossRef]
38. Widjaja, W.; Tan, J.; Maitz, P.K.M.M. Efficacy of dermal substitute on deep dermal to full thickness burn injury: A systematic review. *ANZ J. Surg.* **2017**, *87*, 446–452. [CrossRef]
39. Ucare. *Bioengineering Skin Substitutes—Medical Policy 2016*; Ucare Medical Policy-Policy Number: 2016M0011B; Ucare: Minneapolis, MN, USA, 2016.
40. Mohebichamkhorami, F.; Alizadeh, A. Skin Substitutes: An Updated Review of Products from Year 1980 to 2017. *J. Appl. Biotechnol. Reports* **2017**, *4*, 615–623.
41. Boyce, S.T.; Lalley, A.L. Tissue engineering of skin and regenerative medicine for wound care. *Burns Trauma* **2018**, *6*, 1–10. [CrossRef]
42. Ma, P.X. Scaffolds for tissue fabrication. *Mater. Today* **2004**, *7*, 30–40. [CrossRef]
43. Gibot, L.; Galbraith, T.; Huot, J.; Auger, F.A. A preexisting microvascular network benefits in vivo revascularization of a microvascularized tissue-engineered skin substitute. *Tissue Eng. Part A* **2010**, *16*, 3199–3206. [CrossRef] [PubMed]
44. Hou, Q.; Grijpma, D.W.; Feijen, J. Porous polymeric structures for tissue engineering prepared by a coagulation, compression moulding and salt leaching technique. *Biomaterials* **2003**, *24*, 1937–1947. [CrossRef]
45. Braghirolli, D.I.; Steffens, D.; Pranke, P. Electrospinning for regenerative medicine: A review of the main topics. *Drug Discov. Today* **2014**, *19*, 743–753. [CrossRef]
46. Pörtner, R.; Nagel-Heyer, S.; Goepfert, C.; Adamietz, P.; Meenen, N.M. Bioreactor Design for Tissue Engineering. *J. Biosci. Bioeng.* **2005**, *100*, 235–245. [CrossRef]
47. Helmedag, M.; Weinandy, S.; Marquardt, Y.; Baron, J.M.; Pallua, N. The Effects of Constant Flow Bioreactor Cultivation and Keratinocyte Seeding Densities on Organotypic Skin Grafts Based on a Fibrin Scaffold Corresponding Author. *Tissue Eng. Part A* **2013**, *21*, 1–31.

135. Suzuki, M.; Yakushiji, N.; Nakada, Y.; Satoh, A. Limb Regeneration in Xenopus laevis Froglet. *Sci. World J.* **2006**, *6*, 26–37. [CrossRef] [PubMed]
136. Clinical Trials. Available online: https://clinicaltrials.gov/ (accessed on 10 September 2019).
137. FDA. Available online: https://www.accessdata.fda.gov/scripts/cder/daf/ (accessed on 10 September 2019).
138. Frueh, F.S.; Später, T.; Körbel, C.; Scheuer, C.; Simson, A.C.; Lindenblatt, N.; Giovanoli, P.; Menger, M.D.; Laschke, M.W. Prevascularization of dermal substitutes with adipose tissue-derived microvascular fragments enhances early skin grafting. *Sci. Rep.* **2018**, *8*, 1–9. [CrossRef] [PubMed]

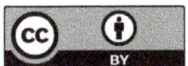

© 2019 by the authors. Licensee MDPI, Basel, Switzerland. This article is an open access article distributed under the terms and conditions of the Creative Commons Attribution (CC BY) license (http://creativecommons.org/licenses/by/4.0/).

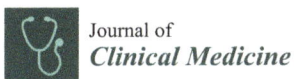

Review

Modular Strategies to Build Cell-Free and Cell-Laden Scaffolds towards Bioengineered Tissues and Organs

Aurelio Salerno [1,*], Giuseppe Cesarelli [1,2], Parisa Pedram [1,2] and Paolo Antonio Netti [1,2,3]

1. Center for Advanced Biomaterials for Healthcare, Istituto Italiano di Tecnologia (IIT@CRIB), 80125 Naples, Italy; Giuseppe.Cesarelli@unina.it (G.C.); Parisa.Pedram@iit.it (P.P.); nettipa@unina.it (P.A.N.)
2. Department of Chemical, Materials and Industrial Production Engineering, University of Naples Federico II, 80125 Naples, Italy
3. Interdisciplinary Research Center on Biomaterials (CRIB), University of Naples Federico II, 80125 Naples, Italy
* Correspondence: asalerno@unina.it

Received: 30 September 2019; Accepted: 28 October 2019; Published: 1 November 2019

Abstract: Engineering three-dimensional (3D) scaffolds for functional tissue and organ regeneration is a major challenge of the tissue engineering (TE) community. Great progress has been made in developing scaffolds to support cells in 3D, and to date, several implantable scaffolds are available for treating damaged and dysfunctional tissues, such as bone, osteochondral, cardiac and nerve. However, recapitulating the complex extracellular matrix (ECM) functions of native tissues is far from being achieved in synthetic scaffolds. Modular TE is an intriguing approach that aims to design and fabricate ECM-mimicking scaffolds by the bottom-up assembly of building blocks with specific composition, morphology and structural properties. This review provides an overview of the main strategies to build synthetic TE scaffolds through bioactive modules assembly and classifies them into two distinct schemes based on microparticles (µPs) or patterned layers. The µPs-based processes section starts describing novel techniques for creating polymeric µPs with desired composition, morphology, size and shape. Later, the discussion focuses on µPs-based scaffolds design principles and processes. In particular, starting from random µPs assembly, we will move to advanced µPs structuring processes, focusing our attention on technological and engineering aspects related to cell-free and cell-laden strategies. The second part of this review article illustrates layer-by-layer modular scaffolds fabrication based on discontinuous, where layers' fabrication and assembly are split, and continuous processes.

Keywords: additive manufacturing; bioprinting; drug delivery; microparticles; scaffold; soft lithography; vascularization

1. Introduction to Tissue Engineering Scaffolds and Bottom-Up Fabrication

Traumas, diseases and population ageing are major reasons for damage and failure of human body tissues and organs, which require medical treatments for their restoration or replacement. Despite the intrinsic body capability of repairing small injuries given sufficient time, to date, tissue growth in large (centimeter-size) defects requires complex, expensive and patient-painful autografts, allografts or xenografts [1,2]. In the case of bone, autograft and allograft implantation produces the best clinical results, but it requires secondary surgery and has a limited supply. The main advantage of a xenograft is its abundant supply and no need for secondary surgery, but poor implantation results and problems of infection from donors are critical issues [2]. Besides, the neo-tissue generated within the interstitial spaces of these grafts is often different from the native tissue and requires large remodeling time for the complete biological and biomechanical integration with surrounding tissues. For these reasons, the development of novel solutions for tissues and organs bioengineering is extremely demanding in the medical field.

Tissue engineering (TE), an important biomedical engineering field, aims to solve this important challenge by combining scaffolds and bioactive molecules for the artificial reconstruction of functional, three-dimensional (3D) tissues and organs [3]. Biomedical scaffolds are porous, implantable biomaterials, shaped to promptly restore the natural tissue anatomy and mechanical functions. The scaffolds must also be capable of controlling foreign body reaction and new-tissue formation by targeted presentation and delivery of key molecules, e.g., anti-inflammatory, growth factors, and proteins. Indeed, these molecules help scaffolds to reduce inflammation, recruit and direct differentiation of stem cells from surrounding tissues and ultimately, promote functional tissue integration in situ [4–6].

Scaffolds design and fabrication have evolved greatly in the past twenty years due to the large knowledge accumulated on materials design, processing and characterization of cell/scaffold interactions. In the natural tissues, cells and extracellular matrix (ECM) organize into 3D structures from sub-cellular to tissue level. Consequently, to engineer functional tissues and organs successfully, scaffolds must capture the essence of this cells/ECM organization and must provide a porous structure able to facilitate cells distribution and guide 3D tissue regeneration [7–9]. Scaffolds pore size and shape, pore wall morphology, porosity, surface area and pore interconnectivity, are probably the most important architectural parameters, as they have been shown to directly impact cells migration and colonization, new ECM biosynthesis and organization, oxygen and nutrients transport to cells, as well as metabolic wastes removal in the whole cell/scaffold construct [10–16]. The scaffold material must be selected and/or designed with a degradation and resorption rate such that scaffold strength is retained until the tissue-engineered transplant is fully remodeled by the host tissue and can assume its own structural role [17,18]. More importantly, controlling mechanical properties at cellular and sub-cellular levels is important to emulate as closely as possible the in vivo cell behavior and tissue growth [19,20]. Nevertheless, controlling the morphological and biomechanical properties of porous scaffolds is not enough for the success of scaffolds-based therapies, as there is also the need to load matricellular and soluble molecules inside scaffolds' matrix as biochemical regulators of cells behavior [21]. Indeed, it is reported that porous scaffolds releasing biochemical signals following a precise dose and time intervals to target sites stimulate cells' functions (e.g., adhesion, proliferation and migration) [22–25], promote the biosynthesis of new ECM [26] and, ultimately, guide tissue growth, morphogenesis [27] and vascularization [28–30].

Increasing scaffolds' design complexity is therefore extremely demanding and scientists face some important challenges, such as: (1) engineering of scaffold microarchitecture to mimic the ECM structure, (2) imprinting topological and biochemical patterns inside scaffolds pores to guide cells' growth and tissue morphogenesis, and (3) developing automated processes for the precise and reliable control of scaffolds' features and geometry.

Porous bioactive scaffolds can be fabricated by combining biomaterials and growth factors through different processing techniques. This review focuses the attention on modular approaches where samples are built by the "bottom-up" assembly of smaller units or "modules", each one specifically designed for distinct tasks [31–33]. Bottom up approaches have the potential to build scaffolds mimicking the complex molecular and structural microenvironment of the native ECM of every kind of tissues by the proper assembly of micro- and nano-structured modules with well-defined morphological and biochemical properties [34].

Several processing techniques are available for modules fabrication, including fluidic emulsion [35], electrofluidodynamic processes [36], and advanced computer aided manufacturing [37,38]. All of these approaches offer, nowadays, a wide library of materials, each one characterized by different composition, shape, nano- and micro-topography, and porous architecture. The assembly of individual modules, such as microparticles (μPs) or patterned layers, by packing, stacking, and printing, allows for achieving multifunctional scaffolds for tissue and organ bioengineering. As will be discussed in the next sections, cell-free or cell-laden μPs can be packed together in a mold giving rise to a sintered matrix by contact points union [39]. Sintering can be obtained by heat or proper plasticizers, in the case of cell-free samples, and by promoting cells/cells and cells/ECM interlocking to obtain hybrid structures [34]. µPs can also be used as cell and/or drug carriers to be loaded inside hydrogel pastes for printing more ordered and complex structures [40]. Layer-by-layer scaffolds' fabrication uses medical imaging combined with computer-aided design (CAD) and automated scaffolds' manufacturing processes to produce customized cell-free or cell-laden scaffolds characterized by a highly controlled structure and reliable properties. This broad category of fabrication techniques includes discontinuous processes, based on the assembly (stacking/sintering) of layered structures obtained by mold replication methods [37]. Alternatively, continuous processes, named additive manufacturing (AM), are used to construct scaffolds by joining/printing biomaterials and cells [38].

The focus of this review is to describe and discuss the advancement of current bottom-up techniques for creating adaptive scaffolds built from µPs or prepared using layer-by-layer assembly techniques, focusing on cell-free and cell-laden strategies. The advantages of each approach to controlling scaffolds' microstructural properties and drug release capability will be discussed, outlining some of the most promising results achieved for regenerating different tissues and organs, such as bone and cartilage, blood vessels, and derma.

2. Microparticles (µPs) as Building Blocks for Modular Tissue Engineering Scaffolds

Nowadays, µPs are essential elements of clinical and regenerative medicine applications such as cell culture µ-scaffolds for in vivo cell delivery and in vitro tissue biofabrication, and drug delivery carriers for biosensing and diagnostic purposes [41–43]. Both synthetic and natural polymeric biomaterials have been investigated for µPs design and engineering. Indeed, chemical and physical polymers properties can be easily manipulated to design and fabricate µPs with tailored morphological properties, size-shape distribution, and degradation rate. Furthermore, scaffolds prepared from synthetic polymeric µPs offer better chemical stability and mechanical properties than those prepared by using natural polymers, especially for load bearing applications. Common examples of the main synthetic polymers for µPs' fabrication which can be mentioned are PCL, poly-lactic acid (PLA), polylactic-co-glycolic acid (PLGA), poly-ethylene glycol (PEG), and their composites with ceramic fillers like calcium phosphate, alumina, and hydroxyapatite [4,44–48]. Natural polymers, conversely, have a chemical composition and structure resembling that of native biological tissues. This aspect is extremely fascinating for µPs' fabrication as it makes it possible to achieve materials faithfully replicating the ECM microenvironment functions. Natural polymeric µPs can be classified into two main groups: protein-based, such as silk, collagen, and fibrin, and polysaccharide-based, like agarose, chitosan, and hyaluronic acid. These kinds of µPs have advantages like excellent biocompatibility, immunogenicity, and degradation rate that can be tuned by varying µPs' materials composition, molecular weight, and crosslinking degree. In the next section, an overview will be provided about µPs' fabrication, highlighting the most advanced techniques to control µPs' composition, structure, and size-shape distribution. Furthermore, the use of µPs as building blocks for cell-free and cell-laden scaffolds fabrication and their use as µ-scaffolds for in vitro cell culture and tissue production will be described in detail.

2.1. µPs Fabrication by Advanced Processes

Several conventional methods are used to prepare µPs, such as phase separation, spray drying, and batch emulsion techniques. The resulting polymeric material is often characterized by heterogeneous size distribution and limited control over their shape [49,50]. To overcome these limitations and achieve even highly complex µPs morphology and composition, new advanced techniques were implemented for µPs' fabrication in the past decades, as highlighted in Figure 1. Microfluidics is a revolutionary technique that manipulates fluids into microscale channels for fluid mixing, merging, splitting, and reaction [51]. Microfluidic emulsion is one of the most investigated techniques for the high-throughput production of monodisperse modular microstructures variable in size, shape, and composition. Microfluidic devices are generally made of transparent and chemically strong devices obtained by assembling glass capillaries or patterning channels in a silicone elastomer, e.g., polydimethylsiloxane (PDMS), through soft lithography methods (Figure 1a,b) [52]. Oil-in-water single emulsions generated with the assistance of the co-flow devices schematized in Figure 1a,b enabled the production of uniform and size-controlled droplets by simple modulation of flow rate of continuous and disperse phases. These droplets can be conveniently converted into uniform beads (Figure 1c) or beads with core-shell, patchy, and Janus architectures (Figure 1d) by the adequate choice of solutions' compositions and controlling the solvent evaporation and phase separation mechanism [45,53]. For instance, using PLGA/PCL as model materials, the authors showed that the core-shell, patchy, and Janus types of particles can be produced with a high yield and a narrow size distribution by precisely controlling interfacial tensions and spreading coefficients between immiscible phases of the generated droplets. As a direct consequence, µPs' hydrophilicity, degradation rate, and drug delivery properties can be tuned depending on the specific application [45].

The formation of multiple emulsions within these microfluidic devices may enable the fabrication of µPs with multiples cores and drug delivery capability (Figure 1e). More importantly, these methods are able to improve loading efficiency of hydrophobic polymeric µPs by changing their polarity [54]. Microfluidic flow-focusing devices were fabricated to generate droplets of different sizes and shapes and narrow size distribution in either PDMS or glass capillary devices [55]. Indicating the diameter of an undeformed (regular) spherical droplet as dS = $(6V/\pi)1/3$, non-spherical droplets are obtained when dS is larger than at least one of the dimensions of the outlet channel, as the confinement hinder shape relaxation of droplets into spheres after breakup. As a direct consequence, in wide channels, when w > dS (w = width) while the height h < dS, the drops assume a discoid shape with rounded borders (Figure 1f). For channels with both h and w smaller than dS, the droplet makes contact with all channel walls and assumes a rod-like morphology (Figure 1g). As shown in Figure 1h, microfluidic approaches were also used for preparing porous µPs with a large surface area, good mechanical strength, and high interconnectivity to be suitable as µ-scaffolds for cells' culture [53]. This was achieved by injecting an unstable water-in-oil emulsion, made of gelatin and poly (vinyl alcohol) (PVA) as discontinuous phase in a PLGA solution in dichloromethane that served as continuous phase. The resultant water-oil-in-water droplets were subsequently solidified by solvent extraction and evaporation in a collection phase (water), generating porous µPs.

Lithography-based processes, such as those reported in Figure 1, are the subsequent example to manufacture precisely shaped polymeric µPs. Flow-lithography processes (e.g., continuous or stop-flow-lithography) enable for continuously synthesizing a variety of different shapes and sizes using several oligomers and produce multifunctional Janus particles. These approaches use ultraviolet (UV) light combined with light-transparent PDMS devices for the selective photopolymerization of a fluidic bead with the aid of proper masks (Figure 1i). Particles' shape in the x–y plane is determined by the transparency masks pattern (Figure 1j–l); whereas the z-plane projection is dependent on the height of the channel used and the thickness of the oxygen inhibition layer [47]. For instance, polyethylene glycol diacrylate (PEGDA) microgels were synthesized with tunable shapes such as triangles, squares, and hexagons, showing good fidelity to the original mask features (Figure 1j–l) [47]. The fundamental limitations of the flow-lithography technique are mainly dependent on the optical resolution and the depth-of-field of the microscope objective used as well, as it requires a short polymerization time or slow flow rate to avoid smearing of the patterned feature in the hydrogels. The main limitation of this technique is the use of prepolymer solutions with high concentrations of monomer and/or photoinitiator, necessary for reducing µPs' setting time that may induce a possible cytotoxic effect. A stop-flow-lithography (SFL) process was recently proposed to overcome this limitation. This process involves stopping the liquid flow, polymerizing the patterned solution, and the flowing of the particles out of the device. This workflow proved suitable for fabricating cell-laden PEGDA particles with controlled shapes and size for TE (Figure 1m,n) [56]. Nevertheless, flow-lithography processes are mainly limited to materials that can polymerize under UV light (hydrogels) and therefore, cannot be used for synthetic materials such as thermoplastic polymers.

Recent advances in micro/nanotechnology have allowed fabrication of µPs made of thermoplastic polymers with uniform sizes and well-defined shapes and composition, which are otherwise impossible to fabricate using conventional µPs' manufacturing methods, providing new building blocks libraries for modular TE. In particular, soft-lithography techniques involve the use of elastomeric PDMS stamps with topological microfeatures to fabricate µPs with precise control over size and geometry in a simple, versatile, and cost-effective modality (Figure 1o) [57–59]. After solvent evaporation, the dried polymer is deposited on selective portions of the mold in the form of particles, and it is removed from the PDMS mold by stamping it onto a PVA sacrificial layer at temperatures and pressures in the range of 80–120 °C and 30–90 KPa, respectively [58]. The µPs are released from the mold by dissolving the PVA layer in water. The versatility of these fabrication methods has been demonstrated using materials of biomedical interest including thermoplastic polymers such as PCL and PLGA (Figure 1p–r) [59], polyethylene glycol dimethacrylate (PEGDMA) hydrogels, and chitosan. An advancement in this fabrication technique was reported recently by McHugh and co-workers that developed a microfabrication method, termed StampEd Assembly of polymer Layers (SEAL), for fabricating modular micrometric structures, such as injectable pulsatile drug-delivery PLGA µPs with complex geometry at a high resolution (Figure 1s,t) [60]. In another study, de Alteriis and co-workers used microspheres to obtain shaped µPs by a soft-lithography approach [46]. This was achieved by positioning PLGA microspheres into PDMS mold cavities with different shapes and deforming them under gentle process conditions, i.e., at room temperature using a solvent/non-solvent vapor mixture. By this approach, it was also possible to preserve the microstructure and bioactivity of molecules loaded inside the µPs (Figure 1u). In conclusion, all of the discussed advanced µPs' fabrication methods may open new avenues for the fabrication of multifunctional building blocks for modular TE applications.

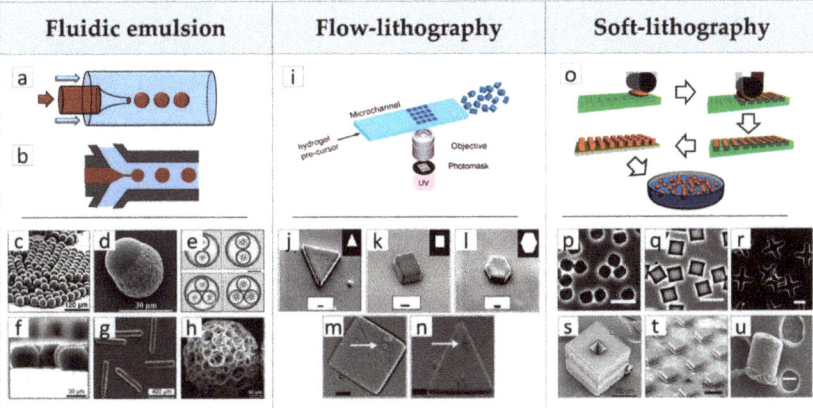

Figure 1. Microfluidic emulsion: Fabrication of microparticles (µPs) with advanced processes. (**a**) Co-flow and (**b**) flow-focusing pictures of fluidic emulsion devices. Effect of processing conditions on µPs morphology, composition and structure: (**c**) spherical monodisperse µPs, (**d**) Janus µPs, (**e**) core-shell µPs with dual and triple cores, (**f**) disks and (**g**) rods µPs obtained by controlling the dimension of the outlet channel, (**h**) highly porous polylactic-co-glycolic acid (PLGA) spherical µPs prepared by double emulsion. Flow-lithography: (**i**) Picture of the flow-lithography continuous process for making shape-controlled µPs by exposure of precursor solution to patterned ultraviolet (UV) light. Morphology of (**j**) triangles, (**k**) squares and (**l**) hexagons µPs prepared by the continuous flow-lithography process. Single-cell encapsulated within (**m**) square and (**n**) triangular µPs prepared by the stop-flow-lithography (SFL) process. Soft-lithography: (**o**) Schematic drawing of the soft-lithography and lift-out molding fabrication protocol of µPs: (**p**,**q**,**r**) effect of mold type on µPs shape. Morphology of µPs obtained by the StampEd Assembly of polymer Layers (SEAL) process before (**s**) and (**t**) after sealing. (**u**) Morphology of vascular endothelial growth factor (VEGF)-loaded PLGA microsphere after solvent vapor shaping

process. **c, f, g** Reproduced with permission from Reference [55] (Xu, Angewandte Chemie International Edition; Published by John Wiley and Sons, 2005); **d** Reproduced with permission from Reference [45] (Cao, RCS. Advances; published by Royal Society of Chemistry, 2015); **e, i** Reproduced with permission from Reference [54] (Baah, Microfluid Nanofluid; published by Springer Nature, 2014); **h** Reproduced with permission from Reference [53] (Choi, Small; published by John Wiley and Sons, 2010); **j, l** Reproduced with permission from Reference [47] (Dendukuri, Nature Materials; published by Springer Nature, 2006); **m, n** Reproduced with permission from Reference [56] (Panda, Lab Chip; published by Royal Society of Chemistry, 2008); **o** Reproduced with permission from Reference [57] (Canelas, Nanomed Nanobiotechnol; published by John Wiley and Sons, 2009); **p, q, r** Reproduced with permission from Reference [59] (Guan, Biomaterials; published by Elsevier Ltd, 2006); **s, t** Reproduced with permission from Reference [60] (Kevin J. McHugh, Science; published by American Association for the Advancement of Science, 2017); **u** Reproduced with permission from Reference [46] (Renato de Alteriis, Scientific Reports; published by Springer Nature, 2015).

2.2. μPs as Building Blocks for In Vitro and In Vivo Modular Tissue Engineering (TE) Scaffolds

The use of μPs for engineering biological tissues may follow two main approaches. In the first approach, named cell-free, μPs are used as building blocks and assembled together to form a sintered porous scaffold. Therefore, the scaffold can be used for in vitro cell culture studies before in vivo implantation. Alternatively, the scaffold is directly implanted in vivo to deliver bioactive molecules and to promptly restore tissue anatomy and functions. In the second approach, named cell-laden, μPs are used as μ-scaffolds for in vitro cell expansion and proliferation. The as-obtained cell-laden μ-scaffolds are subsequently assembled in vitro inside bioreactors to stimulate cell biosynthesis and material degradation, finally leaving a biological tissue replicating native tissues' composition and structure. Both approaches require building blocks assembly into 3D large (centimeter scale) structures by two main ways: random and ordered assembly [61]. The following sections will describe techniques of μPs' assembly for cell-free and cell-laden TE strategies, bringing to light some of the most relevant results achieved to date.

2.2.1. Porous Scaffolds Prepared by the Random/Ordered Assembly of μPs

The literature review has evidenced a plethora of works reporting the design and fabrication of scaffolds by using biodegradable and biocompatible μPs, demonstrating the possibility to achieve tailored porous structure, full interconnected porosity, high mechanical stiffness and, ultimately, drug loading and controlled release features. In a typical process, researchers prepared bioactive and biodegradable μPs using traditional or advanced methods, such as those described in the previous section. The μPs were then poured into appropriate molds and sintered together to form a continuous matrix. As shown in Figure 2a, the resultant scaffolds have a particles-aggregated structure while their size and shape replicated the mold (cylinder) geometry [4].

A scaffold's morphology as well as its pore structures were correlated to the size and shape of the μPs and the sintering process. Sintering depended on the motion of polymeric chains from the μPs surface to contact points that leads to chain inter-diffusion and the subsequent formation of connecting necks between μPs. This mechanism depends on polymer plasticization and can be promoted by heat, organic solvents, or high-pressure fluids [62–67]. For instance, PCL scaffolds were fabricated using thermal sintering of spherical μPs with two different size ranges, smaller (300–500 μm) and larger (500–630 μm) at 60 °C for 1 h. A double emulsion process was also implemented for bovine serum albumin (BSA) encapsulation inside the depots of smaller (50–180 μm) PCL particles for drug delivery purposes. The authors reported the decrease of scaffolds' porosity and pore size as well as the increase of compression moduli with the decrease of μPs' size. This effect is ascribable to an enhanced μPs' compaction and a concomitant higher number of fusion points between smaller μPs [4]. However, low porosity and pore size may result in decreased cell adhesion and colonization. The use of porous μPs enable to overcome this limitation and achieve higher scaffolds' porosity. This aspect was studied by

Qutachi and co-workers, who fabricated highly porous PLGA µPs by the double emulsion technique, where phosphate buffered saline (PBS) was used as the internal aqueous phase. Hydrolysis treatment on µPs using 30% 0.25 M NaOH:70% absolute ethanol enabled the formation of a double-scale sintered matrix at body temperature that can therefore be used as a minimally invasive injectable scaffold (Figure 2b) [62].

The optimization of the sintering step is a critical aspect for scaffolds prepared by µPs' assembly. Indeed, sintering not only affects the integrity of the scaffold structure, but also influences some key properties, such as porosity and mechanical stiffness. Borden et al. addressed this aspect for melt-sintered scaffolds [68], while Brown et al. [69] and Hyeong Jeon et al. [63] addressed it for solvent-sintered scaffolds and for a high-pressure CO_2 sintering, respectively. As shown in Figure 2c, the mechanical properties of PLGA scaffolds increased with the increase of fusion time from 2 to 4 h, while higher treatment times produced the complete collapse of the pore structure due to the extensive polymer melting. Overall, these scaffolds, with a range in modulus from 137.44 to 296.87 MPa, appeared to be capable of sustaining loads in the mid-range of cancellous bone [68]. The solvent/non-solvent chemical sintering, is an alternative strategy for sintering a wide range of polymeric µPs at a low temperature for developing TE scaffolds and drug delivery vehicles [69]. Polymers such as polyphosphazenes, exhibiting glass transition temperatures from −8 to 41 °C, and PLGA were tested to optimize solvent/non-solvent mixtures and the treatment time based on the affinity between polymer and solvent mixtures. The authors reported that the solvent/non-solvent sintering technique produced scaffolds with median pore size and porosity similar to the heat-sintered microspheres [69]. Nevertheless, the use of potentially toxic organic solvents is a critical issue for this approach. A low-temperature organic solvent-free approach was proposed for µPs' sintered scaffolds fabrication [62,63]. This approach used high-pressurized CO_2 to produce scaffolds from a large variety of polymeric materials, such as PCL, PLGA, and PLA [63]. For instance, it was reported that the optimal CO_2 pressure for PLGA scaffolds was in the 15–25 MPa range, and that sintering increased with pressure due to the enhanced polymer plasticization, representing a useful way to tune scaffolds' porosity and mechanical properties [63].

As pointed out in the Introduction section, engineering tissues and organs requires combinations of biomaterials, cells, and bioactive signaling cues. The design of bioactive molecules releasing scaffolds has to consider that the spatial patterning of bioactive signals is vital to some of the most fundamental aspects of life, from embryogenesis to wound healing, all involving concentration gradients of signaling molecules that have to be replicated by scaffolds. µPs have been long studied as drug delivery systems for a variety of molecules as they enable an easy control of the release kinetics of loaded therapeutics. Alendronate (AL)- and dexamethasone (Dex)-loaded PLGA-based scaffolds were proposed by Shi and co-workers for bone regeneration [70]. These molecules were chosen as AL is a bisphosphonate able to promote the activity and maturation of osteoblasts and mesenchymal stem cells (MSCs) differentiation, while Dex is a glucocorticoid with osteogenic properties. Scaffolds' capability to release AL and Dex up to two months in a sustained fashion resulted in a marked osteogenic differentiation of MSCs in vitro and in vivo, as evidenced by significantly higher expression of bone-related proteins and genes, such as alkaline phosphatase activity (ALP), type-I collagen, osteocalcin, and bone morphogenic protein (BMP)-2, if compared to unloaded scaffold. Additionally, drug-loaded scaffolds showed significantly higher new bone formation at eight weeks implantation into rabbit femurs bone defects [70]. Jaklenec et al. used PLGA µPs loaded with dyes to demonstrate the feasibility of creating spatially controlled particles' distribution inside porous scaffolds (Figure 2d) [71]. In another study, Singh and co-workers developed a two-syringe pumping device for the controlled deposition of functional microspheres to create gradients of releasing molecules for interfacial tissues' regeneration [72]. By controlling suspensions composition and flow rates during pumping, it was possible to engineer multiple gradient configurations, such as the bi-layered and multi-layered concentration profiles. The authors further used this technique to prepare a PLGA microspheres scaffold containing opposing gradients of BMP-2 and transforming growth factor (TGFb1) for osteochondral interface TE (Figure 2e) [73]. After six weeks of in vitro culture, MSCs-seeded scaffolds evidence regionalized gene expression of major osteogenic and chondrogenic markers.

Overall, scaffolds based on the assembly of µPs are versatile for a wide range of TE applications, from soft to hard tissues. For instance, the use of synthetic polymers resulted in high mechanical stiffness and a slow degradation rate for in vivo load-bearing implantation, such as bone [74] and osteochondral tissue [75]. Conversely, soft biopolymeric chitosan µPs scaffolds were proposed as a 3D, functional neuronal networks' regeneration platform [76]. Even if all of these studies clearly evidenced the potential of µPs-based scaffolds in TE applications, some key issues are still to be addressed for their successful clinical translation. As previously discussed, biological tissues are characterized by hierarchical-ordered architectures at both nano- and micro-metric size scales, that can be replicated only in part by µPs' random assembly. Furthermore, µPs-based scaffolds require multiple steps of fabrication, from µPs' fabrication up to assembly and sintering. Therefore, the possibility to reduce scaffolds' fabrication time by automated processes will be a great step towards clinical implementation.

One of the most investigated methods to obtain ordered scaffolds from sintered µPs is selective laser sintering (SLS). As shown in Figure 2f–h, this powder-based AM technique enabled patient-specific implantable scaffolds with interconnected multi-scaled porosity [77]. SLS employs a CO_2 laser beam to selectively sinter a powder bead, based on a computer-aided design (CAD) scaffold model. Du and co-workers fabricated PCL and PCL-hydroxyapatite scaffolds for bone TE [78]. Both in vitro and in vivo evaluations demonstrated that these scaffolds not only promoted cell adhesion, supported cell proliferation, and induced cell differentiation in vitro, but also evidenced in vivo bone formation and vascularization. This effect was higher for composite scaffold as the hydroxyapatite increased surface roughness and positively charged the PCL surface. The same authors also explored the fabrication of bioinspired multilayer scaffolds mimicking the complex hierarchical architecture of the osteochondral tissue that was used to repair osteochondral defects of a rabbit model [78]. It is, however, important to point out that SLS techniques create ordered structures (Figure 2g) inside randomly assembled µPs (Figure 2h), while they cannot manipulate µPs and allow their precise positioning inside the scaffold structure. One of the first attempts to solve this aspect and to fabricate porous µPs'-sintered scaffolds with highly ordered pore structure at the µPs-scale was recently proposed by Rossi and co-workers [79]. The authors prepared PCL µPs with size in the 425–500 µm range and used alignment PDMS molds for precise particle positioning and sintering. Final scaffolds were achieved by the stacking of three µPs layers followed by a solvent bonding step (Figure 2i). If compared to randomly assembled scaffolds, the ordered scaffolds showed a better vascularization in the inner core, as evidenced by the deeper blood vessel penetration and the larger diameter of the infiltrating vessels [79]. This approach was tested with large µPs (500 µm), as smaller µPs require the implementation of new advanced automated manufacturing. Nevertheless, these recent results pave the way on the importance on µPs' scaffold design features and provide the basis for the future development in this extremely promising scaffold design research field.

2.2.2. Porous µPs as µ-Scaffolds for In Vitro Tissue Building

In the past decade, researchers in TE have focused the attention on the possibility of recreating large implantable living and functional tissues in vitro by assembling cell-laden µ-scaffolds. The advantage of this approach relies on the fact that porous micro-sized scaffolds can be designed and modularly assembled to guide the correct spatial composition and organization of the de-novo synthesized cell/ECM construct. Furthermore, by this approach, it is possible to overcome limitations related to cells culturing in 3D thick scaffolds, such as cells' seeding efficiency and oxygen and nutrients' transport inside the scaffold core. The capability of recreating in vitro fully biologic centimeter-sized tissues was validated for a large variety of applications. For instance, Urciuolo and co-workers [80] have studied the fabrication of a dermis-equivalent tissue by culturing human dermal fibroblasts (HDFs) onto gelatin µ-scaffolds. The developed process involved two main steps: (Step 1) dynamic cell-seeding of fibroblasts on porous µ-scaffolds using a spinner flask bioreactor for up to nine days to obtain micro-tissue precursors (µTPs). (Step 2) assembly of µTPs and maturation in a specifically designed chamber for up to 28 days [80]. Following this strategy, a 3D functional dermal tissue has been created and used as a base platform to study natural and pathologic tissue morphogenesis mechanisms, such as follicle-like structure formation [81] and tissue vascularization [82], as well as to study dermis remodeling and epidermis senescence after UV radiation exposure [83]. The feasibility of using cell-laden µ-scaffolds to fabricate highly complex biomimetic tissues was also explored in the case of bone [84], cardiac tissue [85], and liver tissues [86]. For example, Chen et al. cultured human amniotic MSCs onto gelatin µ-scaffolds for up to eight days, after which, cells were induced to undergo osteogenic differentiation in the same culture flask and cultured for up to 28 days. These bone-like µ-tissues were finally used as building blocks to fabricate a macroscopic cylindrical bone construct (2 cm in diameter, 1 cm height) evidencing good cell viability and homogenous distribution of cellular content (Figure 2j) [87]. The modularity of this approach was explored by Scott et al., who combined human liver cancer cell line, HepG2, and different types of PEG µPs to study the effect of porosity and drug delivery on cells' behavior (Figure 2k) [88]. In particular, the authors considered three types of PEG microspheres: the first type provided µ-scaffolds mechanical support, the second type provided controlled delivery of the sphingosine 1-phosphate (S1P), an angiogenesis-promoting molecule, and the third type served as a slowly dissolving non-cytotoxic porogen. After components' centrifugation into a mold and incubation at 37 °C overnight, µPs fused together and, within two days of culture, macropores formed thanks to the dissolution of the porogenic particles. The S1P delivery combined with the structural properties allowed HepG2 cells' migration through the scaffolds' macropores (Figure 2j).

AM processes are successfully used to obtain cell-laden µ-scaffolds with ordered structures for biomedical applications. Among these techniques, bioprinting is the most popular as it allows the fabrication of living constructs with custom-made architectures by the controlled deposition of cell-laden µ-scaffolds bioinks [40,89]. In a recent study, Levato and co-workers seeded MSCs onto PLA µ-scaffolds via static culture or spinner flask expansion and loaded these samples in gelatin methacrylamide-gellan gum bioinks [40]. The optimization of the composite material formulation and printing conditions enabled the fabrication of highly ordered constructs with enhanced mechanical properties and high cell-seeded densities (Figure 2l). Process flexibility was also validated by designing and fabricating bi-layered osteochondral scaffolds (Figure 2l). Tan et al. presented a similar approach for the recreation of vascular tubular tissues, based on the micropipette extrusion bioprinting method (Figure 2m) [89]. The selected bioink was made of cell-laden PLGA porous microspheres encapsulated within agarose-collagen hydrogels. Furthermore, the authors demonstrated the possibility to use concomitantly C2C12 and Rat2 cell-laden µ-scaffolds.

Manipulation of cell-laden µ-scaffolds at the micro-scale was also investigated to obtain precisely designed 3D structures for TE. The µ-scaffolds were soaked in an inert medium (mineral oil) while their assembly was obtained by geometrical constraints, specifically by the use of guiding structures or by more complex mechanisms, such as magnetic actuation. The picture in Figure 2n highlights 3D structures obtained by assembling cell-laden µ-scaffolds fabricated by soft-lithography (Figure 1) and starting from a UV-photo-cross-linkable metacrylated gelatin solution [90]. The assembly process was controlled by geometrical constraint or by using a syringe needle swiped uniaxially against the linear array of ring-shaped µ-scaffolds [90]. Liu and co-workers combined µ-scaffolds shape and magnetic field for the construction of artificial bioarchitectures [91]. Magnetite-alginate-chitosan composite microcapsule robots characterized by magnetization along the central axis were magnetically actuated to grab the building components during the transportation and assembly processes. Position and orientation remote control of the cell-laden µ-scaffolds offered a non-invasive and dynamical manipulation system for the creation of complex 3D structures for TE.

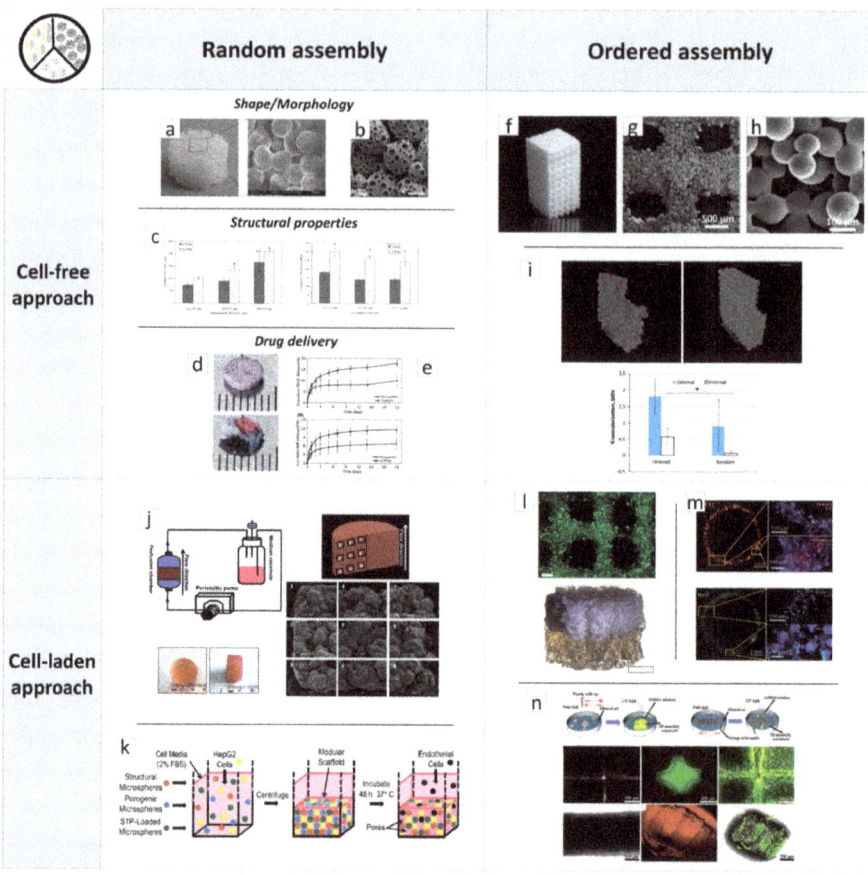

Figure 2. Overview of µPs applications in tissue engineering (TE) scaffold-based strategies classified by random (left column) and ordered (right column) assemblies, cell-free (first row) and cell-laden (second row) approaches. (**a**) morphology of µPs' sintered polycaprolactone (PCL) scaffold obtained by thermal sintering. (**b**) Morphology of porous µPs' sintered PLGA scaffold obtained by chemical sintering. (**c**) Effect of µPs' diameter and thermal sintering time on mean pore size and compressive modulus of PLGA-sintered scaffolds. (**d**) Optical images of sintered scaffolds with homogeneous and heterogeneous spatial distribution of loaded µPs. (**e**) Release profiles of bone morphogenic protein (BMP)-2 and transforming growth factor (TGF) b1 from µPs'-sintered scaffolds for osteochondral interface TE. (**f**) Optical image of ordered scaffold obtained by selective laser sintering (SLS) and made of PCL µPs. (**g,h**) morphology of SLS scaffold evidencing the order and random structures, respectively. (**i**) Comparison of random and ordered PCL scaffolds on degree of vascularization in vivo. Results proved that the internal vascularization of the ordered scaffolds has significantly better vascularization in the inner core if compared to the random scaffold. (**j**) Culture device used to generate three-dimensional (3D) bone in vitro by cell-laden µPs' assembly and morphological and optical visualization of corresponding tissue. (**k**) Assembly of cells and multifunctional poly-ethylene glycol (PEG) µPs to study cells migration in vitro as a function of scaffolds porosity and sphingosine 1-phosphate (S1P) release. (**l,m**) Porous scaffolds obtained by µPs' printing for osteochondral and vascular tissues repair, respectively. (**n**) Schematic of assembly processes of cell-laden µ-scaffolds obtained by soft-lithography process and resulting cell-laden constructs. **a** Reproduced with permission from Reference [4] (Luciani, Biomaterials; published by Elsevier Ltd., 2008); **b** Reproduced with permission from Reference [62] (Qutachi, Acta

Biomaterialia; published by Elsevier Ltd., 2014); **c** Reproduced with permission from Reference [68] (Borden, Biomaterials; published by Elsevier Science Ltd., 2002); **d** Reproduced with permission from Reference [71] (Jaklenec, Biomaterials; published by Elsevier Ltd., 2008); **e** Reproduced with permission from Reference [73] (Dormer, Annals of Biomedical Engineering; published by Springer Nature, 2010); **f–h** Reproduced with permission from Reference [77] (Du, Colloids and Surfaces B: Biointerfaces; published by Elsevier B.V, 2015); **i** Reproduced with permission from Reference [79] (Rossi, Journal of Materials Science Materials in Medicine; published by Springer Nature, 2016); **j** Reproduced with permission from Reference [87] (Chen, Biomaterials; published by Elsevier Ltd., 2011); **k** Reproduced with permission from Reference [88] (Scott, Acta Biomaterialia; published by Elsevier Ltd., 2009); **l** Reproduced with permission from Reference [40] (Levato, Biofabrication; published by Institute of Physics Publishing, 2014); **m** Reproduced with permission from Reference [89] (Tan, Scientific Reports; published by Springer Nature, 2016); **n** Reproduced with permission from Reference [90] (Xiao, Materials Letters; published by Elsevier Ltd., 2018).

3. Layer-by-Layer Approaches for Scaffolds' Fabrication

A valid alternative to modular μPs-based scaffolds is micro/nanostructured modular scaffolds obtained by layer-by-layer assembly processes, as layers' assembly into 3D modular scaffolds enables the fabrication of geometrically and topographically complex architectures. The layer-by-layer scaffolds' fabrication approaches that are the subject of this review are divided into two groups: discontinuous and continuous processes. Discontinuous processes involve layers' fabrication and assembly in two distinct processing steps. Conversely, the continuous processes steps are almost totally automated and take place simultaneously. This part of the review will outline and discuss some of the most useful and efficient techniques for layer-by-layer scaffolds' fabrication, highlighting the most promising results in tissue and organ regeneration.

3.1. Discontinuous Processes

Discontinuous processes involve the separate fabrication of scaffolds' layers followed by their assembly into 3D structures. These two steps often increase processing times but take advantage of the possibility to use micro/nanofabrication technologies for scaffolds' features creation. This was mainly achieved by replication methods, such as those highlighted in Figure 3, where layers are obtained by replicating the features of master molds. As shown, replication methods can be divided into two main groups based on mold type, namely elastomeric (PDMS) and rigid molds, and two sub-groups, depending on polymers processing (solution/temperature plasticization). We also report suitable assembly techniques for the fabricated layers considering the absence (cell-free)/presence of biological matter (cell-laden). However, we would like to point out herein that layers' fabrication and assembly are not confined to only one set of methods and could be combined properly depending on the application.

Common methods to fabricate two-dimensional (2D) layers involved the deposition of pre-polymer or polymer solutions onto PDMS mold by casting or spin-coating, followed by a consolidation step. For instance, Gallego et al. have presented a multilayer micromolding technique to fabricate and assemble PCL scaffolds [92]. Layers were fabricated via spin-coating of a PCL solution in tetrahydrofuran and dimethylsulfoxide (1:3:6 w/w/w ratio) at 4000 rpm for 1 min. Later, solvent was extracted overnight and 10 μm thick PCL layers, with 45×45 μm^2 pores were achieved. One of the previously obtained layers was then transferred onto a glass slide and manually stacked to another layer for 3D scaffold building. By following this approach, the authors obtained up to 100 μm thick PCL scaffolds characterized by 81% porosity, which were suitable for studying the effect of pores size and architecture on cell behavior in vitro. A similar approach was used by Sodha et al. for preparing PCL scaffolds with 200 μm circular or star-shaped pores for retinal transplantation [93].

		2D layers			3D scaffolds	
	Fabrication process	Main features	Composition	Layers assembling/bonding		Main outcomes
Elastomeric mould	Consolidation from solution	Spin coating/ solvent evaporation [92]	✓ Layer thickness: 10 µm ✓ Dual-scale pores: large (45 × 45 µm², square); small (≈1µm, round)	✓ PCL ✓ Cell-free	Manual stacking followed by thermal bonding at 70°C for 2 min under 52 psi pressure	✓ Scaffolds thickness up to 100 µm ✓ 81% porosity ✓ Scaffolds with different layers orientations ✓ Platform for studying in vitro cell/scaffold interactions
		Solution casting/ solvent evaporation [94]	✓ Layer thickness: 25 µm ✓ Dual scale pores: large (100 × 500 µm², rectangular); small (< 100 nm, round)	✓ Poly(NIPAAm-co-HEMAHex)/alginate/ gelatin ✓ Cell-free	Manual stacking followed by thermal bonding at 60°C for 10 min under compression	✓ Anisotropic mechanical properties and high stiffness ✓ Myoblasts elongation and orientation along scaffolds patterning
		Solution casting/ freeze drying [37, 95]	✓ Layer thickness: 500 µm ✓ Dual scale pores: large (≈100 µm, channels); small (10-50µm, round) [37]	✓ Chitosan–gelatin ✓ Cell-free	HUVEC or SMC cell seeding, manual stacking, Cell/ECM mediated bonding	✓ Controlled endothelialisation by interactive HUVEC/SMC layers stacking
			✓ Layer thickness: 2 mm ✓ Dual-scale pores: large (500 µm, liver lobule-like); small (100-200 µm, round) ✓ Porosity (70-90%) [95]	✓ Silk fibroin-gelatin ✓ Cell-free	Stacking mould with alignment wires followed by polymeric solution bonding at RT	✓ Scaffolds thickness up to 3 cm ✓ Complex 3D microfluidic channels design
		Solution casting/ gelation [97, 98]	✓ Layer thickness: 140 µm ✓ Hepatic lobule-like mesh with 300-µm-diameter central pore and smaller cylindrical pores (150 µm distanced) [97]	✓ HepG2 or NIH3T3 cell-laden alginate	Stacking container, Alginate solution bonding with calcium chloride for 30 s	✓ 420 µm thick scaffolds ✓ 3D model for studying cells interaction in co-culture
			✓ Layer thickness: 200 µm ✓ Hexagonal pores (100-250-500 µm) [98]	✓ HUVEC/HepG2 cell-laden collagen	Stacking container, Cell/ECM mediated bonding after 4 days culture	✓ Construct thickness up to 2 mm and customized modular tissue assembly ✓ HUVEC migration and scaffold vascularization model
	Thermal processing	Pre-polymer solution casting + UV crosslinking [99]	✓ Layer thickness: 150-300 µm ✓ Dual scale-pores: channels luminal section and microstructured pores (10 - 20 µm) induced by porogen leaching	✓ POMaC ✓ Cell-free	Stage+microscope alignment and stacking followed by pressing and UV crosslinking for 4 min	✓ Up to 2 cm-thick scaffold ✓ 3D platforms for in vitro and in vivo models of cardiac and hepatic tissues studies
		Microembossing [101, 102]	✓ Layer thickness: 60 µm ✓ 120 µm wide pores	✓ PLGA ✓ Cell-free	hMSCs or mouse ES cells seeding, manual stacking followed by layers pressing and bonding with CO₂ or N₂ at 0.69-1.73 MPa, 37°C for 15 min	✓ Up to 2 cm-thick scaffold ✓ 3D platforms for studying the effect of pore geometry and pore size as well as biomolecules release on tissue growth
		Polymeric solution casting/phase separation [104]	✓ Layer thickness: 20-100 µm ✓ 75% porosity, 2-10 µm rounded pores and 45 µm ridge height.	✓ PLLA ✓ Cell-free	C2C12 pre-myoblast cell seeding, manual stacking by rolling, external fixation without bonding	✓ 4 layers planar or tubular scaffolds ✓ In vitro study of cell behaviour in 3D conditions
Rigid mould	Consolidation from solution	Polymeric solution electrodeposition [105]	✓ Layer thickness: 300 µm ✓ Hepatic lobule structure with 1.5 and 2 mm outer diameter	✓ Ca-Alginate ✓ RLC-1B cell-laden	Stacking mould without bonding	✓ 600 µm scaffolds thickness (2 layers) ✓ In vitro model of liver tissue
		Pre-polymer solution casting followed by thermal curing [106]	✓ Layer thickness: 100 µm ✓ Rectangular pores (500x350 µm²)	✓ APS ✓ Cell-free	Dip coating in pre-polymeric solution and manual stacking followed by curing at 165°C for 2h	✓ 200 µm scaffolds thickness (2 layers) ✓ Struts offset configuration ✓ Design of vascularized myocardial grafts by modular assembly of scaffold and microfluidic base separated by a rapidly degradable interface.
		Pre-polymer solution casting followed by UV crosslinking [107]	✓ 87/125 µm thick layers ✓ Micropores (362 × 564 µm², rectangular)	✓ PLT32o and PGS ✓ Cell-free	Manual stacking with struts offset followed by solvent treatment and bonding	✓ Up to 2 mm thick scaffolds ✓ Elastomeric mechanical properties ✓ In vitro and in vivo Cardiac TE
	Thermal processing	Microembossing [108, 109]	✓ Layer thickness: 20 µm ✓ Layer 1: channels (20 × 30 µm, rectangular) ✓ Layer 2: micropores (20 µm diameter) [108]	✓ PCGA ✓ Cell-free	Layers plasticization by vaporised solvent followed by stacking chamber and pressing for bonding	✓ Up to 60 µm scaffolds thickness ✓ In vitro model to study single cell population
			✓ 500 µm thick layers ✓ Micropores (300 µm diameter) [109]	✓ PCL and SPCL ✓ Cell-free	Layer dipping into polymeric solution followed by manual staking and bonding for 20 min	✓ 1.5 mm scaffolds thickness ✓ 88% porosity ✓ In vitro platform for bone TE

Figure 3. Discontinuous processes overview scheme. Left side: two-dimensional (2D) layers' fabrication processes. Right side: three-dimensional (3D) scaffolds' assembly processes. APS: Poly (ester-amide),1:2 poly (1,3-diamino-2-hydroxypropane-co -polyol sebacate); ECM: Extracellular matrix; ES cells: Embryonic stem cells; hMSC: Human mesenchymal stem cell; HUVEC: Human umbilical vein endothelial cell; NIH3T3: Mouse embryo fibroblast cell line; PCGA: Poly (ε-caprolactone–co-glycolic acid); PCL Polycaprolactone; PGS: Poly (glycerol sebacate); PLGA: Polylactic-co-glycolic acid; PLLA: Poly(L-lactic acid); PLT32o: Poly (limonene thioether); Poly(NIPAAm-co-HEMAHex): Poly (N-isopropylacrylamide–co-2-hydroxyethylmethacrylate-6-hydroxyhexanoate); POMaC: Poly (octamethylene maleate (anhydride) citrate; RLC: Rat liver cells; SMC: Smooth muscle cell; SPCL: Starch-polycaprolactone; TE: Tissue engineering.

A valid alternative to spin-coating consists in solution infiltration through a vacuum. Rosellini et al. [94] in fact fabricated a biomimetic myocardial scaffold, based on a simplified model of an original ECM microarchitecture. Several 25 µm thick layers with 100×500 µm² rectangular pores were successfully fabricated and thermally assembled to promote layers' merging and achieve a mechanically consistent scaffold.

Freeze-drying has been proven as another effective solution-based consolidation method to increase layers' thickness and obtain additional porosity. For example, He and co-workers [95] have fabricated 2 mm thick cylindrical layers by pipetting a silk fibroin/gelatin solution onto a pre-frozen micropatterned PDMS mold. The frozen system is then freeze-dried for at least one day to extract the residual solvent, preserving the fabricated microstructure. Results showed the possibility to modulate layers porosity, in the 70–90% range, and pores size, from 125 to 225 µm by changing the concentration of the polymer in solution, to control cell behavior. A solution-mediated bonding was used to prepare microstructured scaffolds mimicking the liver lobule architecture for liver TE purposes. The use of freeze-drying for polymeric layers' setting was also explored by Wang et al. [37], who fabricated porous scaffolds for vascular TE purposes. The authors used a microfluidic molding method to obtain 500 µm thick chitosan/gelatin layers (100 µm microstructures thickness) pipetting a 1:1 solution between a PDMS mold covered by a glass slide. The final layer was achieved by cooling and freeze-drying. An interesting aspect of their approach was that, before scaffolds' assembly, the layers were seeded with human umbilical vein endothelial cells (HUVECs) or smooth muscle cells (SMCs) with bonding promoted in this case by the cell/cell and cell/ECM interactions. Morphological and histological analysis demonstrated the possibility to create a complete branching vascular network and direct SMCs growth into fiber-like bundles inside the microstructured channels. A similar approach was implemented by He et al., who fabricated agarose/collagen layers by solvent casting and thermal gelation [96]. These layers were seeded with HUVECs/collagen suspension, disposed inside an alignment mold, and bonded with the aid of a thin layer of agarose to obtain a fully perfusable 3D construct.

To explore the advantages of combining layers and cells, Son et al. [97] have presented an evolution of the aforementioned methods using cell-laden solutions and a solution cross-linking assembly method to fabricate a 3D construct which mimics the hepatic liver lobule with sinusoids. To accomplish this purpose, a cell-laden alginate suspension was casted on a plasma-cleaned PDMS mold. Then, the system was incubated into a humidifier with a cross-linking reagent to induce gelation and achieve 8×8.7 mm layers with thicknesses up to 200 µm. The authors fabricated a PDMS chamber for layer stacking and used a small amount of alginate solution and cross-linker at layers' edges for bonding. The results show that layers maintained their structure during cell proliferation, while the manipulation techniques did not result in cell loss. Furthermore, cells show high viability because scaffolds' lateral and central pores ensure oxygen and nutrients' transport in the entire 3D structure. HepG2 cell-loaded constructs exhibited increased hepatic secretion and, when used in combination with mouse embryo fibroblast cell line (NIH3T3), allowed for studying cells interactions in 3D co-culture experiments. This approach was also used to test different porous structures, namely hexagonal pores with size in the 100–500 µm range, and by using collagen as layers' material [98]. A patterned cellulose filter substrate was used for collagen layer manipulation and the scaffold was assembled by alternating cell-free and HUVECs-laden collagen sheets to study cells' migration and scaffold vascularization [98].

Solution-based layers' fabrication was also implemented by using pre-polymer mixtures, which can be consolidated by UV radiation, as reported by Zhang and co-workers, for the microfabrication of the AngioChip scaffold [99]. Layers were fabricated from a mixture of poly (ethylene glycol) dimethyl ether (PEGDM) and poly (octamethylene maleate (anhydride) citrate) (POMaC), that was injected in a patterned PDMS prior to UV cross-linking and solution consolidation. Later, the as-obtained layers (5×3.1 mm^2 surface and 150–300 µm thickness) were demolded, stacked, and bonded by an additional UV treatment. The key feature of this micro-construct is the presence of a built-in endothelialized branched network, suitable to assess cardiac and hepatic tissues' responses to drugs delivered through the internal vasculature. For example, the generation of an angiogenic stimulus (thymosin β4) in vitro allowed endothelial cells' migration through the scaffold micro-holes as a first step of blood vessel formation in vitro. AngioChip also enabled fast anastomosis in vivo and tissue remodeling during the first week.

Processing biomaterials and bioactive molecules from organic solvent solutions require the removal of solvent residues from the final scaffolds, as these residues could be toxic for cells and tissues. In this context, previous researchers have also documented that PDMS could be used as a mold to produce micro-patterned layers from thermally plasticized polymers [100]. Yang et al. [101] have in fact presented several protocols to fabricate PLGA layers (120 µm wide pores and 60 µm thick) by PDMS micro-embossing at a temperature close to the PLGA glass transition temperature. The final porous scaffolds were obtained by stacking layers with the help of an alignment mold followed by compressed CO2 bonding for 1 h. This solvent-free approach was successfully applied to cell-seeded PLGA layers, demonstrating that CO2 bonding ensured proper human MSCs viability and functions [101]. Later, Xie and co-workers also demonstrated the possibility of bonding PLGA layers using N_2, which resulted in enhanced embryonic stem (ES) cells' viability with respect to CO_2 [102].

Although we have explained the motivations that have directed several researchers to choose elastomeric PDMS mold for layers' fabrication, features distortion during the process may be a critical issue. This problem arises because PDMS may swell and deform in contact with a broad range of organic solvents [103] or during compression [101]. As shown in Figure 3, rigid molds are the suitable alternative to overcome this limitation and fabricate layers for TE applications through replication techniques from solution and thermal processing.

Regarding solution-based processes, the first examples we introduce are those presented by Papenburg et al., who fabricated layers of different biocompatible polymers through solution casting/phase separation on a silicon mold [104]. Morphological analysis evidenced 80% porosity and high pore interconnection, low closed isolated pores, and a minor dense outer layer. However, this process leads to films with micropattern dimensions differing to the mold pattern because of film shrinking during the solvent extraction process [104]. Manual stacking and residual solvent bonding enabled the achievement of 3D scaffolds. In a further work, settled layers were seeded with C2C12 pre-myoblasts cells and rolled up to form a hollow cylinder without bonding to evaluate the effect of static and dynamic culture conditions on nutrient transport and cell behavior in vitro [104].

Recently, Liu et al. proposed an electrodeposition process for the preparation of rat liver cell (RLC-18)-laden alginate layers for an in vitro liver application [105]. The process involves the casting of a solution onto a rigid mold, fabricated through photolithographic techniques, with an architecture mimicking the hepatic lobule morphology. Then, the solution was electrodeposited for 15 s to obtain 300 μm thick cell-laden hydrogel layers, whose cells remain viable during all the microfabrication steps and proliferate over time. Two layers were subsequently stacked in an appropriate mold, similar to the process described in Reference [97], to obtain a 3D scaffold.

As for the "Angiochip" device [99], cell-free scaffolds for vascular TE purposes represent interesting examples of modules fabricated by solution consolidation [106,107]. In the work by Ye and co-workers, a modular strategy was proposed to build a slowly degradable poly(ester-amide),1:2 poly (1,3-diamino-2-hydroxypropane-co -polyol sebacate) (APS) bilayer scaffold connected to a microfluidic base through a rapidly degradable porous poly (glycerol sebacate) (PGS) module fabricated by an acrylic template [106]. As-obtained four-layer scaffolds increased the 3D permeability to oxygen and nutrients in vitro and degraded in vivo with a rate suitable to enhance scaffold vascularization. The fabrication of layer-by-layer heart scaffolds by photo-cross-linkable poly (limonene thioether) (PLT32o) prepolymer was reported by Fisher et al., with the aim to provide long in vivo half-life [107]. Layers with rectangular micropores (362×564 μm^2) were obtained by replica molding (REM) of polycarbonate molds and were assembled to form 3D scaffolds with elastomeric mechanical behavior and were able to retain structural integrity until one month in vivo.

Micro-embossing in rigid molds is the last discontinuous process described in this section. This process was widely used by Ryu and co-workers, who fabricated silicon molds to realize patterned layers with interconnecting structures made of thermoplastic materials such as PLGA, poly (p-dioxanone), and Monocryl® [108]. Morphological analyses showing the possibility of embossing structures of different aspect ratios were presented and discussed. Technological points of interest for the process, mainly mold-microstructures detachment and modulation of polymers bulk properties were also addressed. Porous scaffolds were fabricated by layers' stacking and bonding using a novel solvent vapor-mediated assembly process. Briefly, two layers were placed in an assembly chamber at a pre-defined temperature followed by a solvent vapor injection. Layers bonding was then achieved bringing the layers in contact under pressure. By this approach, it was possible to preserve layers' features and eventually incorporate bioactive molecules. As a result, 60 μm thick scaffolds with rectangular pores (20×30 μm) were achieved and tested as a 3D platform for single-cells' culture and characterization. In another work, Lima et al. [109] produced PCL and starch-polycaprolactone (SPCL) thicker layers (500 μm) with 300 μm circular pores and 300 thick pillars using a stainless-steel mold. Layers were manually stacked and bonded by using a PCL solution in chloroform, finally achieving 1.5 mm thick scaffolds with 88% porosity for in vitro bone TE.

3.2. Continuous Processes

Scaffolds' fabrication has evolved significantly by continuous processes due to the impressive evolution in the fields of materials science, cells engineering, and AM materials/cells processing platforms. AM are bottom-up processes where the basic components are assembled layer-by-layer to make objects from 3D model data. For example, the common workflow starts with the 3D virtual reconstruction of the defect to regenerate and can end with a patient-specific scaffold implantation to the site of injury [110]. To date, several AM systems available in market are capable of performing multiple operations simultaneously in the same work, e.g., extruding a synthetic polymer strand from a nozzle and embedding a cell-laden hydrogel in a predefined position. In addition, other important features of AM are scaffolds' reproducibility and consistency, as well as the possibility to create complex shaped 3D structures that are necessary for patient-specific treatments.

Regarding the application fields, AM techniques have still proven versatile and of great impact in regenerating several tissues. Indeed, the level of control offered by these techniques is a key technological aspect to increase our knowledge regarding biophysical and biochemical cues governing tissues' formation and functions. Through this section, we will show relevant results published in recent literature about AM scaffolds, pointing out advantages of the implemented manufacture technique and promising results.

Bone is a dynamic tissue characterized by heterogeneous and anisotropic structures and compositions that are required to support biomechanical and biological bone functions. The hierarchical structure of bone is composed of nanostructures made of organic (e.g., collagen) fibers and inorganic (HA) crystals that form the macroscopic cortical and cancellous bone structures passing through a series of intermediate microstructures, like lamellae, osteons, and harvesian channels. Scaffolds for bone regeneration must mimic bone morphology and structure. Concomitantly, these scaffolds must promote bone deposition (ostoconductive) and must be capable of delivering growth factors, such as BMPs and TGFs, to promote recruited cells' osteogenic differentiation (osteoinductive).

Advances in bone scaffolds' fabrication by AM processes have tried to replicate bone biological and biomechanical complexities. An example of this biomimetic approach is proposed by Kang and co-workers, who developed an innovative AM platform named "integrated tissue–organ printer" (ITOP) [110]. The ITOP is equipped with multi-cartridges capable of printing concomitantly synthetic polymers and cell-laden hydrogels with a resolution down to 2 μm for biomaterials and down to 50 μm for cells (Figure 4a). These features were used to fabricate a calvarial bone construct (8 mm diameter × 1.2 mm thickness) made of a PCL and tricalcium phosphate (TCP) nanoparticles blend and stem cells-loaded hydrogels, embedded in predefined positions (Figure 4b). After 10 days of in vitro osteogenic culture, the bioprinted bone is implanted in a calvarial bone defect region to study maturation up to five months. Histological (Figure 4c) and immunohistological images clearly show new bone formation even in the defect central portion; moreover, the presence of blood vessels demonstrates the absence of tissue necrosis confirming regeneration effectiveness. These promising results suggested the potential utility of printed living tissue constructs in translational applications.

Other recent examples have demonstrated, in vivo, successful calvarial bone regeneration using printed scaffolds made of hydroxyapatite (HA) or PCL/PLGA/HA composite, respectively [111,112]. Furthermore, the advantage of printing techniques to process multiple bioinks in a single scaffold was used to bioactivate the scaffold with BMP-2 peptide or μ-RiboNucleic Acid (μ-RNA) conjugates to enhance stem cells' osteoinduction to stimulate in vivo bone formation.

The regeneration of interface tissues, as osteocartilagenous anatomical regions, requires scaffolds displaying compositional and structural complexity that are only achievable with AM processes. In this context, an interesting fabrication approach is presented by Mekhileri and co-workers [113]. The authors have combined a commercial printer (BioScaffolder) with a custom-made device capable of handling pre-loaded μ-tissues (Figure 4d). The fabricated polymer strands are about 225 μm with a maximum resolution of 25 μm. μ-tissues could be positioned in scaffolds' pores once the fabrication process is finished or could be integrated during the fabrication process (inset of Figure 4d), demonstrating the possibility to fabricate large hybrid constructs with a predetermined architecture and mechanical stability. μ-tissues were produced with dimension of 700 μm to 1.4 mm, without undifferentiated or necrotic cells in the central regions at 28 days of in vitro culture and the chosen dimension was 1 mm for the integration into scaffolds due to design and handling considerations. Using this approach, the authors presented a proof of concept scaffold for joint resurfacing purposes (Figure 4e,f), in which two different natural hydrogels' microspheres were used to simulate the biphasic bone and cartilage portions. The process enabled the manipulation and positioning of the μ-tissues inside the scaffold (Figure 4g), while adjacent μ-tissues fusion is observed at 35 days of in vitro culture in chondrogenic differentiation media (Figure 4h).

A wide range of materials was used for AM purposes in this field, with encouraging results. For example, Gao and co-workers [114] have synthesized a strong copolymer hydrogel with large stretchability (up to 860%) and high compressive strength (up to 8.4 MPa). The material had a rapid thermoreversible sol-gel transition behavior that makes it suitable for graded scaffold printing. Furthermore, this gradient hydrogel scaffold printed with TGF β1 and β-tricalciumphosphate for chondral and bone layers respectively, promotes simultaneous regeneration of cartilage and subchondral bone in a rat model [114]. In another work, Deng and co-workers [115] used 3D printing process to prepare lithium (Li)- and silicon (Si)-containing scaffolds to study the effect of ions' release on osteochondral tissue repair in rabbits. The release of Li and Si ions synergistically exerted a positive effect on cartilage through the activation of hypoxia-inducible factor (HIF-1α) pathway and preservation of chondrocytes from an osteoarthritic environment. Concomitantly, Li and Si ions released from the scaffold improve subchondral bone reconstruction through activating Wnt signal pathways.

The versatility of AM techniques in terms of materials choice and structure design enabled the use of additive manufactured scaffolds in other important fields, such as cardiac and nerve tissues' regeneration. One of the most interesting works concerns a scaffold for cardiac remodeling after myocardial infarction, which is proposed by Yang and co-workers [116]. This device was fabricated by employing the fused deposition modeling (FDM) technology, whose typical resolution is of hundreds of microns [117], to obtain a stacked construction of PGS/PCL blend with regular crisscrossed strands and interconnected micropores (Figure 4i). The PGS/PCL scaffolds exhibited improved elasticity and toughness, if compared to raw PCL and PGS scaffolds respectively, and mechanical properties similar to heart tissue. Moreover, the PGS/PCL mixture was filled with NaCl particles with the goal to leach them out to generate an additional interconnected microporosity for oxygen and nutrients' transport and neovascularization. The study was conducted to first assess the in vitro and in vivo scaffolds' behavior, demonstrating an interesting therapeutic effect in rodents with respect to scaffold-free and PCL or PGS scaffolds implanted after myocardial infarction (Figure 4j), and later to study an annular-shaped scaffold whose results indicate a promising application for preventing ventricular dilation (Figure 4k). Moreover, those 3D-printed PGS/PCL scaffolds possess interesting shape-memory properties after rolling, folding, and compression. This feature holds promise for minimal invasiveness delivery via, for example, a catheter or mini-thoracotomy, in case of future surgical translation.

Another interesting example in this field is that of Boffito and co-workers [118], who have used a custom-made AM equipment to fabricate polyurethane (PU) scaffolds seeded with human cardiac progenitor cells (CPCs). PU scaffolds grafted with laminin-1 supported CPCs differentiation in cardiomyocytes while preliminary in vivo subcutaneous implantation experiments evidenced a minimal inflammatory response and adequate angiogenesis, suggesting their future use as implantable patches for myocardial TE.

Regarding the neural TE field, here we reported the results of the study of Koffler and co-workers [119], who have developed a "microscale continuous projection printing method" (μCPP) (Figure 4l) to fabricate, in a very short time (less than 2 s), a 2 mm-thick biomimetic scaffold for spinal cord injury repair (Figure 4m,n). Materials used for fabrication were mixtures of PEG and gelatin methacrylate. This material, in fact retained its structure over four weeks in vivo and exhibited an acceptable inflammatory response. The chosen material was then processed to obtain scaffolds mimicking the spinal cord structure (Figure 4m,n) and which were seeded with neural progenitor cells (NPCs) before implantation. After six weeks in vivo, injured host axons regenerate into 3D biomimetic scaffolds and synapse onto NPCs implanted into the device (Figure 4o). Furthermore, implanted NPCs extend axons out of the scaffold and into the host spinal cord below the injury to restore synaptic transmission and significantly improve spinal cord functionality.

The advantage of NPCs-laden 3D-printed biocompatible scaffold on nerve tissue repair is also highlighted in Reference [120], where clusters of induced pluripotent stem cell (iPSC)-derived spinal NPCs and oligodendrocyte progenitor cells (OPCs) are placed in precise positions within 3D-printed hydrogel scaffolds during assembly. A combination of transplanted neuronal and glial cells enhance functional axonal connections' formation across areas of the damaged central nervous system. Finally, the combination of cells and growth factor therapies, such as scaffolds releasing neurotrophin-3 growth factor [121], may represent a possible further step towards complete nerve tissue repair.

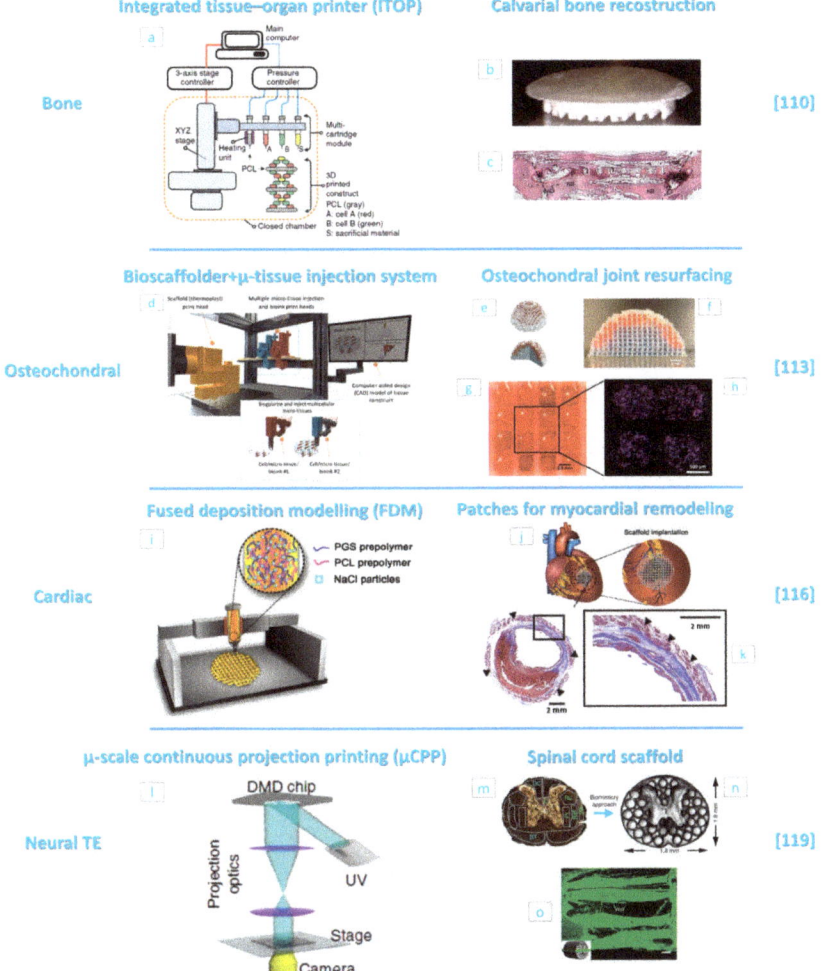

Figure 4. (**a**) Integrated tissue–organ printer (ITOP) system components and materials. (**b**) Photograph of the printed calvarial bone construct. (**c**) Histological image of the printed calvarial construct after in vivo implantation. (**d**) Image of the bioscaffolder + micro-tissue injection system (inset: working

concept overview of the micro-tissue injection system) used for the preparation of the osteochondral joint resurfacing device. (**e**) Computer-aided design (CAD) images and (**f**) optical image of an assembled hemispherical construct. (**g**) Image of µ-tissues in 3D printed PCL fibers and (**h**) resulting 4′,6-diamidino-2-phenylindole (DAPI) (blue) and Aggrecan (purple) antibodies staining of the construct showing cells distribution and µ-tissues fusion at 35 days of in vitro chondrogenic culture. (**i**) Fused deposition modeling (FDM) machine overview and materials for the elastic cardiac patch fabrication. (**j**) Illustration of the scaffold implantation site after induced myocardial infarction in rats. (**k**) Representative Masson's trichrome stained heart section four weeks after implantation. Black boxes denote higher magnification area of the left panel. Black arrows indicate the annular-shaped PGS-PCL scaffolds. Scale bars: 2.0 mm. (**l**) Microscale continuous projection printing (µCPP) system used to fabricate PEG–gelatin methacrylate scaffolds loaded with neural progenitor cells (NPCs) for nerve regeneration. (**m**) Spinal cord structure evidencing fascicles regions (motor systems are shown in green and sensory systems are shown in blue) and (**n**) corresponding scaffold. (**o**) Image of the NPCs-loaded scaffold after four weeks in vivo showing channels filled with green fluorescent protein (GFP)-expressing NPCs. (**a–c**) Reproduced with permission from Reference [110] (Kang, Nature Biotechnology; published by Springer Nature, 2016). (**d–h**) Reproduced with permission from Reference [113] (Mekhileri, Biofabrication; published by IOP Publishing, 2018). (**i–k**) Reproduced with permission from Reference [116] (Yang, Advanced Healthcare Materials; published by John Wiley and Sons, 2019). (**l–o**) Reproduced with permission from Reference [119] (Koffler, Nature Medicine; published by Springer Nature, 2019).

4. Conclusions

Over the last decade, there has been an impressive advancement on scaffolds-based formulations and strategies for bioengineer functional tissues and organs in vitro and in vivo. In this context, bottom-up approaches based on the rational assembly of modular units, in the form of cell-free/cell-laden µPs and/or layers, are, nowadays, the most promising and used approaches. Polymeric µPs offer the advantage in scaffolds' design of morphology and shape control, full pores interconnectivity, high mechanical properties, and biomolecules encapsulation and release. Furthermore, cell-laden µ-scaffolds demonstrated the capability to self-assemble in vitro to form µTPs made up of endogenous ECM and tunable in size and shape. These µTPs can be further assembled in large 3D patches. After µPs degradation, the resulting tissue can be used for in vitro study of complex tissue morphogenesis or for screening normal and dysfunctional tissues' response to specific biophysical and biochemical factors.

Soft-lithography and AM techniques enabled the CAD of cell-free scaffolds and cell-laden constructs down to nano-scale resolution, thereby overcoming limitations related to in vitro cell seeding and micro-architectural features' control. Although it was possible the fabrication of patient-specific devices suitable for clinical implantation, the regeneration of even complex biological tissues aided by these scaffolds is still far from being achieved and requires extensive research efforts on materials design and processing, automated systems integration, and processing times acceleration.

In conclusion, all the results highlighted in this work indicate that the next decades challenge will be to obtain a technology platform that enables users to fabricate ECM-mimicking architectures capable of controlling cell activities and directing their fate for clinical translation and successful engineering of tissues and organs.

Author Contributions: Conceptualization, A.S. and P.A.N.; writing—original draft preparation, A.S., G.C. and P.P.; writing—review and editing, A.S., G.C., P.P. and P.A.N.; visualization, A.S., G.C. and P.P.

Funding: This research received no external funding.

Conflicts of Interest: The authors declare no conflict of interest.

Abbreviations

AL	Alendronate
ALP	Alkaline phosphatase activity
AM	Additive manufacturing
APS	Poly (ester-amide),1:2 poly (1,3-diamino-2-hydroxypropane-co -polyol sebacate)
3D	Three-dimensional
BMP	Bone morphogenic protein
BSA	Bovine serum albumin
CAD	Computer-aided design
CPC	Cardiac progenitor cell
Dex	Dexamethasone
ECM	Extracellular matrix
ES cells	Embryonic stem cells
FDM	Fused deposition modeling
HA	Hydroxyapatite
HDF	Human dermal fibroblast
HIF	Hypoxia-inducible factor
hMSC	Human mesenchymal stem cell
HUVEC	Human umbilical vein endothelial cell
ITOP	Integrated tissue–organ printer
µCPP	Microscale continuous projection printing method
µP	Microparticle
µTP	Micro-tissue precursor
MSC	Mesenchymal stem cell
NIH3T3	Mouse embryo fibroblast cell line
NPC	Neural progenitor cell
OPC	Oligodendrocyte progenitor cell
Pa	Pascal
PBS	Phosphate-buffered saline
PCGA	Poly (ε-caprolcatone–co-glycolic acid)
PCL	Polycaprolactone
PDMS	Polydimethylsiloxane
PEG	Poly-ethylene glycol
PEGDM	Poly (ethylene glycol) dimethyl ether
PEGDA	Polyethylene glycol diacrylate
PEGDMA	Polyethylen glycol dimethacrylate
PGS	Poly (glycerol sebacate)
PLA	Poly-lactic acid
PLGA	Polylactic-co-glycolic acid
PLLA	Poly(L-lactic acid)
PLT32o	Poly (limonene thioether)
Poly(NIPAAm-co-HEMAHex)	Poly (N-isopropylacrylamide–co-2-hydroxyethylmethacrylate-6-hydroxyhexanoate)
POMaC	Poly (octamethylene maleate (anhydride) citrate
PSC	Pluripotent stem cell
PU	Polyurethane
PVA	Poly (vinyl alcohol)
REM	Replica molding
RLC	Rat liver cells
RNA	RiboNucleic Acid
S1P	Sphingosine 1-phosphate
SEAL	StampEd Assembly of polymer Layers
SLS	Selective laser sintering
SMC	Smooth muscle cell
SPCL	Starch-polycaprolactone

TCP	Tricalcium phosphate
TE	Tissue engineering
TGF	Transforming growth factor
UV	Ultraviolet
VEGF	Vascular endothelial growth factor

References

1. O'Brien, F.J. Biomaterials & scaffolds for tissue engineering. *Mater. Today* **2011**, *14*, 88–95.
2. Trappmann, B.; Gautrot, J.E.; Connelly, J.T.; Strange, D.G.T.; Li, Y.; Oyen, M.L.; Stuart, M.A.C.; Boehm, H.; Li, B.; Vogel, V.; et al. Extracellular-matrix tethering regulates stem-cell fate. *Nat. Mater.* **2012**, *11*, 642–649. [CrossRef] [PubMed]
3. Stratton, S.; Shelke, N.B.; Hoshino, K.; Rudraiah, S.; Kumbar, S.G. Bioactive polymeric scaffolds for tissue engineering. *Bioact. Mater.* **2016**, *1*, 93–108. [CrossRef] [PubMed]
4. Luciani, A.; Coccoli, V.; Orsi, S.; Ambrosio, L.; Netti, P.A. PCL microspheres based functional scaffolds by bottom-up approach with predefined microstructural properties and release profiles. *Biomaterials* **2008**, *29*, 4800–4807. [CrossRef] [PubMed]
5. Netti, P.A. *Biomedical Foams for Tissue Engineering Applications*; Woodhead Publishing series in biomaterials; Woodhead Publishing: Cambridge, UK, 2014; ISBN 978-0-85709-703-3.
6. Moioli, E.K.; Clark, P.A.; Xin, X.; Lal, S.; Mao, J.J. Matrices and scaffolds for drug delivery in dental, oral and craniofacial tissue engineering. *Adv. Drug Deliv. Rev.* **2007**, *59*, 308–324. [CrossRef]
7. Schantz, J.-T.; Chim, H.; Whiteman, M. Cell Guidance in Tissue Engineering: SDF-1 Mediates Site-Directed Homing of Mesenchymal Stem Cells within Three-Dimensional Polycaprolactone Scaffolds. *Tissue Eng.* **2007**, *13*, 2615–2624. [CrossRef]
8. Iannone, M.; Ventre, M.; Pagano, G.; Giannoni, P.; Quarto, R.; Netti, P.A. Defining an optimal stromal derived factor-1 presentation for effective recruitment of mesenchymal stem cells in 3D: Optimal SDF-1 Presentation for MSCs Recruitment. *Biotechnol. Bioeng.* **2014**, *111*, 2303–2316. [CrossRef]
9. Sundararaghavan, H.G.; Saunders, R.L.; Hammer, D.A.; Burdick, J.A. Fiber alignment directs cell motility over chemotactic gradients. *Biotechnol. Bioeng.* **2013**, *110*, 1249–1254. [CrossRef]
10. Ma, J.; Both, S.K.; Yang, F.; Cui, F.-Z.; Pan, J.; Meijer, G.J.; Jansen, J.A.; van den Beucken, J.J.J.P. Concise Review: Cell-Based Strategies in Bone Tissue Engineering and Regenerative Medicine. *STEM CELLS Transl. Med.* **2014**, *3*, 98–107. [CrossRef]
11. Badylak, S.F.; Taylor, D.; Uygun, K. Whole-Organ Tissue Engineering: Decellularization and Recellularization of Three-Dimensional Matrix Scaffolds. *Annu. Rev. Biomed. Eng.* **2011**, *13*, 27–53. [CrossRef]
12. Loh, Q.L.; Choong, C. Three-Dimensional Scaffolds for Tissue Engineering Applications: Role of Porosity and Pore Size. *Tissue Eng. Part B Rev.* **2013**, *19*, 485–502. [CrossRef] [PubMed]
13. Reinwald, Y.; Johal, R.; Ghaemmaghami, A.; Rose, F.; Howdle, S.; Shakesheff, K.; Howdle, S.; Shakesheff, K. Interconnectivity and permeability of supercritical fluid-foamed scaffolds and the effect of their structural properties on cell distribution. *Polymers* **2014**, *55*, 435–444. [CrossRef]
14. Harley, B.A.C.; Kim, H.-D.; Zaman, M.H.; Yannas, I.V.; Lauffenburger, D.A.; Gibson, L.J. Microarchitecture of Three-Dimensional Scaffolds Influences Cell Migration Behavior via Junction Interactions. *Biophys. J.* **2008**, *95*, 4013–4024. [CrossRef] [PubMed]
15. Bai, F.; Wang, Z.; Lu, J.; Liu, J.; Chen, G.; Lv, R.; Wang, J.; Lin, K.; Zhang, J.; Huang, X. The Correlation between the Internal Structure and Vascularization of Controllable Porous Bioceramic Materials In Vivo: A Quantitative Study. *Tissue Eng. Part A* **2010**, *16*, 3791–3803. [CrossRef]
16. Perez, R.A.; Mestres, G. Role of pore size and morphology in musculo-skeletal tissue regeneration. *Mater. Sci. Eng. C* **2016**, *61*, 922–939. [CrossRef]
17. Hutmacher, D.W. Scaffolds in tissue engineering bone and cartilage. *Biomaterials* **2000**, *21*, 2529–2543. [CrossRef]
18. Zhang, H.; Zhou, L.; Zhang, W. Control of Scaffold Degradation in Tissue Engineering: A Review. *Tissue Eng. Part B Rev.* **2014**, *20*, 492–502. [CrossRef]
19. Huang, J.; Gräter, S.V.; Corbellini, F.; Rinck, S.; Bock, E.; Kemkemer, R.; Kessler, H.; Ding, J.; Spatz, J.P.; Rinck-Jahnke, S. Impact of Order and Disorder in RGD Nanopatterns on Cell Adhesion. *Nano Lett.* **2009**, *9*, 1111–1116. [CrossRef]

20. Sun, A.X.; Lin, H.; Fritch, M.R.; Shen, H.; Alexander, P.G.; Dehart, M.; Tuan, R.S. Chondrogenesis of human bone marrow mesenchymal stem cells in 3-dimensional, photocrosslinked hydrogel constructs: Effect of cell seeding density and material stiffness. *Acta Biomater.* **2017**, *58*, 302–311. [CrossRef]
21. Swinehart, I.T.; Badylak, S.F. Extracellular matrix bioscaffolds in tissue remodeling and morphogenesis: ECM Bioscaffolds in Development and Healing. *Dev. Dyn.* **2016**, *245*, 351–360. [CrossRef]
22. Chaudhuri, O.; Gu, L.; Klumpers, D.; Darnell, M.; Bencherif, S.A.; Weaver, J.C.; Huebsch, N.; Lee, H.; Lippens, E.; Duda, G.N.; et al. Hydrogels with tunable stress relaxation regulate stem cell fate and activity. *Nat. Mater.* **2016**, *15*, 326–334. [CrossRef] [PubMed]
23. Baker, B.M.; Trappmann, B.; Wang, W.Y.; Sakar, M.S.; Kim, I.L.; Shenoy, V.B.; Burdick, J.A.; Chen, C.S. Cell-mediated fibre recruitment drives extracellular matrix mechanosensing in engineered fibrillar microenvironments. *Nat. Mater.* **2015**, *14*, 1262–1268. [CrossRef] [PubMed]
24. Subbiah, R.; Guldberg, R.E. Materials Science and Design Principles of Growth Factor Delivery Systems in Tissue Engineering and Regenerative Medicine. *Adv. Healthc. Mater.* **2019**, *8*, 1801000. [CrossRef] [PubMed]
25. Lee, K.; Silva, E.A.; Mooney, D.J. Growth factor delivery-based tissue engineering: General approaches and a review of recent developments. *J. R. Soc. Interface* **2011**, *8*, 153–170. [CrossRef] [PubMed]
26. Fusco, S.; Panzetta, V.; Embrione, V.; Netti, P.A. Crosstalk between focal adhesions and material mechanical properties governs cell mechanics and functions. *Acta Biomater.* **2015**, *23*, 63–71. [CrossRef] [PubMed]
27. Hoffman-Kim, D.; Mitchel, J.A.; Bellamkonda, R.V. Topography, cell response, and nerve regeneration. *Annu. Rev. Biomed. Eng.* **2010**, *12*, 203–231. [CrossRef]
28. Carmeliet, P.; Conway, E.M. Growing better blood vessels. *Nat. Biotechnol.* **2001**, *19*, 1019–1020. [CrossRef]
29. Richardson, T.P.; Peters, M.C.; Ennett, A.B.; Mooney, D.J. Polymeric system for dual growth factor delivery. *Nat. Biotechnol.* **2001**, *19*, 1029–1034. [CrossRef]
30. Patel, Z.S.; Young, S.; Tabata, Y.; Jansen, J.A.; Wong, M.E.; Mikos, A.G. Dual delivery of an angiogenic and an osteogenic growth factor for bone regeneration in a critical size defect model. *Bone* **2008**, *43*, 931–940. [CrossRef]
31. Nichol, J.W.; Khademhosseini, A. Modular Tissue Engineering: Engineering Biological Tissues from the Bottom Up. *Soft Matter* **2009**, *5*, 1312–1319. [CrossRef]
32. Elbert, D.L. Bottom-up tissue engineering. *Curr. Opin. Biotechnol.* **2011**, *22*, 674–680. [CrossRef] [PubMed]
33. Kesireddy, V.; Kasper, F.K. Approaches for building bioactive elements into synthetic scaffolds for bone tissue engineering. *J. Mater. Chem. B* **2016**, *4*, 6773–6786. [CrossRef] [PubMed]
34. Leferink, A.; Schipper, D.; Arts, E.; Vrij, E.; Rivron, N.; Karperien, M.; Mittmann, K.; Van Blitterswijk, C.; Moroni, L.; Truckenmuller, R. Engineered Micro-Objects as Scaffolding Elements in Cellular Building Blocks for Bottom-Up Tissue Engineering Approaches. *Adv. Mater.* **2014**, *26*, 2592–2599. [CrossRef] [PubMed]
35. Huang, C.-C.; Wei, H.-J.; Yeh, Y.-C.; Wang, J.-J.; Lin, W.-W.; Lee, T.-Y.; Hwang, S.-M.; Choi, S.-W.; Xia, Y.; Chang, Y.; et al. Injectable PLGA porous beads cellularized by hAFSCs for cellular cardiomyoplasty. *Biomaterials* **2012**, *33*, 4069–4077. [CrossRef] [PubMed]
36. Maya, I.C.; Guarino, V. Introduction to electrofluidodynamic techniques. Part I. In *Electrofluidodynamic Technologies (EFDTs) for Biomaterials and Medical Devices*; Elsevier BV: Amsterdam, The Netherlands, 2018; pp. 1–17.
37. Wang, L.; Chen, Y.; Qian, J.; Tan, Y.; Huangfu, S.; Ding, Y.; Ding, S.; Jiang, B. A bottom-up method to build 3d scaffolds with predefined vascular network. *J. Mech. Med. Boil.* **2013**, *13*, 1340008. [CrossRef]
38. Giannitelli, S.; Accoto, D.; Trombetta, M.; Rainer, A. Current trends in the design of scaffolds for computer-aided tissue engineering. *Acta Biomater.* **2014**, *10*, 580–594. [CrossRef]
39. Cheng, D.; Hou, J.; Hao, L.; Cao, X.; Gao, H.; Fu, X.; Wang, Y. Bottom-up topography assembly into 3D porous scaffold to mediate cell activities. *J. Biomed. Mater. Res. B Appl. Biomater.* **2016**, *104*, 1056–1063. [CrossRef]
40. Levato, R.; Visser, J.; Planell, J.A.; Engel, E.; Malda, J.; Mateos-Timoneda, M.A. Biofabrication of tissue constructs by 3D bioprinting of cell-laden microcarriers. *Biofabrication* **2014**, *6*, 035020. [CrossRef]
41. Xu, Y.; Kim, C.-S.; Saylor, D.M.; Koo, D. Polymer degradation and drug delivery in PLGA-based drug-polymer applications: A review of experiments and theories. *J. Biomed. Mater. Res. B Appl. Biomater.* **2017**, *105*, 1692–1716. [CrossRef]
42. Cho, D.-I.D.; Yoo, H.J. Microfabrication Methods for Biodegradable Polymeric Carriers for Drug Delivery System Applications: A Review. *J. Microelectromech. Syst.* **2015**, *24*, 10–18. [CrossRef]

43. Edmondson, R.; Broglie, J.J.; Adcock, A.F.; Yang, L. Three-Dimensional Cell Culture Systems and Their Applications in Drug Discovery and Cell-Based Biosensors. *ASSAY Drug Dev. Technol.* **2014**, *12*, 207–218. [CrossRef] [PubMed]
44. Salerno, A.; Levato, R.; Mateos-Timoneda, M.A.; Engel, E.; Netti, P.A.; Planell, J.A. Modular polylactic acid microparticle-based scaffolds prepared via microfluidic emulsion/solvent displacement process: Fabrication, characterization, and in vitro mesenchymal stem cells interaction study. *J. Biomed. Mater. Res. A* **2013**, *101A*, 720–732. [CrossRef] [PubMed]
45. Cao, X.; Li, W.; Ma, T.; Dong, H. One-step fabrication of polymeric hybrid particles with core–shell, patchy, patchy Janus and Janus architectures via a microfluidic-assisted phase separation process. *RSC Adv.* **2015**, *5*, 79969–79975. [CrossRef]
46. De Alteriis, R.; Vecchione, R.; Attanasio, C.; De Gregorio, M.; Porzio, M.; Battista, E.; Netti, P.A. A method to tune the shape of protein-encapsulated polymeric microspheres. *Sci. Rep.* **2015**, *5*, 12634. [CrossRef]
47. Dendukuri, D.; Pregibon, D.C.; Collins, J.; Hatton, T.A.; Doyle, P.S. Continuous-flow lithography for high-throughput microparticle synthesis. *Nat. Mater.* **2006**, *5*, 365–369. [CrossRef] [PubMed]
48. Vallet-Regí, M.; Salinas, A.J. Ceramics as bone repair materials. In *Bone Repair Biomaterials*; Elsevier: Amsterdam, The Netherlands, 2019; pp. 141–178, ISBN 978-0-08-102451-5.
49. Xia, Y.; Pack, D.W. Uniform biodegradable microparticle systems for controlled release. *Chem. Eng. Sci.* **2015**, *125*, 129–143. [CrossRef]
50. Campos, E.; Branquinho, J.; Carreira, A.S.; Carvalho, A.; Coimbra, P.; Ferreira, P.; Gil, M.H. Designing polymeric microparticles for biomedical and industrial applications. *Eur. Polym. J.* **2013**, *49*, 2005–2021. [CrossRef]
51. Ma, S.; Mukherjee, N. Microfluidics Fabrication of Soft Microtissues and Bottom-Up Assembly. *Adv. Biosyst.* **2018**, *2*, 1800119. [CrossRef]
52. Li, W.; Zhang, L.; Ge, X.; Xu, B.; Zhang, W.; Qu, L.; Choi, C.-H.; Xu, J.; Zhang, A.; Lee, H.; et al. Microfluidic fabrication of microparticles for biomedical applications. *Chem. Soc. Rev.* **2018**, *47*, 5646–5683. [CrossRef]
53. Choi, S.-W.; Yeh, Y.-C.; Zhang, Y.S.; Sung, H.-W.; Xia, Y. Uniform beads with controllable pore sizes for biomedical applications. *Small* **2010**, *6*, 1492–1498. [CrossRef]
54. Baah, D.; Floyd-Smith, T. Microfluidics for particle synthesis from photocrosslinkable materials. *Microfluid. Nanofluid.* **2014**, *17*, 431–455. [CrossRef]
55. Xu, S.; Nie, Z.; Seo, M.; Lewis, P.; Kumacheva, E.; Stone, H.A.; Garstecki, P.; Weibel, D.B.; Gitlin, I.; Whitesides, G.M. Generation of Monodisperse Particles by Using Microfluidics: Control over Size, Shape, and Composition. *Angew. Chem.* **2005**, *117*, 3865. [CrossRef]
56. Panda, P.; Ali, S.; Lo, E.; Chung, B.G.; Hatton, T.A.; Khademhosseini, A.; Doyle, P.S. Stop-flow lithography to generate cell-laden microgel particles. *Lab Chip* **2008**, *8*, 1056–1061. [CrossRef] [PubMed]
57. Canelas, D.A.; Herlihy, K.P.; DeSimone, J.M. Top-down particle fabrication: Control of size and shape for diagnostic imaging and drug delivery: Top-down particle fabrication. *Wiley Interdiscip. Rev. Nanomed. Nanobiotechnol.* **2009**, *1*, 391–404. [CrossRef] [PubMed]
58. Higuita, N.; Dai, Z.; Kaletunç, G.; Hansford, D.J. Fabrication of pH-sensitive microparticles for drug delivery applications using soft lithography techniques. In Proceedings of the Mater. Res. Soc. Symp. Proc. **2008**, *1095*, 7–12.
59. Guan, J.; Ferrell, N.; Lee, L.J.; Hansford, D.J. Fabrication of polymeric microparticles for drug delivery by soft lithography. *Biomaterials* **2006**, *27*, 4034–4041. [CrossRef] [PubMed]
60. McHugh, K.J.; Nguyen, T.D.; Linehan, A.R.; Yang, D.; Behrens, A.M.; Rose, S.; Tochka, Z.L.; Tzeng, S.Y.; Norman, J.J.; Anselmo, A.C.; et al. Fabrication of fillable microparticles and other complex 3D microstructures. *Science* **2017**, *359*, 1138–1142. [CrossRef]
61. Wang, H.; Leeuwenburgh, S.C.G.; Li, Y.; Jansen, J.A. The Use of Micro- and Nanospheres as Functional Components for Bone Tissue Regeneration. *Tissue Eng. Part B Rev.* **2012**, *18*, 24–39. [CrossRef]
62. Qutachi, O.; Vetsch, J.R.; Gill, D.; Cox, H.; Scurr, D.J.; Hofmann, S.; Müller, R.; Quirk, R.A.; Shakesheff, K.M.; Rahman, C.V. Injectable and porous PLGA microspheres that form highly porous scaffolds at body temperature. *Acta Biomater.* **2014**, *10*, 5090–5098. [CrossRef]
63. Jeon, J.H.; Bhamidipati, M.; Sridharan, B.; Scurto, A.M.; Berkland, C.J.; Detamore, M.S. Tailoring of processing parameters for sintering microsphere-based scaffolds with dense-phase carbon dioxide. *J. Biomed. Mater. Res. B Appl. Biomater.* **2013**, *101B*, 330–337. [CrossRef]

64. Bhamidipati, M.; Sridharan, B.; Scurto, A.M.; Detamore, M.S. Subcritical CO2 sintering of microspheres of different polymeric materials to fabricate scaffolds for tissue engineering. *Mater. Sci. Eng. C* **2013**, *33*, 4892–4899. [CrossRef] [PubMed]
65. Ghanbar, H.; Luo, C.; Bakhshi, P.; Day, R.; Edirisinghe, M. Preparation of porous microsphere-scaffolds by electrohydrodynamic forming and thermally induced phase separation. *Mater. Sci. Eng. C* **2013**, *33*, 2488–2498. [CrossRef] [PubMed]
66. Mikael, P.E.; Amini, A.R.; Basu, J.; Arellano-Jimenez, M.J.; Laurencin, C.T.; Sanders, M.M.; Carter, C.B.; Nukavarapu, S.P. Functionalized carbon nanotube reinforced scaffolds for bone regenerative engineering: Fabrication, in vitro and in vivo evaluation. *Biomed. Mater.* **2014**, *9*, 35001. [CrossRef] [PubMed]
67. Lv, Q.; Nair, L.; Laurencin, C.T. Fabrication, characterization, and in vitro evaluation of poly(lactic acid glycolic acid)/nano-hydroxyapatite composite microsphere-based scaffolds for bone tissue engineering in rotating bioreactors. *J. Biomed. Mater. Res. A* **2009**, *91A*, 679–691. [CrossRef]
68. Borden, M. Structural and human cellular assessment of a novel microsphere-based tissue engineered scaffold for bone repair. *Biomaterials* **2003**, *24*, 597–609. [CrossRef]
69. Brown, J.L.; Nair, L.S.; Laurencin, C.T. Solvent/non-solvent sintering: A novel route to create porous microsphere scaffolds for tissue regeneration. *J. Biomed. Mater. Res. Part B Appl. Biomater.* **2008**, *86*, 396–406. [CrossRef]
70. Shi, X.; Ren, L.; Tian, M.; Yu, J.; Huang, W.; Du, C.; Wang, D.-A.; Wang, Y. In vivo and in vitro osteogenesis of stem cells induced by controlled release of drugs from microspherical scaffolds. *J. Mater. Chem.* **2010**, *20*, 9140. [CrossRef]
71. Jaklenec, A.; Wan, E.; Murray, M.E.; Mathiowitz, E. Novel scaffolds fabricated from protein-loaded microspheres for tissue engineering. *Biomaterials* **2008**, *29*, 185–192. [CrossRef]
72. Singh, M.; Morris, C.P.; Ellis, R.J.; Detamore, M.S.; Berkland, C. Microsphere-Based Seamless Scaffolds Containing Macroscopic Gradients of Encapsulated Factors for Tissue Engineering. *Tissue Eng. Part C Methods* **2008**, *14*, 299–309. [CrossRef]
73. Dormer, N.H.; Singh, M.; Wang, L.; Berkland, C.J.; Detamore, M.S. Osteochondral interface tissue engineering using macroscopic gradients of bioactive signals. *Ann. Biomed. Eng.* **2010**, *38*, 2167–2182. [CrossRef]
74. Jiang, T.; Nukavarapu, S.P.; Deng, M.; Jabbarzadeh, E.; Kofron, M.D.; Doty, S.B.; Abdel-Fattah, W.I.; Laurencin, C.T. Chitosan–poly (lactide-co-glycolide) microsphere-based scaffolds for bone tissue engineering: In vitro degradation and in vivo bone regeneration studies. *Acta Biomater.* **2010**, *6*, 3457–3470. [CrossRef] [PubMed]
75. Gupta, V.; Lyne, D.V.; Laflin, A.D.; Zabel, T.A.; Barragan, M.; Bunch, J.T.; Pacicca, D.M.; Detamore, M.S. Microsphere-Based Osteochondral Scaffolds Carrying Opposing Gradients of Decellularized Cartilage And Demineralized Bone Matrix. *ACS Biomater. Sci. Eng.* **2017**, *3*, 1955–1963. [CrossRef]
76. Tedesco, M.T.; Di Lisa, D.; Massobrio, P.; Colistra, N.; Pesce, M.; Catelani, T.; Dellacasa, E.; Raiteri, R.; Martinoia, S.; Pastorino, L. Soft chitosan microbeads scaffold for 3D functional neuronal networks. *Biomaterials* **2018**, *156*, 159–171. [CrossRef] [PubMed]
77. Du, Y.; Liu, H.; Shuang, J.; Wang, J.; Ma, J.; Zhang, S. Microsphere-based selective laser sintering for building macroporous bone scaffolds with controlled microstructure and excellent biocompatibility. *Colloids Surf. B Biointerfaces* **2015**, *135*, 81–89. [CrossRef] [PubMed]
78. Du, Y.; Liu, H.; Yang, Q.; Wang, S.; Wang, J.; Ma, J.; Noh, I.; Mikos, A.G.; Zhang, S. Selective laser sintering scaffold with hierarchical architecture and gradient composition for osteochondral repair in rabbits. *Biomaterials* **2017**, *137*, 37–48. [CrossRef]
79. Rossi, L.; Attanasio, C.; Vilardi, E.; De Gregorio, M.; Netti, P.A. Vasculogenic potential evaluation of bottom-up, PCL scaffolds guiding early angiogenesis in tissue regeneration. *J. Mater. Sci. Mater. Electron.* **2016**, *27*, 107. [CrossRef]
80. Urciuolo, F.; Imparato, G.; Totaro, A.; Netti, P.A. Building a Tissue in Vitro from the Bottom Up: Implications in Regenerative Medicine. *Methodist DeBakey Cardiovasc. J.* **2013**, *9*, 213–217. [CrossRef]
81. Casale, C.; Imparato, G.; Urciuolo, F.; Netti, P.A. Endogenous human skin equivalent promotes in vitro morphogenesis of follicle-like structures. *Biomaterials* **2016**, *101*, 86–95. [CrossRef]
82. Mazio, C.; Casale, C.; Imparato, G.; Urciuolo, F.; Attanasio, C.; De Gregorio, M.; Rescigno, F.; Netti, P.A. Pre-vascularized dermis model for fast and functional anastomosis with host vasculature. *Biomaterials* **2019**, *192*, 159–170. [CrossRef]

83. Casale, C.; Imparato, G.; Urciuolo, F.; Rescigno, F.; Scamardella, S.; Escolino, M.; Netti, P.A. Engineering a human skin equivalent to study dermis remodelling and epidermis senescence in vitro after UVA exposure. *J. Tissue Eng. Regen. Med.* **2018**, *12*, 1658–1669. [CrossRef]
84. Totaro, A.; Salerno, A.; Imparato, G.; Domingo, C.; Urciuolo, F.; Netti, P.A. PCL-HA microscaffolds for in vitro modular bone tissue engineering: PCL-HA microscaffolds for bone tissue engineering. *J. Tissue Eng. Regen. Med.* **2017**, *11*, 1865–1875. [CrossRef] [PubMed]
85. Totaro, A.; Urciuolo, F.; Imparato, G.; Netti, P.A. Engineered cardiac micromodules for the in vitro fabrication of 3D endogenous macro-tissues. *Biofabrication* **2016**, *8*, 025014. [CrossRef] [PubMed]
86. Yajima, Y.; Yamada, M.; Utoh, R.; Seki, M. Collagen Microparticle-Mediated 3D Cell Organization: A Facile Route to Bottom-up Engineering of Thick and Porous Tissues. *ACS Biomater. Sci. Eng.* **2017**, *3*, 2144–2154. [CrossRef]
87. Chen, M.; Wang, X.; Ye, Z.; Zhang, Y.; Zhou, Y.; Tan, W.-S. A modular approach to the engineering of a centimeter-sized bone tissue construct with human amniotic mesenchymal stem cells-laden microcarriers. *Biomaterials* **2011**, *32*, 7532–7542. [CrossRef]
88. Scott, E.A.; Nichols, M.D.; Kuntz-Willits, R.; Elbert, D.L. Modular scaffolds assembled around living cells using poly(ethylene glycol) microspheres with macroporation via a non-cytotoxic porogen. *Acta Biomater.* **2010**, *6*, 29–38. [CrossRef] [PubMed]
89. Tan, Y.J.; Tan, X.; Yeong, W.Y.; Tor, S.B. Hybrid microscaffold-based 3D bioprinting of multi-cellular constructs with high compressive strength: A new biofabrication strategy. *Sci. Rep.* **2016**, *6*, 39140. [CrossRef] [PubMed]
90. Xiao, W.; Xi, H.; Li, J.; Wei, D.; Li, B.; Liao, X.; Fan, H. Fabrication and assembly of porous micropatterned scaffolds for modular tissue engineering. *Mater. Lett.* **2018**, *228*, 360–364. [CrossRef]
91. Liu, Y.; Li, G.; Lu, H.; Yang, Y.; Liu, Z.; Shang, W.; Shen, Y. Magnetically Actuated Heterogeneous Microcapsule-Robot for the Construction of 3D Bioartificial Architectures. *ACS Appl. Mater. Interfaces* **2019**, *11*, 25664–25673. [CrossRef]
92. Gallego, D.; Ferrell, N.; Sun, Y.; Hansford, D.J. Multilayer micromolding of degradable polymer tissue engineering scaffolds. *Mater. Sci. Eng. C* **2008**, *28*, 353–358. [CrossRef]
93. Sodha, S.; Wall, K.; Redenti, S.; Klassen, H.; Young, M.J.; Tao, S.L. Microfabrication of a Three-Dimensional Polycaprolactone Thin-Film Scaffold for Retinal Progenitor Cell Encapsulation. *J. Biomater. Sci. Polym. Ed.* **2011**, *22*, 443–456. [CrossRef]
94. Rosellini, E.; Vozzi, G.; Barbani, N.; Giusti, P.; Cristallini, C. Three-dimensional microfabricated scaffolds with cardiac extracellular matrix-like architecture. *Int. J. Artif. Organs* **2010**, *33*, 885–894. [CrossRef] [PubMed]
95. He, J.; Liu, Y.; Hao, X.; Mao, M.; Zhu, L.; Li, D. Bottom-up generation of 3D silk fibroin–gelatin microfluidic scaffolds with improved structural and biological properties. *Mater. Lett.* **2012**, *78*, 102–105. [CrossRef]
96. He, J.; Zhu, L.; Liu, Y.; Li, D.; Jin, Z. Sequential assembly of 3D perfusable microfluidic hydrogels. *J. Mater. Sci. Mater. Electron.* **2014**, *25*, 2491–2500. [CrossRef] [PubMed]
97. Son, J.; Bae, C.Y.; Park, J.-K. Freestanding stacked mesh-like hydrogel sheets enable the creation of complex macroscale cellular scaffolds. *Biotechnol. J.* **2016**, *11*, 585–591. [CrossRef]
98. Son, J.; Bang, M.S.; Park, J.-K. Hand-Maneuverable Collagen Sheet with Micropatterns for 3D Modular Tissue Engineering. *ACS Biomater. Sci. Eng.* **2019**, *5*, 339–345. [CrossRef]
99. Zhang, B.; Lai, B.F.L.; Xie, R.; Huyer, L.D.; Montgomery, M.; Radisic, M. Microfabrication of AngioChip, a biodegradable polymer scaffold with microfluidic vasculature. *Nat. Protoc.* **2018**, *13*, 1793–1813. [CrossRef]
100. Lee, B.-K.; Lee, B.-Y. Investigation of thermoplastic hot embossing process using soft polydimethylsiloxane (PDMS) micromold. *J. Mech. Sci. Technol.* **2015**, *29*, 5063–5067. [CrossRef]
101. Yang, Y.; Xie, Y.; Kang, X.; Lee, L.J.; Kniss, D.A. Assembly of Three-Dimensional Polymeric Constructs Containing Cells/Biomolecules Using Carbon Dioxide. *J. Am. Chem. Soc.* **2006**, *128*, 14040–14041. [CrossRef]
102. Xie, Y.; Yang, Y.; Kang, X.; Li, R.; Volakis, L.I.; Zhang, X.; Lee, L.J.; Kniss, D.A. Bioassembly of three-dimensional embryonic stem cell-scaffold complexes using compressed gases. *Biotechnol. Prog.* **2009**, *25*, 535–542. [CrossRef]
103. Wang, Y.; Balowski, J.; Phillips, C.; Phillips, R.; Sims, C.E.; Allbritton, N.L. Benchtop micromolding of polystyrene by soft lithography. *Lab Chip* **2011**, *11*, 3089–3097. [CrossRef]
104. Papenburg, B.J.; Liu, J.; Higuera, G.A.; Barradas, A.M.; De Boer, J.; Van Blitterswijk, C.A.; Wessling, M.; Stamatialis, D. Development and analysis of multi-layer scaffolds for tissue engineering. *Biomaterials* **2009**, *30*, 6228–6239. [CrossRef] [PubMed]

105. Liu, Z.; Lu, M.; Takeuchi, M.; Yue, T.; Hasegawa, Y.; Huang, Q.; Fukuda, T. In vitro mimicking the morphology of hepatic lobule tissue based on Ca-alginate cell sheets. *Biomed. Mater.* **2018**, *13*, 035004. [CrossRef] [PubMed]
106. Ye, X.; Lu, L.; Kolewe, M.E.; Hearon, K.; Fischer, K.M.; Coppeta, J.; Freed, L.E. Scalable units for building cardiac tissue. *Adv. Mater.* **2014**, *26*, 7202–7208. [CrossRef] [PubMed]
107. Fischer, K.M.; Morgan, K.Y.; Hearon, K.; Sklaviadis, D.; Tochka, Z.L.; Fenton, O.S.; Anderson, D.G.; Langer, R.; Freed, L.E. Poly (Limonene Thioether) Scaffold for Tissue Engineering. *Adv. Healthc. Mater.* **2016**, *5*, 813–821. [CrossRef] [PubMed]
108. Ryu, W.; Hammerick, K.E.; Kim, Y.B.; Kim, J.B.; Fasching, R.; Prinz, F.B. Three-dimensional biodegradable microscaffolding: Scaffold characterization and cell population at single cell resolution. *Acta Biomater.* **2011**, *7*, 3325–3335. [CrossRef] [PubMed]
109. Lima, M.J.; Pirraco, R.P.; Sousa, R.A.; Neves, N.M.; Marques, A.P.; Bhattacharya, M.; Correlo, V.M.; Reis, R.L. Bottom-up approach to construct microfabricated multi-layer scaffolds for bone tissue engineering. *Biomed. Microdevices* **2014**, *16*, 69–78. [CrossRef]
110. Kang, H.-W.; Lee, S.J.; Ko, I.K.; Kengla, C.; Yoo, J.J.; Atala, A. A 3D bioprinting system to produce human-scale tissue constructs with structural integrity. *Nat. Biotechnol.* **2016**, *34*, 312–319. [CrossRef]
111. Chen, G.; Sun, Y.; Lu, F.; Jiang, A.; Subedi, D.; Kong, P.; Wang, X.; Yu, T.; Chi, H.; Song, C.; et al. A three-dimensional (3D) printed biomimetic hierarchical scaffold with a covalent modular release system for osteogenesis. *Mater. Sci. Eng. C* **2019**, *104*, 109842. [CrossRef]
112. Moncal, K.K.; Aydin, R.S.T.; Abu-Laban, M.; Heo, D.N.; Rizk, E.; Tucker, S.M.; Lewis, G.S.; Hayes, D.; Ozbolat, I.T. Collagen-infilled 3D printed scaffolds loaded with miR-148b-transfected bone marrow stem cells improve calvarial bone regeneration in rats. *Mater. Sci. Eng. C* **2019**, *105*, 110128. [CrossRef]
113. Mekhileri, N.V.; Lim, K.S.; Brown, G.C.J.; Mutreja, I.; Schon, B.S.; Hooper, G.J.; Woodfield, T.B.F.; Lim, K. Automated 3D bioassembly of micro-tissues for biofabrication of hybrid tissue engineered constructs. *Biofabrication* **2018**, *10*, 024103. [CrossRef]
114. Gao, F.; Xu, Z.; Liang, Q.; Liu, B.; Li, H.; Wu, Y.; Zhang, Y.; Lin, Z.; Wu, M.; Ruan, C.; et al. Direct 3D Printing of High Strength Biohybrid Gradient Hydrogel Scaffolds for Efficient Repair of Osteochondral Defect. *Adv. Funct. Mater.* **2018**, *28*, 1706644. [CrossRef]
115. Deng, C.; Yang, Q.; Sun, X.; Chen, L.; Feng, C.; Chang, J.; Wu, C. Bioactive scaffolds with Li and Si ions-synergistic effects for osteochondral defects regeneration. *Appl. Mater. Today* **2018**, *10*, 203–216. [CrossRef]
116. Yang, Y.; Lei, D.; Huang, S.; Yang, Q.; Song, B.; Guo, Y.; Shen, A.; Yuan, Z.; Li, S.; Qing, F.; et al. Elastic 3D-Printed Hybrid Polymeric Scaffold Improves Cardiac Remodeling after Myocardial Infarction. *Adv. Healthc. Mater.* **2019**, *8*, e1900065. [CrossRef] [PubMed]
117. Zhang, B.; Seong, B.; Nguyen, V.; Byun, D. 3D printing of high-resolution PLA-based structures by hybrid electrohydrodynamic and fused deposition modeling techniques. *J. Micromech. Microeng.* **2016**, *26*, 25015. [CrossRef]
118. Boffito, M.; Di Meglio, F.; Mozetic, P.; Giannitelli, S.M.; Carmagnola, I.; Castaldo, C.; Nurzynska, D.; Sacco, A.M.; Miraglia, R.; Montagnani, S.; et al. Surface functionalization of polyurethane scaffolds mimicking the myocardial microenvironment to support cardiac primitive cells. *PLoS ONE* **2018**, *13*, e0199896. [CrossRef]
119. Koffler, J.; Zhu, W.; Qu, X.; Platoshyn, O.; Dulin, J.N.; Brock, J.; Graham, L.; Lu, P.; Sakamoto, J.; Marsala, M.; et al. Biomimetic 3D-printed scaffolds for spinal cord injury repair. *Nat. Med.* **2019**, *25*, 263–269. [CrossRef]
120. Joung, D.; Truong, V.; Neitzke, C.C.; Guo, S.-Z.; Walsh, P.J.; Monat, J.R.; Meng, F.; Park, S.H.; Dutton, J.R.; Parr, A.M.; et al. 3D Printed Stem-Cell Derived Neural Progenitors Generate Spinal Cord Scaffolds. *Adv. Funct. Mater.* **2018**, *28*, 1801850. [CrossRef]
121. Chen, X.; Zhao, Y.; Li, X.; Xiao, Z.; Yao, Y.; Chu, Y.; Farkas, B.; Romano, I.; Brandi, F.; Dai, J. Functional Multichannel Poly (Propylene Fumarate)-Collagen Scaffold with Collagen-Binding Neurotrophic Factor 3 Promotes Neural Regeneration After Transected Spinal Cord Injury. *Adv. Healthc. Mater.* **2018**, *7*, 1800315. [CrossRef]

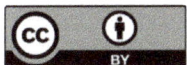

© 2019 by the authors. Licensee MDPI, Basel, Switzerland. This article is an open access article distributed under the terms and conditions of the Creative Commons Attribution (CC BY) license (http://creativecommons.org/licenses/by/4.0/).

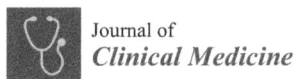

Review

Induced Pluripotent Stem Cells as Vasculature Forming Entities

Antonio Palladino [1], Isabella Mavaro [2,3], Carmela Pizzoleo [2,3], Elena De Felice [4], Carla Lucini [2], Paolo de Girolamo [2], Paolo A. Netti [3,5] and Chiara Attanasio [2,3,5,*]

[1] CESMA—Centro Servizi Metrologici e Tecnologici Avanzati, University of Naples Federico II, 80146 Naples, Italy; a.palladino1986@gmail.com
[2] Department of Veterinary Medicine and Animal Productions, University of Naples Federico II, I-80137 Naples, Italy; isabellamavaro@live.it (I.M.); carmela.pizzoleo@iit.it (C.P.); lucini@unina.it (C.L.); degirola@unina.it (P.d.G.)
[3] Interdepartmental Center for Research in Biomaterials (CRIB) University of Naples Federico II, I-80125 Naples, Italy; nettipa@unina.it
[4] School of Biosciences and Veterinary Medicine, University of Camerino, 62032 Camerino, MC, Italy; elena.defelice@unicam.it
[5] Center for Advanced Biomaterials for Healthcare, Istituto Italiano di Tecnologia, 80125 Naples, Italy
* Correspondence: chiara.attanasio@unina.it; Tel.: +39-08-1253-6099

Received: 27 September 2019; Accepted: 23 October 2019; Published: 25 October 2019

Abstract: Tissue engineering (TE) pursues the ambitious goal to heal damaged tissues. One of the most successful TE approaches relies on the use of scaffolds specifically designed and fabricated to promote tissue growth. During regeneration the guidance of biological events may be essential to sustain vasculature neoformation inside the engineered scaffold. In this context, one of the most effective strategies includes the incorporation of vasculature forming cells, namely endothelial cells (EC), into engineered constructs. However, the most common EC sources currently available, intended as primary cells, are affected by several limitations that make them inappropriate to personalized medicine. Human induced Pluripotent Stem Cells (hiPSC), since the time of their discovery, represent an unprecedented opportunity for regenerative medicine applications. Unfortunately, human induced Pluripotent Stem Cells-Endothelial Cells (hiPSC-ECs) still display significant safety issues. In this work, we reviewed the most effective protocols to induce pluripotency, to generate cells displaying the endothelial phenotype and to perform an efficient and safe cell selection. We also provide noteworthy examples of both in vitro and in vivo applications of hiPSC-ECs in order to highlight their ability to form functional blood vessels. In conclusion, we propose hiPSC-ECs as the preferred source of endothelial cells currently available in the field of personalized regenerative medicine.

Keywords: induced pluripotent stem cells; tissue engineering; angiogenesis; tissue regeneration; from bench to bedside

---

1. Introduction

The main goal of tissue engineering (TE) is to replace tissues and, more ambitiously, organs damaged by a large variety of insults. To this aim, TE relies on the combination of biocompatible scaffolds, suitable cellular sources and correct sets of signaling molecules. The integration of these factors is required for a successful and long-lasting regeneration process. The field is continuously evolving and the number of both in vitro and in vivo studies has grown exponentially over the last two decades. Despite this substantial increase still a very small fraction of bioengineered products is currently used for clinical applications.

The reason behind this discrepancy is mainly related to factors that cause graft failure, thus influencing the clinical translatability. It has been widely demonstrated that graft failure is mostly caused by the inadequate onset of a functional vasculature within the implanted scaffold. The insufficient vascularization of the neoforming tissue leads to a lack of integration of the construct with the host tissue due to insufficient metabolic supply and waste disposal [1]. In this scenario, different strategies have been developed, relying on the use of bioactive molecules [2], specific architectures [3] and topographic signals [4,5]. Concerning the support to vascular growth with bioactive factors [6] it has been proven that, in some cases, the host vasculature itself is unable to extend into the core of scaffolds exceeding 200 µm in thickness [7].

A possible approach to overcome this drawback is based on the incorporation of vasculature forming cells, namely endothelial cells (Figure 1), into the scaffold, as it has been already successfully performed in the case of bioengineered tissues [8,9] and organs [10]. ECs for scaffold vascularization could be derived from multiple sources. Doubtless, in most studies, the cells used are human umbilical vein endothelial cells (HUVECs), which hold several features that make them an attractive source of primary human ECs. They are retrieved from the umbilical cord, a tissue which is usually discarded, and is thus relatively abundant and easy to isolate [11]. In addition, a large set of assays has been set-up and widely validated. This means that a broad range of standardized tools to study angiogenic and antiangiogenic factors is available. Furthermore, a developing understanding of the cascade of molecular and cellular mechanisms of angiogenesis is crucial [12]. On the other hand, HUVECs show high heterogeneity depending on the donor, beyond the rapid loss of endothelial phenotype that they show when they are kept in culture [13]. The latter issue is extremely limiting in the view of an autologous cell transplant. Therefore, alternative EC sources are urgently needed for tissue engineering applications.

In addition, adult tissues such as skin, adipose tissue and aorta or coronary arteries could also provide ECs [14]. From the beginning of the 2000s, several studies using mouse models have indicated that microvascular endothelial cells isolated from human dermal tissue (HDMECs) are able to generate a functional vascular network anastomosed with the host vasculature [15,16]. In the following years, several works using scaffold entrapped growth factors in combination with HDMECs further confirmed the ability of these cells to form a fully functional vascular network [17]. Thus, ECs derived from adult tissues represent a good alternative to HUVECs. However, these cells suffer some major limitations that impair their translatability into the clinic. In particular, tissue procurement requires a procedure that is invasive for the patient; in addition, the in vitro proliferative potential of the isolated cells is very low. These limitations demonstrate the necessity to find an alternative source of cells suitable to be used in regenerative medicine.

Advances in vascular biology shed light on putative HUVEC substitutes: Asahara et al. showed the presence of Endothelial progenitor cells in 1997 [18], and a few years later, in 2000, Lin et al. identified these cells in peripheral blood, indicating them as Endothelial colony forming cells (ECFCs) [19]. ECFCs show a full set of endothelial cell markers. Beyond the molecular similarity to adult endothelial cells, ECFCs also hold a functional competence specific to ECs. In fact, in vitro studies demonstrate that ECFCs are capable to form more efficient vascular networks when embedded in a collagen matrix in comparison to other EC sources [20]. Within the in vivo setting, ECFCs display the ability to integrate and form perfused blood vessels when injected into immunocompromised mice [21,22]. Furthermore, Fuchs reported that these cells are able to guide the vascularization of an engineered bone tissue equivalent [23]. Although, starting from their first identification, the use of ECFCs has constantly increased [24], this EC source also implies severe restrictions. Indeed, if on one hand ECFCs are an efficient source of autologous ECs, on the other their use is strongly limited by their amount in the peripheral blood, where only 0.05–0.2 cells/Ml can be retrieved [25]. In addition, Mund et al. indicated the absence of specific markers, which is a further significant hindrance to the widespread use of these cells [26]. Overall, these concerns strongly discourage the isolation of ECFCs for tissue engineering purposes [26]. In this context, the best source of ECs is probably represented by embryonic stem cells (ESCs) derived from the Inner Cell Mass (ICM) of the blastocysts. ESCs are able to remain undifferentiated and to indefinitely proliferate in vitro, while maintaining the potential to differentiate into derivatives of all three embryonic germ layers [27]. The use of human ESCs is strongly hampered by ethical concerns since the withdrawal of ICM results in the disruption of a human embryo. In this respect, even though several in vivo studies demonstrate their validity in forming new vessels, ESCs do not represent the ideal source of endothelial cells suitable for biomedical applications [28,29]. A remarkable breakthrough in cellular biology research was the discovery of induced pluripotent stem cells (iPSC) made by Takahashi in 2006 [30]. In adult life, multipotent stem cells can differentiate and replace almost all damaged tissues. Multipotency confers the ability to differentiate into cell lines belonging to the same germ layer. Pluripotent cells show a wider differentiation range; the germ layer of origin makes them even more exploitable for TE purposes. Yamanaka et al. [30] set up a method to reprogram mouse fibroblasts into iPSC by retroviral delivery of four reprogramming factors (OSKM factors: OCT-3/4, Sox2, Klf4 and c-Myc) while Takahashi et al., in 2007, improved the reprogramming method in order to obtain iPSC from human somatic cells (hiPSCs) [31]. The advent of iPSC represented a real milestone in the field of vascular biology since 2009, when Taura et al. collected the first evidence of the possibility to generate endothelial cells starting from iPSC (iPSC-EC) [32]. IPSC-ECs could be a valuable source of cells in regenerative medicine for several reasons [33]. These cells display the same pluripotency of ESCs, based on their gene expression profile, overcoming all the limitations that hampered embryonic stem cell usage [34,35]. Further iPSCs can be easily generated from patients; therefore, they can provide an autologous source of cells for regenerative medicine applications able to bypass the issue of host immune rejection. Moreover, iPSCs, as they are derived from adult somatic cells, do not present strong ethical concerns as ESCs do.

Among the various advantages, the most promising one is to have a tissue specific EC source; in fact, iPSC-EC display the same plasticity of immature ECs [36]. Evidence collected in independent studies demonstrates that, when exposed to tissue-specific cues, iPSC-ECs generate mature ECs able to almost completely resemble the characteristics of resident ECs [37,38]. On the other hand, a well-defined selection of iPSC is required, since, once implanted, they can easily induce teratoma formation [39]. In this paper, we aimed to display the potential of iPSC-ECs in vascular biology and regenerative medicine by analyzing the behavior of these cells both in vitro and in vivo. Furthermore, we critically reviewed the advances concerning the protocols set-up to generate and select these cells in order to overcome the most important safety issues.

2. Pluripotency Induction

The first method used to confer pluripotency to a somatic cell has been the nuclear transfer into an oocyte [40]. Pluripotency can be alternatively acquired by fusing a somatic cell to an ESC [41,42]. These findings indicate that both oocytes and embryonic stem cells possess factors able to confer pluripotency. Takahashi et al. identified putative pluripotency-associate genes, and among them, selected a minimum set of four genes responsible of the pluripotent state: OCT-3/4, Sox2, Klf4 and c-Myc [31] (Figure 2). These transcription factors, re-expressed into somatic cells, promote pluripotency, also affecting self-renewal and cell cycle progression [43–45].

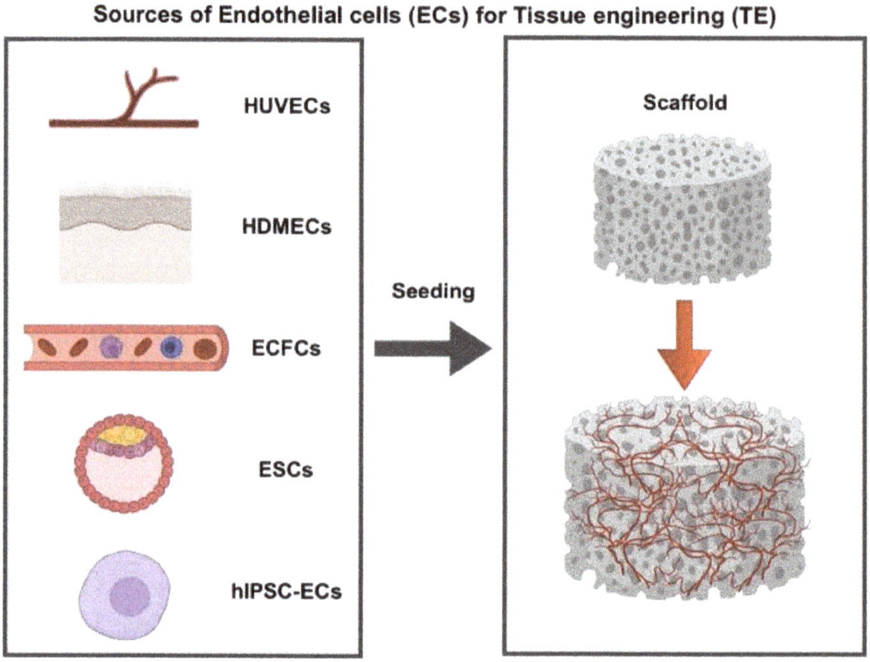

Figure 1. Sources of endothelial cells (ECs) used in scaffold-based approaches for tissue engineering (TE). HUVECs: Human Umbilical Vein Endothelial Cells, HDMECs: Human Dermal Microvascular Endothelial Cells, ECFCs: Endothelial Colony Forming Cells, ESCs: Embryonic Stem Cells, hIPSC-ECs: Endothelial Cells derived from Human Induced Pluripotent Stem Cells.

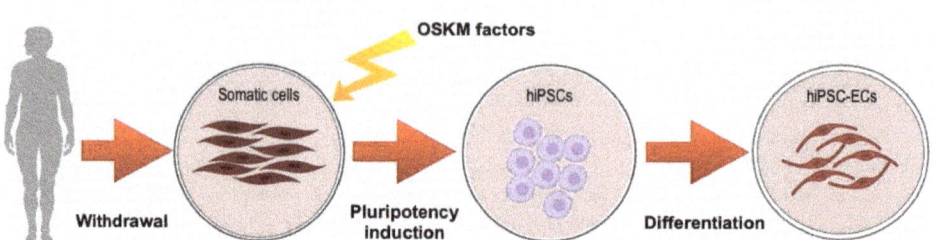

Figure 2. Schematic representation of human Induced Pluripotent Stem Cells-EndothelialCells (hiPSC-ECs) generation. Firstly, somatic cells are collected from the patient, then pluripotency is induced by the re-expression of four genes identified by Yamanaka et al. in 2006: OCT-3/4, Sox2, Klf4 and c-Myc (OSKM factors) which are normally inactive in somatic cells. Afterwards, induced Pluripotent Stem Cells (iPSCs) differentiation is induced towards mature Endothelial Cells (ECs).

To induce pluripotency the OSKM factors were introduced in somatic cells by means of viral transfection. In particular, Takahashi and Yamanaka groups, by means of Murine Leukemia Virus (MuLV) and a lentivirus delivery, were able to generate induced pluripotent cells [30]. The construct carried out by the retrovirus consisted in a single polycistronic unit under the control of an inducible promoter, while lentivirus was necessary to deliver the viral construct. This approach leads to the expression of the genetic material as soon as the inducible factor persists. Therefore, when the induction is complete, the polycistronic unit is switched off. The method described relies on the integration of the retrovirus into the genome. Genome integration is itself a limitation of this induction approach. In this context, Okita et al. demonstrated that genomic integration of reprogramming factors increases the rate of tumor formation in chimeric mice [46]. This reprogramming method is dangerous because it may cause mutations in the site of insertion and, in addition, it shows a low induction efficiency. All these aspects strongly limit the translation of the induced pluripotent cells into the clinic.

Other reprogramming approaches could represent a safer alternative for clinical applications (Figure 3). In the context of integrating methods, a non-viral approach such as the transfection of linear DNA introduced by liposomes or direct electroporation can be used [47]. An intriguing approach to overcome viral delivery was developed by using PiggyBac (PB) transposon [48]. PB delivery is based on a kind of "cut and paste" mechanism by which the PB is co-transfected together with PB trasposase, causing a transgene cut from the PB vector, as well as the integration into the genomic TTAA sites. After this, the cut and paste mechanism includes a second transfection of the PB trasposase to remove the transgene from the insertion site. PB was also shown to be able to successful reprogram human somatic cells into iPSCs [49]. Despite the low efficiency, this method can be enhanced by adding butyrate to cell culture by 15- to 51-fold [50]. This approach, by involving innocuous vectors, is undoubtedly preferred to viral ones. Although PB can be considered a step forward in the development of a safe delivery method, the integration of transgene into the host DNA can cause genomic interruptions with uncontrollable downstream consequences [51].

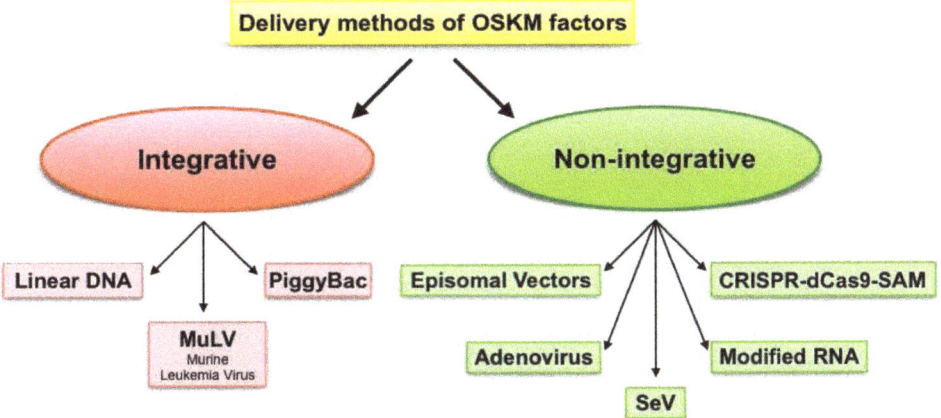

Figure 3. Diagram representing the different approaches to deliver reprogramming factors OSKM (Oct-3/4, Sox2, Klf4 and c-Myc) to somatic cells. The Integrative approaches: Linear DNA, MuLV (Murine Leukemia Virus), PiggyBac. The Non-Integrative approaches: Episomal Vectors, Adenovirus, SeV (Sendai Virus), Modified RNA and CRISPR-dCas9 Synergistic Activation Mediators (SAM).

However, non-integrative approaches are the only option suitable for the clinic in order to avoid side effects of the integrating delivery techniques.

Among others, the first choice of a non-integrative strategy is adenoviral delivery. The adenoviruses used to deliver factors are defective for replication machinery. Stadtfeld et al. indicated that such adenoviruses can reprogram somatic cells, and that no traces of integration are detected afterwards [52]. However, this approach suffers from a low infection efficiency [53]. An intriguing option in the field of non-integrative approaches was reported by Yu et al., who derived human iPS cells from fibroblasts completely free of vectors and transgene sequences by a single transfection with oriP/EBNA1 (Epstein-Barr nuclear antigen-1)-based episomal vectors [54].

Episomal vectors stem from the Epstein-Barr virus and are plasmids well suited for the introduction of reprogramming factors into human somatic cells, since they can be transfected without the need of viral packaging, and can be subsequently removed by culturing the cells without the need of drug selection [54]. The oriP/EBNA1 vectors replicate only once per cell cycle, and they can be recognized by drug selection as stable episomes in about 1% of the cells transfected [55]. The absence of drug selection causes episome loss in the ~5% of cells per cell generation due to defects in plasmid synthesis and partitioning which make the isolation of cells free of plasmids very easy [56]. Unfortunately, the efficiency of iPSC generation by episomal reprogramming remains low [57]. In 2011, Okita et al. considerably improved the efficiency (10–100 fold) of the procedure by suppressing p53 and by using non-transforming L-Myc instead of c-Myc, during the reprogramming process [58]. However, the use of the p53 short-harpin RNA (shRNA) is problematic for translational purposes, since the interference with p53 pathway may antagonize the antitumoral function of the gene [59]. In 2009, Fusaki used a Sendai virus (SeV) as a vector to generate transgene-free iPSCs in different conditions [60]. Sendai virus is a negative-strand RNA virus, differently from other RNA viruses it replicates into the cytoplasm of infected cells and does not integrate into the host genome [61]. This characteristic makes Sendai virus-based vectors the safest viral-based tool to generate iPSCs since they are considered "zero footprint" and are diluted from the infected cells with the physiological cell division [62]. To maximize reprogramming efficiency during several steps, the use of inactivated feeders, but also the use of animal-derived products, was required; however, exposure of human cells to products of animal origin increases the risks of non-human pathogen transmission and immune rejection [63]. Macarthur et al. made a step forward into a safe generation of iPSCs in 2012 [64]. These authors were able to generate, by SeV infection, transgene-free human iPSCs in feeder-free and xeno-free conditions, even though they noticed a decrease in reprogramming efficiency [64]. However, since Sendai virus vectors can reprogram with high efficiency, they were able to obtain enough colonies for further expansion.

In a recent comparison between non-integrative methods to generate iPSC, Schlaeger indicated that the SeV reprogramming approach is the most efficient and reliable, with a low workload and a complete absence of viral sequences in most lines at higher passages [65]. However, no clinical grade SeV reprogramming vectors are available. Thus, in the view of clinical applications, SeV still presents major concerns.

In this scenario the gold standard non-integrative approach is the one proposed by Warren in 2010 [66], who used modified RNA to deliver reprogramming factors. These modifications included the replacement of the 5′ cap with a synthetic one. In this protocol, RNA is complexed with cationic vehicle to facilitate cell uptake by endocytosis. Moreover, to prevent host ribonucleasic degradation and improve constructs half-life, the common cytidine and uridine bases are replaced respectively with 5 methylcitidine and pseudouridine. By these means, the authors were able to produce iPSCs [67,68]. A reprogramming method recently proposed is the one based on CRISPR-Cas9 fused to a synergistic activator mediator (SAM) [69]. This system is based on an engineered Cas9 protein (dCas9) serving as RNA-guided-DNA binding domain fused to a transcriptional activator domain (VP64). This chimeric activator complex can be directed towards promoter regions guided by specific single-guide RNAs (sgRNAs) [70]. Based on this approach Weltner et al., in 2018, generated iPSCs by targeting the promoters of OSKM factors [71].

3. Protocols to Induce Mature EC Phenotype

It is well known that for clinical use, it is mandatory to generate cells able to show a high degree of commitment. This requirement fulfills not only functional issues, but also safety ones, in order to prevent teratoma formation after implantation. Thus, a prerequisite to exploit iPSC-ECs in the clinical setting is the development of defined protocols to guide their differentiation into functional endothelial cells. The ideal induction protocol should be reproducible, easy to perform and relatively quick in order to allow yielding an adequate quantity of homogeneous cells [72]. Current induction strategies include embryonic bodies (EB) generation [73,74], differentiation on monolayers [75] and co-culture with primary cells (Figure 4).

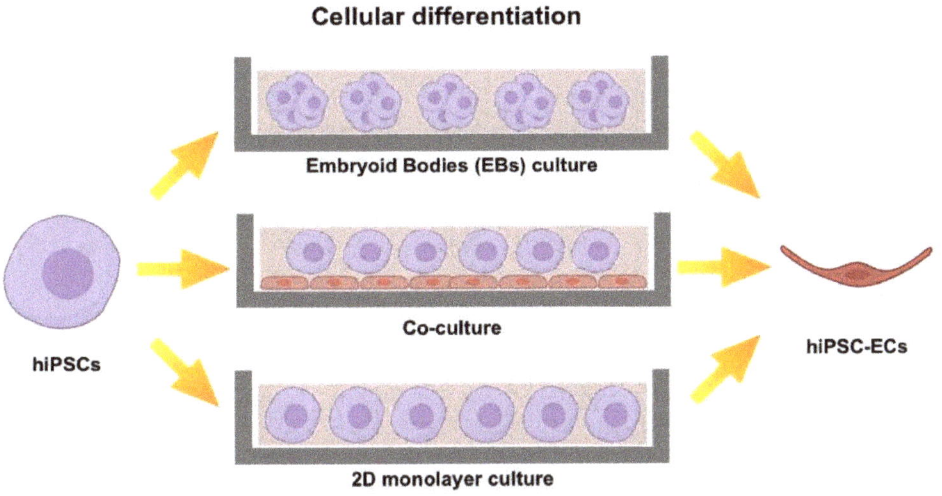

Figure 4. Illustration of the main strategies used to differentiate hiPSC into hiPSC-ECs. Embryoid Bodies (EBs): cultured in suspension hiPSCs tend to auto-aggregate in embryoid bodies. Co-culture: hiPSCs are co-cultured with cells able to guide their differentiation into the mature phenotype. Two-dimensional (2D) monolayer culture: hiPSCs are seeded on matrix-coated plates where they are induced to differentiate.

IPSCs tend to self-assemble into three-dimensional (3D) structures (EB) when grown in suspension. From EBs, cell aggregates encompassing all three germ layers develop, and afterwards, within the positive mesodermal, EB cells tend to form vascular structures [36]. This method is affected by low efficiency (1–5%) [76] and slow production rate [77]; however, differentiation can be improved by adding proper growth factors to the culture medium [78,79]. Another approach involves a co-culture with primary cell lines able to induce iPSC-EC differentiation toward mature ECs. In detail, Choi et al. directed hiPSCs into mature ECs in the presence of OP9, a mouse bone marrow stromal cell line [80]. The authors speculated that these cells regulate iPSC induction via a paracrine signaling.

Monolayer differentiation holds a significantly higher efficiency that depends on external factors, such as medium constituents, showing a final yield that is still too low in the view of clinical applications [81]. To date, the best protocols showing the highest EC yields were developed by culturing a monolayer of hiPSCs on a matrix-coated culture plate and by treating them with different molecules or growth factors in a timed fashion in order to guide the progressive differentiation of hiPSCs toward the EC lineage [82]. In this context, GSK3 inhibitors play an important role among the set of molecules necessary to induce the differentiation of pluripotent cells into mature ECs [83]. In particular, vascular progenitors derive during human development from latero-posterior mesoderm [84]. To specify mesoderm [85,86], Wnt signaling, which is activated by GSK3 inhibition, is required [87]. In view of this, several authors have exploited GSK3 inhibitors to differentiate hiPSCs into ECs. Patsch et al. [72] exposed a monolayer of hiPSC to GSK3 inhibitor CHIR-99021 (CHIR) [88] and to mesoderm inducer bone morphogenetic protein 4 (BMP4). The combination of these two molecules led to the production of mature ECs in a relatively short time (six days) with 80% efficiency.

However, mesoderm induction is only the first step of differentiation. The second part starts upon mesodermal commitment by exposing the cells to factors that further induce the mature vascular phenotype. Gu [89] set up a protocol through which, after 4 days of treatment with VEGF and bFGF, he produced mature ECs in only 8 days. These cells, when tested, were molecularly and functionally similar to native ECs.

Paik et al. [90] added VEGF, bFGF and BMP4 to an already established protocol to produce mature ECs from hiPSCs within 12 days. Although this protocol requires more time compared to other ones reported in literature, the aim of this study was different. In fact, these cells were used to draw an RNA signature at different stage of differentiation.

The last step included in the differentiation protocol is the purification of positive cells. This step is essential to fish out a homogenous subset of cells and to ensure the safety needed for the future cell implantation and engraftment.

Cell sorting is usually performed by using magnetic beads on which surface specific antibodies are adsorbed [91]. These antibodies are directed against mature endothelial markers such as CD31 or VE-cadherin (also known as CD144).

4. Behavioral Differences Between iPSC and Primary ECs During In Vitro Culture

The significant vasculogenic potential of iPSC-ECs in vitro has been highlighted in several studies. Among the most noteworthy, there is the one carried out by Clayton et al., who compared three lines of endothelial cells: iPSC, induced Endothelial Cells (iECs) and cells derived from Human Coronary Artery (HCAECs) [92]. IPSC-ECs were obtained from neonatal fibroblasts through a retroviral overexpression of Oct4, SOX2, KLF4 and c-Myc and differentiated into endothelial cells. To score cell behavior concerning tubulogenesis, the authors measured cell migration and inflammatory response. Among the three cell lines (iECs, HCAECs and iPSC-ECs), the iPSC-ECs showed the best rate of vascular network formation. This result was also confirmed by cell migration assay and inflammatory response evaluation [92]. In a different study, Adams et al. compared iPSC-ECs to HUVECs by generating a human endothelium and by measuring the functional contribution of both the cell lines [93].

The results indicated that the inflammatory response, particularly the expression of cytokines and adhesion molecules as well as the number of transmigrating leukocytes, expressed by iPSC-ECs were similar to those reported for primary cells (HUVECs).

In the same study, the authors tested the electrical resistance of the cells as an indicator of the barrier function physiologically exerted by the vascular endothelium. Interestingly, iPSC–ECs displayed a lower permeability compared to HUVECs, indicating that these cells are able to create a functional endothelial barrier. This result was also corroborated by the analysis of structural protein organization that showed a better dynamic resistance of iPSC-ECs [93] when exposed to thrombin.

5. Exploring iPSC-ECs Features in 3D Environments

In a recent study, Campisi et al. used iPSC-ECs and primary cultures to develop an innovative 3D model of the microvascular network of the Blood Brain Barrier (BBB), able to replicate the physiologic neurovascular organization of BBB [94]. Indeed, this model displayed a selective microvasculature, with a degree of permeability lower than the one showed by the conventional in vitro models and more similar to the levels measured in rat brain.

The authors based their study on a microfluidic model comparing BBB derived from culturing human iPSC-EC alone and with a co-culture of human pericytes (PCs) and astrocytes (ACs). BBB from triple culture iPSC-ECs together with PCs and ACs showed the best performance in terms of stability and permeability.

These results indicate that iPSC-ECs co-cultured BBB functionally responds to physiological stimuli and that iPSC-ECs are a reliable model to investigate blood vessel properties in vitro [94]. Kurokawa et al. in 2017 developed a variety of methods to create a functional 3D vasculature in vitro. In particular, they compared iPSC-EC derived from CDH5-mCherry iPSCs to primary ECs [95].

After the phenotypic and functional characterization of iPSC-ECs, the authors created a microfluidic device loaded with HUVECs, Endothelial Colony Forming Cell Derived-Endothelial Cells (ECFC-ECs) and fluorescent iPSC-ECs in order to test their proliferative and vasculogenic potential.

Fluorescent iPSC-ECs displayed the physiological functions of endothelial cells when tested in standard culture condition, and a predominant venous phenotype as well as a response to shear stress when cultured into a 3D microfluidic device where they formed a perfusable vascular network. Furthermore, the cell loaded device when used for drug screening purposes showed a different behavior of the newly formed vasculature according to the different molecules used to modulate angiogenesis.

Within the microfluidic device, the authors investigated the performance of a co-culture composed of human lung fibroblasts and iPSC-ECs in comparison to the one displayed when these fibroblasts were cultured with primary ECs. More in details, they featured the characteristics of the 3D vascular network, the parameters related to the vascular barrier function, and the ability of the cells to aggregate into tube-like structures [95]. Additionally, Belair et al. described a model of engineered blood vessel developed using iPSC-EC cultured into a microfluidic device and then investigated iPSC-EC barrier function in response to a wound healing stimulus [96]. They demonstrate that human iPSC-EC reproduce functional properties of primary ECs in two in vitro platforms. After a physiological and phenotypic characterization, the iPSC-ECs and primary endothelial cells (HUVECs) were used for a comparison between Matrigel culture in standard conditions and a 3D culture in capillary-like structures embedded in fibrin. Afterwards, the authors investigated the iPSC-barrier function in response to a wound healing stimulus measured by means of impedance-based platform that records the electrical resistance as a direct indicator of cell junction damage. They generated a barrier by seeding an iPSC-EC monolayer and then assessed the expression of Zona Occludent-1 after a treatment with a low concentration of thrombin to damage the tight junctions. The authors investigated the capacity of iPSC-ECs to express cell adhesion molecules (CAMs) in response to Tumor Necrosis Factor-α stimulation, thus recapitulating EC properties necessary for cell recruitment during wound healing and inflammation. Flow cytometry analysis demonstrated that TNF-α treatment induced upregulation of Intercellular Adhesio Molecule-1 and Melanoma Cell Adhesion Molecule, which are expressed by ECs to promote attachment of immune and progenitor cells to blood vessels. The results indicate that the barrier formed with iPSC-ECs responded to a wound healing stimulus in a way that resembles mature ECs.

In the same study, the iPSC-ECs were seeded in fibrin gels into a microfluidic device and co-cultured with normal human lung fibroblasts. The co-cultured cells assembled into the three dimensional pattern developed inter-connected capillary networks and remarkably formed cord-like structures containing visibly hollow lumens [96].

6. Ability of iPSC-ECs to Induce In Vivo Neovascularization

Over the last decade, the behavior of iPSC-ECs in vivo has been investigated in numerous studies. Already in 2011, Li et al. revealed the ability of hiPSC-ECs to form functional blood vessels by means of tissue-engineered constructs through a Matrigel plug assay performed in immunodeficient Severe Combined Immunodeficient (SCID) mice [97]. The authors isolated endothelial cells from undifferentiated hiPSCs cultured on Matrigel-coated plates that were placed into Petri dishes with differentiation medium. Then, two weeks after the subcutaneous injection of the plugs, they harvested them and performed histological analyses revealing the presence of microvessels containing murine blood cells into their lumen [97]. In order to decrease the risk of teratoma development after implantation, Margariti et al., in 2012, generated partially induced pluripotent stem cells (PiPSC) that clearly showed the ability to differentiate into endothelial cells thanks to specific culture media and conditions. To test vessel patency and perfusion the authors used an ischemic model in SCID mice to which they injected subcutaneously a mix of PiPSC-ECs and Matrigel [98]. Fourteen days after surgery, the authors harvested the plugs and compared PiPSC-ECs with both controls (no cells) and fibroblasts reporting a significantly higher blood flow displayed by the PiPSC group. Moreover, high capillary number, stained with CD31, and a typical vascular architecture were observed in engrafted PiPSC-Ecs compared to the control group, in which the injected fibroblasts formed a random pattern. Finally, the engraftment ability was reported to be improved by using PiPSC-ECs [98]. In another very interesting study, Rufaihah et al. evaluated hiPSC-EC heterogeneity [99]. In particular, they investigated whether these cells could be characterized for each subtype. They obtained all the three principal subtypes by using different concentrations of VEGF and highlighted that arterial and venous hiPSC-ECs cytotypes were predominant. The authors injected subcutaneously into the mid lower abdominal region of SCID mice: Matrigel and bFGF (basic Fibroblast Growth Factor), heterogeneous hiPSC-ECs in Matrigel and bFGF, arterial enriched hiPSC-ECs in Matrigel and bFGF. After 14 days, Matrigel plugs were removed and immunostained with anti-CD31 Ab. Matrigel implants including hiPSC-artECs showed the ability to establish a more extensive vascular network also confirming its human origin through the positivity to human anti-CD31 immunostaining. The same work also demonstrated the onset of a widespread capillary network, especially for the arterial lineage derived from PiPSCs [99]. To further investigate and promote the use of iPSC-ECs in tissue engineering and regeneration, Clayton et al. evaluated the behavior of these cells in comparison to iECs in a mouse hind limb ischemia model. During the surgery, they made an intramuscular injection of either 1×10^6 iPSC-ECs or 1×10^6 iECs [92]. In particular, each treatment was divided into two injections of 25 µl (for a total volume of 50 µL of solution) on each side of the adductor muscle, nearby the area where femoral vessels had been ligated and removed. Afterwards, the authors recorded perfusion data after 0, 1, 2, 4, 7, 10 and 14 days. According to Rufaihah, at day 14 post-injection, blood perfusion was notably increased in mice receiving iPSC-ECs, although in those injected with iECs the enhancement reported at all-time points also demonstrated a high pro-angiogenic response in the short-term, specifically at day 10. Moreover, this work shows that iPSC-ECs and iECs, at day 14, were integrated with the host vasculature. Finally, at the same time-point, iPSC-ECs implanted mice did not exhibit functional increasing of capillary density in the ischemic gastrocnemius muscle with respect to mice treated with iECs [92]. Another work by Tan et al. reported that iPSCs-ECs display a longer lifetime and a higher proangiogenic function when seeded on scaffolds than when administered alone [100].

The authors injected FVB/n mice subcutaneously with: control EBM media, iPSC-ECs, iPSC-EC-seeded scaffolds and scaffolds alone. Scaffolds were composed of poly-caprolactone (PCL) and gelatin. In particular, the authors used scaffolds with a PCL:gelatin ratio of 70:30 (PG73) that supported elevated levels of iPSC-ECs growth. Indeed, by injecting iPSC-ECs seeded on PG73 scaffolds the survival of these cells increased up to 3 days.

Therefore, there was an increase of the total engraftment ability of iPSC-ECs seeded on PG73 in comparison to these cells alone. Finally, it was highlighted a higher degree of blood perfusion when the cells were included into the scaffold [100]. A further significant advance about the capacity to obtain a functional microvasculature from iPSCs has been recently made by Bezenah et al., who compared iPSC-ECs to HUVECs by co-injecting subcutaneously endothelial cells (iPSC-EC or HUVEC) and human lung fibroblasts (NHLFs) included into a fibrin matrix in CB17/SCID mice [101].

iPSC-ECs showed a consistent decrease both in vessel density and number of perfused vessels compared to HUVECs. These cells were able to form patent and perfusable vessels, showing many morphological features comparable to those expressed by HUVECs. In fact, 4, 7 or 14 days after cell injection, the authors demonstrated that iPSC-ECs/NHLF fibrin implants were able to induce vascular morphogenesis, while at days 7 and 14, the constructs exhibited increased vessel diameter and perfusion, thus confirming a high degree of integration with the host vasculature. Furthermore, vessel density increased over time in the group injected with iPSC-ECs compared to the one injected with HUVECs with a peaking value at day 7 and a decrease by day 14 [101]. Furthermore, Foster et al. used ischemic NOD-SCID mice to investigate how to control early decline viability that normally happens in iPSC-ECs after implantation [102]. The authors developed an injectable, recombinant hydrogel for cell transplantation termed SHIELD (Shear-thinning Hydrogel for Injectable Encapsulation and Long-term Delivery) able to reduce cell membrane damage during injection.

They performed intramuscular injections into the gastrocnemius muscle in the following groups of animals: PBS, SHIELD 2.5, iPSC-ECs in PBS solution and iPSC-ECs in SHIELD 2.5 They have chosen SHIELD 2.5, 2.5 wt% PNIPAM, because this formulation allows cells to proliferate over 14 days.

Animals were euthanized 14 days post-treatment and the authors demonstrated that treatment with iPSC-ECs delivered within SHIELD-2.5 resulted in significantly greater arteriole density and improved formation of large microvessels, features that usually play a prominent role in neovascularization [102]. In 2019, Ye et al. focused their attention on the exosomes derived from human iPSC-ECs (hiPSC-EC-Exo) [103]. Exosomes are vesicles containing miRNAs and are able to protect them from RNAases but they also release miRNAs which are highly involved in the regulation of angiogenesis. Indeed, it has been recently demonstrated that paracrine factors obtained from iPSCs transplantation are more effective than iPSCs themselves. Therefore, Ye et al. evaluated the role of hiPSC-EC-Exo in promoting angiogenesis in a mouse model of Peripheral Artery Disease (PAD) [103]. Immediately after the ligation of mice femoral artery, the authors injected intramuscularly either PBS or exosomes (hiPSC-EC-Exo and inhibitory-miR199b-5p-Exo) by direct injection of a total volume of 20 µL into four different sites of the ischemic hind limb. Blood perfusion was monitored at day 0, 7, 14 and 21 post hiPSC-EC-Exo treatment and an additional treatment was performed twice a week thereafter. An increased blood perfusion of ischemic limbs was shown from day 14 onwards. Then, after harvesting muscle tissue, Ye et al., by showing an increased number of CD31 positive cells, demonstrated the enhancement of neovascularization with hiPSC-EC-Exo treatment respect to the vehicle (PBS) and to inhibitory- hiPSC-EC-Exo [103]. In conclusion, to contrast several ischemic pathologies, iPSC-ECs use can bypass the shortage and the low functionality of autologous stem cells in creating a vascular network able to promote tissue regeneration. In addition, iPSC-ECs can be generated in large quantities, because they do not derive from embryos and display minimal immunogenicity. Undoubtedly, the formation of teratomas is a real risk that may result from the use of these cells; however, an approach to reduce this issue can be represented by the one proposed in the work of Margariti who created "partial-iPSC-ECs" that, during differentiation, showed reduced capacity to form teratomas [98].

Finally, the approach related to the integration of scaffolds with iPSC-ECs is very promising, especially for the capacity of the scaffolds to retain cells, implying that a lower number of cells is required to improve new vessel formation in ischemic tissues.

7. Conclusions

The opportunity to produce human pluripotent cells (hiPSCs) from somatic cells is one of the most exciting breakthroughs of this scientific era. HiPSCs are useful to develop patient-specific drug screening and validation methodologies as well as to model human diseases, thus allowing to shape an individualized cell therapy. In view of this, these cells clearly represent the launching pad for an efficient personalized medicine.

First-in-Human (FIH) test have been performed in 2014 to treat age-related macular degeneration [104]. Mandai et al. transplanted an autologous iPSC-derived retinal pigment epithelium (RPE) cell sheet [104]. The study involved two patients. Patient 1 did not show any serious adverse event 25 months after implantation, meaning that the procedure did not trigger the host immune response, nor did it trigger tumor formation [104]. Patient 2 did not complete the procedure due to the detection of deletions in chromosome X patient derived iPSCs. Although tumorigenicity has never been reported in association to these deletions, the team decided to exclude patient 2 from the trial. In any case, the same cells implanted in mice did not develop teratomas. It is evident that iPSCs carry on intrinsic critical points that should be carefully analyzed. Reprogramming itself can lead to genetic and epigenetic dysregulation. As previously mentioned, some reprogramming factors are potent oncogenes [105], and it has been widely reported that the reactivation of these genes is able to cause teratoma formation. Another significant issue that should be addressed is the removal from transplanted iPSC of those cells that are not completely differentiated [106], thus implying a careful selection and an accurate screening of the cells. In this respect, in vivo teratoma assay is still an expensive and time-consuming procedure. A molecular approach based on Quantitative Reverse-Transcription Polymerase Chain Reaction (qRT-PCR) could be useful holding the sensitivity needed to detect undifferentiated cells [107]. More in detail, this assay relies on the detection of Lin28, a pluripotency-associated gene, used to recognize undifferentiated cells.

In conclusion, in this work, we reviewed the potential hold by hIPSC-ECs in providing an efficient alternative to primary cells for regenerative medicine applications. The use of IPSC-EC as vascular forming cells is encouraged by several studies involving the comparison with well-established cell lines both in vitro and in vivo. Due to their abilities, it is not difficult to imagine a widespread use of iPSC-EC as the preferential source of endothelial cells in tissue engineering. However, the main issue concerning the safety of their use in the clinic persists. In view of this, to fully exploit hiPSC-ECs potential, it is mandatory to set up reliable methods for their production in order to fulfill clinical grade requirements. The current protocols to induce pluripotency, guide the cells towards a mature phenotype and effectively select the resulting cells seem to be ready to go from bench to clinical trials [108].

Author Contributions: Conceptualization, C.A. and A.P.; methodology, C.A. and A.P.; validation, C.A., A.P. and I.M.; investigation, A.P and I.M.; resources, P.d.G.; data curation, C.L. and E.D.F.; writing—original draft preparation, A.P., I.M. and C.P.; writing—review and editing, C.A.; supervision, C.A., P.d.G. and P.A.N.; project administration, P.A.N.

Conflicts of Interest: The authors declare no conflict of interest.

References

1. Barabaschi, G.D.G.; Manoharan, V. Engineering Mineralized and Load Bearing Tissues. *Adv. Exp. Med. Biol.* **2015**, *881*, 79–94.
2. Baranski, J.D.; Chaturvedi, R.R.; Stevens, K.R.; Eyckmans, J.; Carvalho, B.; Solorzano, R.D.; Yang, M.T.; Miller, J.S.; Bhatia, S.N.; Chen, C.S. Geometric control of vascular networks to enhance engineered tissue integration and function. *Proc. Natl. Acad. Sci. USA* **2013**, *110*, 7586–7591. [CrossRef]
3. Rossi, L.; Attanasio, C.; Vilardi, E.; De Gregorio, M.; Netti, P.A. Vasculogenic potential evaluation of bottom-up, PCL scaffolds guiding early angiogenesis in tissue regeneration. *J. Mater. Sci. Mater. Med.* **2016**, *27*, 1–11. [CrossRef]
4. Natale, C.F.; Lafaurie-Janvore, J.; Ventre, M.; Babataheri, A.; Barakat, A.I. Focal adhesion clustering drives endothelial cell morphology on patterned surfaces. *J. R. Soc. Interface* **2019**, *16*, 20190263. [CrossRef]
5. Fedele, C.; De Gregorio, M.; Netti, P.A.; Cavalli, S.; Attanasio, C. Azopolymer photopatterning for directional control of angiogenesis. *Acta Biomater.* **2017**, *63*, 317–325. [CrossRef]
6. Lee, K.; Silva, E.A.; Mooney, D.J. Growth factor delivery-based tissue engineering: General approaches and a review of recent developments. *J. R. Soc. Interface* **2011**, *8*, 153–170. [CrossRef]
7. Griffith, C.K.; Miller, C.; Sainson, R.C.A.; Calvert, J.W.; Jeon, N.L.; Hughes, C.C.W.; George, S.C. Diffusion limits of an in vitro thick prevascularized tissue. *Tissue Eng.* **2005**, *11*, 257–266. [CrossRef]
8. Mazio, C.; Casale, C.; Imparato, G.; Urciuolo, F.; Attanasio, C.; De Gregorio, M.; Rescigno, F.; Netti, P.A. Pre-vascularized dermis model for fast and functional anastomosis with host vasculature. *Biomaterials* **2019**, *192*, 159–170. [CrossRef]
9. Li, X.; Cho, B.; Martin, R.; Seu, M.; Zhang, C.; Zhou, Z.; Choi, J.S.; Jiang, X.; Chen, L.; Walia, G.; et al. Nanofiber-hydrogel composite–mediated angiogenesis for soft tissue reconstruction. *Sci. Transl. Med.* **2019**, *11*, 1–12. [CrossRef]
10. Attanasio, C.; Latancia, M.T.; Otterbein, L.E.; Netti, P.A. Update on Renal Replacement Therapy: Implantable Artificial Devices and Bioengineered Organs. *Tissue Eng. Part B Rev.* **2016**, *22*, 330–340. [CrossRef]
11. Cheung, A.L. Isolation and Culture of Human Umbilical Vein Endothelial Cells (HUVEC). *Curr. Protoc. Microbiol.* **2007**, *4*, A–4B.
12. Arnaoutova, I.; George, J.; Kleinman, H.K.; Benton, G. The endothelial cell tube formation assay on basement membrane turns 20: State of the science and the art. *Angiogenesis* **2009**, *12*, 267–274. [CrossRef] [PubMed]
13. Hauser, S.; Jung, F.; Pietzsch, J. Human Endothelial Cell Models in Biomaterial Research. *Trends Biotechnol.* **2017**, *35*, 265–277. [CrossRef] [PubMed]

14. Unger, R.E.; Ghanaati, S.; Orth, C.; Sartoris, A.; Barbeck, M.; Halstenberg, S.; Motta, A.; Migliaresi, C.; Kirkpatrick, C.J. The rapid anastomosis between prevascularized networks on silk fibroin scaffolds generated in vitro with cocultures of human microvascular endothelial and osteoblast cells and the host vasculature. *Biomaterials* **2010**, *31*, 6959–6967. [CrossRef]
15. Nör, J.E.; Peters, M.C.; Christensen, J.B.; Sutorik, M.M.; Linn, S.; Khan, M.K.; Addison, C.L.; Mooney, D.J.; Polverini, P.J. Engineering and characterization of functional human microvessels in immunodeficient mice. *Lab. Investig.* **2001**, *81*, 453–463. [CrossRef]
16. Supp, D.M.; Wilson-Landy, K.; Boyce, S.T. Human dermal microvascular endothelial cells form vascular analogs in cultured skin substitutes after grafting to athymic mice. *FASEB J.* **2002**, *16*, 797–804. [CrossRef]
17. Avolio, E.; Alvino, V.V.; Ghorbel, M.T.; Campagnolo, P. Perivascular cells and tissue engineering: Current applications and untapped potential. *Pharmacol. Ther.* **2017**, *171*, 83–92. [CrossRef]
18. Asahara, T.; Murohara, T.; Sullivan, A.; Silver, M.; Van Der Zee, R.; Li, T.; Witzenbichler, B.; Schatteman, G.; Isner, J.M. Isolation of putative progenitor endothelial cells for angiogenesis. *Science* **1997**, *275*, 964–967. [CrossRef]
19. Lin, Y.; Weisdorf, D.J.; Solovey, A.; Hebbel, R.P. Origins of circulating endothelial cells and endothelial outgrowth from blood. *J. Clin. Investig.* **2000**, *105*, 71–77. [CrossRef]
20. Sieminski, A.L.; Hebbel, R.P.; Gooch, K.J. Improved Microvascular Network. *Tissue Eng.* **2005**, *11*, 1332–1345. [CrossRef]
21. Melero-Martin, J.M.; Khan, Z.A.; Picard, A.; Wu, X.; Paruchuri, S.; Bischoff, J. In vivo vasculogenic potential of human blood-derived endothelial progenitor cells. *Blood* **2007**, *109*, 4761–4768. [CrossRef]
22. Yoder, M.C.; Mead, L.E.; Prater, D.; Krier, T.R.; Mroueh, K.N.; Li, F.; Krasich, R.; Temm, C.J.; Prchal, J.T.; Ingram, D.A. Redefining endothelial progenitor cells via clonal analysis and hematopoietic stem/progenitor cell principals. *Blood* **2007**, *109*, 1801–1809. [CrossRef]
23. Fuchs, S.; Ghanaati, S.; Orth, C.; Barbeck, M.; Kolbe, M.; Hofmann, A.; Eblenkamp, M.; Gomes, M.; Reis, R.L.; Kirkpatrick, C.J. Contribution of outgrowth endothelial cells from human peripheral blood on in vivo vascularization of bone tissue engineered constructs based on starch polycaprolactone scaffolds. *Biomaterials* **2009**, *30*, 526–534. [CrossRef]
24. Wang, K.; Lin, R.Z.; Melero-Martin, J.M. Bioengineering human vascular networks: Trends and directions in endothelial and perivascular cell sources. *Cell. Mol. Life Sci.* **2019**, *76*, 421–439. [CrossRef]
25. Ingram, D.A.; Mead, L.E.; Tanaka, H.; Meade, V.; Fenoglio, A.; Mortell, K.; Pollok, K.; Ferkowicz, M.J.; Gilley, D.; Yoder, M.C. Identification of a novel hierarchy of endothelial progenitor cells using human peripheral and umbilical cord blood. *Blood* **2004**, *104*, 2752–2760. [CrossRef]
26. Mund, J.A.; Estes, M.L.; Yoder, M.C.; Ingram, D.A.; Case, J. Flow cytometric identification and functional characterization of immature and mature circulating endothelial cells. *Arterioscler. Thromb. Vasc. Biol.* **2012** *32*, 1045–1053. [CrossRef]
27. Thomson, J.A.; Kalishman, J.; Golos, T.G.; Durning, M.; Harris, C.P.; Becker, R.A.; Hearn, J.P. Isolation of a primate embryonic stem cell line. *Proc. Natl. Acad. Sci. USA* **1995**, *92*, 7844–7848. [CrossRef]
28. Wang, Z.Z.; Au, P.; Chen, T.; Shao, Y.; Daheron, L.M.; Bai, H.; Arzigian, M.; Fukumura, D.; Jain, R.K.; Scadden, D.T. Endothelial cells derived from human embryonic stem cells form durable blood vessels in vivo. *Nat. Biotechnol.* **2007**, *25*, 317–318. [CrossRef]
29. Kraehenbuehl, T.P.; Ferreira, L.S.; Hayward, A.M.; Nahrendorf, M.; van der Vlies, A.J.; Vasile, E.; Weissleder, R.; Langer, R.; Hubbell, J.A. Human embryonic stem cell-derived microvascular grafts for cardiac tissue preservation after myocardial infarction. *Biomaterials* **2011**, *32*, 1102–1109. [CrossRef]
30. Takahashi, K.; Yamanaka, S. Induction of Pluripotent Stem Cells from Mouse Embryonic and Adult Fibroblast Cultures by Defined Factors. *Cell* **2006**, *126*, 663–676. [CrossRef]
31. Takahashi, K.; Tanabe, K.; Ohnuki, M.; Narita, M.; Ichisaka, T.; Tomoda, K.; Yamanaka, S. Induction of Pluripotent Stem Cells from Adult Human Fibroblasts by Defined Factors. *Cell* **2007**, *131*, 861–872. [CrossRef] [PubMed]
32. Taura, D.; Sone, M.; Homma, K.; Oyamada, N.; Takahashi, K.; Tamura, N.; Yamanaka, S.; Nakao, K. Induction and isolation of vascular cells from human induced pluripotent stem cells—Brief report. *Arterioscler. Thromb. Vasc. Biol.* **2009**, *29*, 1100–1103. [CrossRef] [PubMed]
33. Attanasio, C.; Netti, P.A. *Bioreactors for Cell Culture Systems and Organ Bioengineering*; Elsevier Inc.: Amsterdam, The Netherlands, 2017; ISBN 9780128018361.

34. Maherali, N.; Sridharan, R.; Xie, W.; Utikal, J.; Eminli, S.; Arnold, K.; Stadtfeld, M.; Yachechko, R.; Tchieu, J.; Jaenisch, R.; et al. Directly Reprogrammed Fibroblasts Show Global Epigenetic Remodeling and Widespread Tissue Contribution. *Cell Stem Cell* **2007**, *1*, 55–70. [CrossRef] [PubMed]
35. Wernig, M.; Meissner, A.; Foreman, R.; Brambrink, T.; Ku, M.; Hochedlinger, K.; Bernstein, B.E.; Jaenisch, R. In vitro reprogramming of fibroblasts into a pluripotent ES-cell-like state. *Nature* **2007**, *448*, 318–324. [CrossRef]
36. Yoder, M.C. Differentiation of pluripotent stem cells into endothelial cells. *Curr. Opin. Hematol.* **2015**, *22*, 252–257. [CrossRef]
37. Lippmann, E.S.; Azarin, S.M.; Kay, J.E.; Nessler, R.A.; Wilson, H.K.; Al-Ahmad, A.; Palecek, S.P.; Shusta, E.V. Derivation of blood-brain barrier endothelial cells from human pluripotent stem cells. *Nat. Biotechnol.* **2012**, *30*, 783–791. [CrossRef]
38. Nolan, D.J.; Ginsberg, M.; Israely, E.; Palikuqi, B.; Poulos, M.G.; James, D.; Ding, B.S.; Schachterle, W.; Liu, Y.; Rosenwaks, Z.; et al. Molecular Signatures of Tissue-Specific Microvascular Endothelial Cell Heterogeneity in Organ Maintenance and Regeneration. *Dev. Cell* **2013**, *26*, 204–219. [CrossRef]
39. Stevens, K.R.; Murry, C.E. Human Pluripotent Stem Cell-Derived Engineered Tissues: Clinical Considerations. *Cell Stem Cell* **2018**, *22*, 294–297. [CrossRef]
40. Wilmut, I.; Schnieke, A.E.; McWhir, J.; Kind, A.J.; Campbell, K.H.S. Viable offspring derived from fetal and adult mammalian cells (Reprinted from Nature, vol 385, pg 810-3, 1997). *Cloning Stem Cells* **2007**, *9*, 3–7. [CrossRef]
41. Tada, M.; Takahama, Y.; Abe, K.; Nakatsuji, N.; Tada, T. Nuclear reprogramming of somatic cells by in vitro hybridization with ES cells. *Curr. Biol.* **2001**, *11*, 1553–1558. [CrossRef]
42. Cowan, C.A.; Atienza, J.; Melton, D.A.; Eggan, K. Developmental Biology: Nuclear reprogramming of somatic cells after fusion with human embryonic stem cells. *Science* **2005**, *309*, 1369–1373. [CrossRef] [PubMed]
43. Cole, M.D.; Nikiforov, M.A. Transcriptional activation by the Myc oncoprotein. *Curr. Top. Microbiol. Immunol.* **2006**, *302*, 33–50. [PubMed]
44. Rizzino, A. Sox2 and Oct-3/4: A versatile pair of master regulators that orchestrate the self-renewal and pluripotency of embryonic stem cells. *Wiley Interdiscip. Rev. Syst. Biol. Med.* **2009**, *1*, 228–236. [CrossRef] [PubMed]
45. Boyer, L.A.; Tong, I.L.; Cole, M.F.; Johnstone, S.E.; Levine, S.S.; Zucker, J.P.; Guenther, M.G.; Kumar, R.M.; Murray, H.L.; Jenner, R.G.; et al. Core transcriptional regulatory circuitry in human embryonic stem cells. *Cell* **2005**, *122*, 947–956. [CrossRef] [PubMed]
46. Okita, K.; Ichisaka, T.; Yamanaka, S. Generation of germline-competent induced pluripotent stem cells. *Nature* **2007**, *448*, 313–317. [CrossRef] [PubMed]
47. Gonzales, P.R.; Carroll, A.J.; Korf, B.R. Overview of clinical cytogenetics. *Curr. Protoc. Hum. Genet.* **2016**, *2016*, 8.1.1–8.1.13. [CrossRef]
48. Wilson, M.H.; Coates, C.J.; George, A.L. PiggyBac transposon-mediated gene transfer in human cells. *Mol. Ther.* **2007**, *15*, 139–145. [CrossRef]
49. Woltjen, K.; Michael, I.P.; Mohseni, P.; Desai, R.; Mileikovsky, M.; Hämäläinen, R.; Cowling, R.; Wang, W.; Liu, P.; Gertsenstein, M.; et al. PiggyBac transposition reprograms fibroblasts to induced pluripotent stem cells. *Nature* **2009**, *458*, 766–770. [CrossRef]
50. Mali, P.; Chou, B.K.; Yen, J.; Ye, Z.; Zou, J.; Dowey, S.; Brodsky, R.A.; Ohm, J.E.; Yu, W.; Baylin, S.B.; et al. Butyrate greatly enhances derivation of human induced pluripotent stem cells by promoting epigenetic remodeling and the expression of pluripotency-associated genes. *Stem Cells* **2010**, *28*, 713–720. [CrossRef]
51. Abou-Saleh, H.; Zouein, F.A.; El-Yazbi, A.; Sanoudou, D.; Raynaud, C.; Rao, C.; Pintus, G.; Dehaini, H.; Eid, A.H. The march of pluripotent stem cells in cardiovascular regenerative medicine. *Stem Cell Res. Ther.* **2018**, *9*, 1–31. [CrossRef]
52. Stadtfeld, M.; Nagaya, M.; Utikal, J.; Weir, G.; Hochedlinger, K. Induced pluripotent stem cells generated without viral integration. *Science* **2008**, *322*, 945–949. [CrossRef] [PubMed]
53. Kavyasudha, C.; Macrin, D.; ArulJothi, K.N.; Joseph, J.P.; Harishankar, M.K.; Devi, A. Clinical applications of induced pluripotent stem cells—Stato attuale. In *Advances in Experimental Medicine and Biology*; Springer: Cham, Switzerland, 2018.

54. Junying, Y.; Kejin, H.; Kim, S.O.; Shulan, T.; Stewart, R.; Slukvin, I.I.; Thomson, J.A. Human induced pluripotent stem cells free of vector and transgene sequences. *Science* **2009**, *324*, 797–801.
55. Leight, E.R.; Sugden, B. Establishment of an oriP Replicon Is Dependent upon an Infrequent, Epigenetic Event. *Mol. Cell. Biol.* **2001**, *21*, 4149–4161. [CrossRef] [PubMed]
56. Nanbo, A.; Sugden, A.; Sugden, B. The coupling of synthesis and partitioning of EBV's plasmid replicon is revealed in live cells. *EMBO J.* **2007**, *26*, 4252–4262. [CrossRef] [PubMed]
57. Brouwer, M.; Zhou, H.; Nadif Kasri, N. Choices for Induction of Pluripotency: Recent Developments in Human Induced Pluripotent Stem Cell Reprogramming Strategies. *Stem Cell Rev. Rep.* **2016**, *12*, 54–72. [CrossRef]
58. Okita, K.; Matsumura, Y.; Sato, Y.; Okada, A.; Morizane, A.; Okamoto, S.; Hong, H.; Nakagawa, M.; Tanabe, K.; Tezuka, K.I.; et al. A more efficient method to generate integration-free human iPS cells. *Nat. Methods* **2011**, *8*, 409–412. [CrossRef]
59. Chen, J. The cell-cycle arrest and apoptotic functions of p53 in tumor initiation and progression. *Cold Spring Harb. Perspect. Med.* **2016**, *6*, a026104. [CrossRef]
60. Fusaki, N.; Ban, H.; Nishiyama, A.; Saeki, K.; Hasegawa, M. Efficient induction of transgene-free human pluripotent stem cells using a vector based on Sendai virus, an RNA virus that does not integrate into the host genome. *Proc. Japan Acad. Ser. B Phys. Biol. Sci.* **2009**, *85*, 348–362. [CrossRef]
61. Li, H.-O.; Zhu, Y.-F.; Asakawa, M.; Kuma, H.; Hirata, T.; Ueda, Y.; Lee, Y.-S.; Fukumura, M.; Iida, A.; Kato, A.; et al. A Cytoplasmic RNA Vector Derived from Nontransmissible Sendai Virus with Efficient Gene Transfer and Expression. *J. Virol.* **2000**, *74*, 6564–6569. [CrossRef]
62. Trevisan, M.; Desole, G.; Costanzi, G.; Lavezzo, E.; Palù, G.; Barzon, L. Reprogramming methods do not affect gene expression profile of human induced pluripotent stem cells. *Int. J. Mol. Sci.* **2017**, *18*. [CrossRef]
63. Martin, M.J.; Muotri, A.; Gage, F.; Varki, A. Human embryonic stem cells express an immunogenic nonhuman sialic acid. *Nat. Med.* **2005**, *11*, 228–232. [CrossRef]
64. MacArthur, C.C.; Fontes, A.; Ravinder, N.; Kuninger, D.; Kaur, J.; Bailey, M.; Taliana, A.; Vemuri, M.C.; Lieu, P.T. Generation of human-induced pluripotent stem cells by a nonintegrating RNA Sendai virus vector in feeder-free or xeno-free conditions. *Stem Cells Int.* **2012**, *2012*, 564612. [CrossRef] [PubMed]
65. Schlaeger, T.M.; Daheron, L.; Brickler, T.R.; Entwisle, S.; Chan, K.; Cianci, A.; DeVine, A.; Ettenger, A.; Fitzgerald, K.; Godfrey, M.; et al. A comparison of non-integrating reprogramming methods. *Nat. Biotechnol.* **2015**, *33*, 58. [CrossRef] [PubMed]
66. Warren, L.; Manos, P.D.; Ahfeldt, T.; Loh, Y.H.; Li, H.; Lau, F.; Ebina, W.; Mandal, P.K.; Smith, Z.D.; Meissner, A.; et al. Highly efficient reprogramming to pluripotency and directed differentiation of human cells with synthetic modified mRNA. *Cell Stem Cell* **2010**, *7*, 618–630. [CrossRef] [PubMed]
67. Yakubov, E.; Rechavi, G.; Rozenblatt, S.; Givol, D. Reprogramming of human fibroblasts to pluripotent stem cells using mRNA of four transcription factors. *Biochem. Biophys. Res. Commun.* **2010**, *394*, 189–193. [CrossRef]
68. Mandal, P.K.; Rossi, D.J. Reprogramming human fibroblasts to pluripotency using modified mRNA. *Nat. Protoc.* **2013**, *8*, 568–582. [CrossRef]
69. Brodehl, A.; Ebbinghaus, H.; Deutsch, M.-A.; Gummert, J.; Gärtner, A.; Ratnavadivel, S.; Milting, H. Human Induced Pluripotent Stem-Cell-Derived Cardiomyocytes as Models for Genetic Cardiomyopathies. *Int. J. Mol. Sci.* **2019**, *20*, 4381. [CrossRef] [PubMed]
70. Konermann, S.; Brigham, M.D.; Trevino, A.E.; Joung, J.; Abudayyeh, O.O.; Barcena, C.; Hsu, P.D.; Habib, N.; Gootenberg, J.S.; Nishimas, H.; et al. Genome-scale transcriptional activation by an engineered CRISPR-Cas9 complex. *Nature* **2015**, *517*, 583–588. [CrossRef]
71. Weltner, J.; Balboa, D.; Katayama, S.; Bespalov, M.; Krjutškov, K.; Jouhilahti, E.M.; Trokovic, R.; Kere, J.; Otonkoski, T. Human pluripotent reprogramming with CRISPR activators. *Nat. Commun.* **2018**, *9*, 1–12. [CrossRef]
72. Patsch, C.; Challet-Meylan, L.; Thoma, E.C.; Urich, E.; Heckel, T.; O'Sullivan, J.F.; Grainger, S.J.; Kapp, F.G.; Sun, L.; Christensen, K.; et al. Generation of vascular endothelial and smooth muscle cells from human pluripotent stem cells. *Nat. Cell Biol.* **2015**, *17*, 994–1003. [CrossRef]
73. James, D.; Nam, H.S.; Seandel, M.; Nolan, D.; Janovitz, T.; Tomishima, M.; Studer, L.; Lee, G.; Lyden, D.; Benezra, R.; et al. Expansion and maintenance of human embryonic stem cell-derived endothelial cells by TGFB inhibition is Id1 dependent. *Nat. Biotechnol.* **2010**, *28*, 161. [CrossRef] [PubMed]

74. Levenberg, S.; Golub, J.S.; Amit, M.; Itskovitz-Eldor, J.; Langer, R. Endothelial cells derived from human embryonic stem cells. *Proc. Natl. Acad. Sci. USA* **2002**, *99*, 4391–4396. [CrossRef] [PubMed]
75. Kane, N.M.; Xiao, Q.; Baker, A.H.; Luo, Z.; Xu, Q.; Emanueli, C. Pluripotent stem cell differentiation into vascular cells: A novel technology with promises for vascular re(generation). *Pharmacol. Ther.* **2011**, *129*, 29–49. [CrossRef] [PubMed]
76. Li, Z.; Suzuki, Y.; Huang, M.; Cao, F.; Xie, X.; Connolly, A.J.; Yang, P.C.; Wu, J.C. Comparison of Reporter Gene and Iron Particle Labeling for Tracking Fate of Human Embryonic Stem Cells and Differentiated Endothelial Cells in Living Subjects. *Stem Cells* **2008**, *26*, 864–873. [CrossRef]
77. Levenberg, S.; Zoldan, J.; Basevitch, Y.; Langer, R. Endothelial potential of human embryonic stem cells. *Blood* **2007**, *110*, 806–814. [CrossRef]
78. Yu, J.; Huang, N.F.; Wilson, K.D.; Velotta, J.B.; Huang, M.; Li, Z.; Lee, A.; Robbins, R.C.; Cooke, J.P.; Wu, J.C. NAChRs mediate human embryonic stem cell-derived endothelial cells: Proliferation, apoptosis, and angiogenesis. *PLoS ONE* **2009**, *4*, e7040. [CrossRef]
79. Rufaihah, A.J.; Huang, N.F.; Jamé, S.; Lee, J.C.; Nguyen, H.N.; Byers, B.; De, A.; Okogbaa, J.; Rollins, M.; Reijo-Pera, R.; et al. Endothelial cells derived from human iPSCS increase capillary density and improve perfusion in a mouse model of peripheral arterial disease. *Arterioscler. Thromb. Vasc. Biol.* **2011**, *31*, e72–e79. [CrossRef]
80. Choi, K.-D.; Yu, J.; Smuga-Otto, K.; Salvagiotto, G.; Rehrauer, W.; Vodyanik, M.; Thomson, J.; Slukvin, I. Hematopoietic and Endothelial Differentiation of Human Induced Pluripotent Stem Cells. *Stem Cells* **2009**, *27*, 559–567. [CrossRef]
81. Orlova, V.V.; Drabsch, Y.; Freund, C.; Petrus-Reurer, S.; Van Den Hil, F.E.; Muenthaisong, S.; Ten Dijke, P.; Mummery, C.L. Functionality of endothelial cells and pericytes from human pluripotent stem cells demonstrated in cultured vascular plexus and zebrafish xenografts. *Arterioscler. Thromb. Vasc. Biol.* **2014**, *34*, 177–186. [CrossRef]
82. Lin, Y.; Gil, C.H.; Yoder, M.C. Differentiation, evaluation, and application of human induced pluripotent stem cell?derived endothelial cells. *Arterioscler. Thromb. Vasc. Biol.* **2017**, *37*, 2014–2025. [CrossRef]
83. Woll, P.S.; Morris, J.K.; Painschab, M.S.; Marcus, R.K.; Kohn, A.D.; Biechele, T.L.; Moon, R.T.; Kaufman, D.S. Wnt signaling promotes hematoendothelial cell development from human embryonic stem cells. *Blood* **2008**, *111*, 122–131. [CrossRef] [PubMed]
84. Yamashita, J.; Itoh, H.; Hirashima, M.; Ogawa, M.; Nishikawa, S.; Yurugi, T.; Naito, M.; Nakao, K.; Nishikawa, S.I. Flk1-positive cells derived from embryonic stem cells serve as vascular progenitors. *Nature* **2000**, *408*, 92–96. [CrossRef] [PubMed]
85. Dias, T.P.; Fernandes, T.G.; Diogo, M.M.; Cabral, J.M.S. Multifactorial Modeling Reveals a Dominant Role of Wnt Signaling in Lineage Commitment of Human Pluripotent Stem Cells. *Bioengineering* **2019**, *6*, 71. [CrossRef] [PubMed]
86. Chu, L.-F.; Mamott, D.; Ni, Z.; Bacher, R.; Liu, C.; Swanson, S.; Kendziorski, C.; Stewart, R.; Thomson, J.A. An In Vitro Human Segmentation Clock Model Derived from Embryonic Stem Cells. *Cell Rep.* **2019**, *28*, 2247–2255. [CrossRef] [PubMed]
87. Davidson, K.C.; Adams, A.M.; Goodson, J.M.; McDonald, C.E.; Potter, J.C.; Berndt, J.D.; Biechele, T.L.; Taylor, R.J.; Moon, R.T. Wnt/β-catenin signaling promotes differentiation, not self-renewal, of human embryonic stem cells and is repressed by Oct4. *Proc. Natl. Acad. Sci. USA* **2012**, *109*, 4485–4490. [CrossRef] [PubMed]
88. Fábián, Z.; Ramadurai, S.; Shaw, G.; Nasheuer, H.P.; Kolch, W.; Taylor, C.; Barry, F. Basic fibroblast growth factor modifies the hypoxic response of human bone marrow stromal cells by ERK-mediated enhancement of HIF-1α activity. *Stem Cell Res.* **2014**, *12*, 646–658. [CrossRef]
89. Gu, M.; Shao, N.Y.; Sa, S.; Li, D.; Termglinchan, V.; Ameen, M.; Karakikes, I.; Sosa, G.; Grubert, F.; Lee, J.; et al. Patient-Specific iPSC-Derived Endothelial Cells Uncover Pathways that Protect against Pulmonary Hypertension in BMPR2 Mutation Carriers. *Cell Stem Cell* **2017**, *20*, 490–504. [CrossRef]
90. Paik, D.T.; Tian, L.; Lee, J.; Sayed, N.; Chen, I.Y.; Rhee, S.; Rhee, J.W.; Kim, Y.; Wirka, R.C.; Buikema, J.W.; et al. Large-scale single-cell RNA-seq reveals molecular signatures of heterogeneous populations of human induced pluripotent stem cell-derived endothelial cells. *Circ. Res.* **2018**, *123*, 443–450. [CrossRef]
91. Miltenyi, S.; Müller, W.; Weichel, W.; Radbruch, A. High gradient magnetic cell separation with MACS. *Cytometry* **1990**, *11*, 231–238. [CrossRef]

92. Clayton, Z.E.; Yuen, G.S.C.; Sadeghipour, S.; Hywood, J.D.; Wong, J.W.T.; Huang, N.F.; Ng, M.K.C.; Cooke, J.P.; Patel, S. A comparison of the pro-angiogenic potential of human induced pluripotent stem cell derived endothelial cells and induced endothelial cells in a murine model of peripheral arterial disease. *Int. J. Cardiol.* **2017**, *234*, 81–89. [CrossRef]
93. Adams, W.J.; Zhang, Y.; Cloutier, J.; Kuchimanchi, P.; Newton, G.; Sehrawat, S.; Aird, W.C.; Mayadas, T.N.; Luscinskas, F.W.; García-Cardeña, G. Functional vascular endothelium derived from human induced pluripotent stem cells. *Stem Cell Rep.* **2013**, *1*, 105–113. [CrossRef] [PubMed]
94. Campisi, M.; Shin, Y.; Osaki, T.; Hajal, C.; Chiono, V.; Kamm, R.D. 3D self-organized microvascular model of the human blood-brain barrier with endothelial cells, pericytes and astrocytes. *Biomaterials* **2018**, *180*, 117–129. [CrossRef] [PubMed]
95. Kurokawa, Y.K.; Yin, R.T.; Shang, M.R.; Shirure, V.S.; Moya, M.L.; George, S.C. Human Induced Pluripotent Stem Cell-Derived Endothelial Cells for Three-Dimensional Microphysiological Systems. *Tissue Eng. Part C Methods* **2017**, *23*, 474–484. [CrossRef] [PubMed]
96. Belair, D.G.; Whisler, J.A.; Valdez, J.; Velazquez, J.; Molenda, J.A.; Vickerman, V.; Lewis, R.; Daigh, C.; Hansen, T.D.; Mann, D.A.; et al. Human Vascular Tissue Models Formed from Human Induced Pluripotent Stem Cell Derived Endothelial Cells. *Stem Cell Rev. Reports* **2015**, *11*, 511–525. [CrossRef] [PubMed]
97. Li, Z.; Hu, S.; Ghosh, Z.; Han, Z.; Wu, J.C. Functional characterization and expression profiling of human induced pluripotent stem cell- and embryonic stem cell-derived endothelial cells. *Stem Cells Dev.* **2011**, *20*, 1701–1710. [CrossRef] [PubMed]
98. Margariti, A.; Winkler, B.; Karamariti, E.; Zampetaki, A.; Tsai, T.N.; Baban, D.; Ragoussis, J.; Huang, Y.; Han, J.D.J.; Zeng, L.; et al. Direct reprogramming of fibroblasts into endothelial cells capable of angiogenesis and reendothelialization in tissue-engineered vessels. *Proc. Natl. Acad. Sci. USA* **2012**, *109*, 13793–13798. [CrossRef]
99. Rufaihah, A.J.; Huang, N.F.; Kim, J.; Herold, J.; Volz, K.S.; Park, T.S.; Lee, J.C.; Zambidis, E.T.; Reijo-Pera, R.; Cooke, J.P. Human induced pluripotent stem cell-derived endothelial cells exhibit functional heterogeneity. *Am. J. Transl. Res.* **2013**, *5*, 21–35.
100. Tan, R.P.; Chan, A.H.P.; Lennartsson, K.; Miravet, M.M.; Lee, B.S.L.; Rnjak-Kovacina, J.; Clayton, Z.E.; Cooke, J.P.; Ng, M.K.C.; Patel, S.; et al. Integration of induced pluripotent stem cell-derived endothelial cells with polycaprolactone/gelatin-based electrospun scaffolds for enhanced therapeutic angiogenesis. *Stem Cell Res. Ther.* **2018**, *9*, 1–15. [CrossRef]
101. Bezenah, J.R.; Rioja, A.Y.; Juliar, B.; Friend, N.; Putnam, A.J. Assessing the ability of human endothelial cells derived from induced-pluripotent stem cells to form functional microvasculature in vivo. *Biotechnol. Bioeng.* **2019**, *116*, 415–426. [CrossRef]
102. Foster, A.A.; Dewi, R.E.; Cai, L.; Hou, L.; Strassberg, Z.; Alcazar, C.A.; Heilshorn, S.C.; Huang, N.F. Protein-engineered hydrogels enhance the survival of induced pluripotent stem cell-derived endothelial cells for treatment of peripheral arterial disease. *Biomater. Sci.* **2018**, *6*, 614–622. [CrossRef]
103. Ye, M.; Ni, Q.; Qi, H.; Qian, X.; Chen, J.; Guo, X.; Li, M.; Zhao, Y.; Xue, G.; Deng, H.; et al. Exosomes derived from human induced pluripotent stem cells-endothelia cells promotes postnatal angiogenesis in mice bearing ischemic limbs. *Int. J. Biol. Sci.* **2019**, *15*, 158–168. [CrossRef] [PubMed]
104. Mandai, M.; Watanabe, A.; Kurimoto, Y.; Hirami, Y.; Morinaga, C.; Daimon, T.; Fujihara, M.; Akimaru, H.; Sakai, N.; Shibata, Y.; et al. Autologous induced stem-cell-derived retinal cells for macular degeneration. *N. Engl. J. Med.* **2017**, *376*, 1038–1046. [CrossRef]
105. Rossignol, J. Will Undifferentiated Induced Pluripotent Stem Cells Ever have Clinical Utility? *J. Stem Cell Res. Ther.* **2014**, *4*, 10–12. [CrossRef]
106. Ramírez, M.A.; Pericuesta, E.; Fernández-González, R.; Pintado, B.; Gutiérrez-Adán, A. Inadvertent presence of pluripotent cells in monolayers derived from differentiated embryoid bodies. *Int. J. Dev. Biol.* **2007**, *51*, 397–407. [CrossRef] [PubMed]
107. Kuroda, T.; Yasuda, S.; Kusakawa, S.; Hirata, N.; Kanda, Y.; Suzuki, K.; Takahashi, M.; Nishikawa, S.I.; Kawamata, S.; Sato, Y. Highly sensitive in vitro methods for detection of residual undifferentiated cells in retinal pigment epithelial cells derived from human iPS cells. *PLoS ONE* **2012**, *7*, e37342. [CrossRef] [PubMed]

108. Kimbrel, E.A.; Lanza, R. Current status of pluripotent stem cells: Moving the first therapies to the clinic. *Nat. Rev. Drug Discov.* **2015**, *14*, 681–692. [CrossRef]

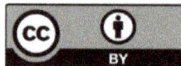

© 2019 by the authors. Licensee MDPI, Basel, Switzerland. This article is an open access article distributed under the terms and conditions of the Creative Commons Attribution (CC BY) license (http://creativecommons.org/licenses/by/4.0/).

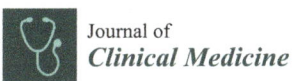 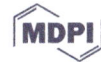

Article

3D Bioprinted Human Cortical Neural Constructs Derived from Induced Pluripotent Stem Cells

Federico Salaris [1,2], Cristina Colosi [1], Carlo Brighi [1], Alessandro Soloperto [1], Valeria de Turris [1], Maria Cristina Benedetti [2], Silvia Ghirga [1], Maria Rosito [1], Silvia Di Angelantonio [1,3,*] and Alessandro Rosa [1,2,*]

1. Center for Life Nano Science, Istituto Italiano di Tecnologia, Viale Regina Elena 291, 00161 Rome, Italy; federico.salaris@uniroma1.it (F.S.); cristinacolosi@gmail.com (C.C.); carlo.brighi@uniroma1.it (C.B.); alessandro.soloperto@iit.it (A.S.); valeria.deturris@iit.it (V.d.T.); silvia.ghirga@uniroma1.it (S.G.); maria.rosito@iit.it (M.R.)
2. Department of Biology and Biotechnology Charles Darwin, Sapienza University of Rome, P.le A. Moro 5, 00185 Rome, Italy; benedetti.1690350@studenti.uniroma1.it
3. Department of Physiology and Pharmacology, Sapienza University of Rome, P.le A. Moro 5, 00185 Rome, Italy
* Correspondence: silvia.diangelantonio@uniroma1.it (S.D.A.); alessandro.rosa@uniroma1.it (A.R.); Tel.: +39-0649910971 (S.D.A.); +39-0649255218 (A.R.)

Received: 6 September 2019; Accepted: 24 September 2019; Published: 2 October 2019

Abstract: Bioprinting techniques use bioinks made of biocompatible non-living materials and cells to build 3D constructs in a controlled manner and with micrometric resolution. 3D bioprinted structures representative of several human tissues have been recently produced using cells derived by differentiation of induced pluripotent stem cells (iPSCs). Human iPSCs can be differentiated in a wide range of neurons and glia, providing an ideal tool for modeling the human nervous system. Here we report a neural construct generated by 3D bioprinting of cortical neurons and glial precursors derived from human iPSCs. We show that the extrusion-based printing process does not impair cell viability in the short and long term. Bioprinted cells can be further differentiated within the construct and properly express neuronal and astrocytic markers. Functional analysis of 3D bioprinted cells highlights an early stage of maturation and the establishment of early network activity behaviors. This work lays the basis for generating more complex and faithful 3D models of the human nervous systems by bioprinting neural cells derived from iPSCs.

Keywords: 3D bioprinting; biofabrication; 3D cultures; iPSCs; cortical neurons; calcium imaging; patch clamp

1. Introduction

In three-dimensional (3D) bioprinting, cells and biocompatible materials are used as a biological ink (bioink) that can be organized in the 3D space with the goal of generating constructs mimicking organs and tissues. Recent advancements in biofabrication techniques have opened the possibility to apply 3D bioprinting methodologies to human pluripotent stem cells (hPSCs), including embryonic stem cells (ESCs) and induced pluripotent stem cells (iPSCs). The interest in using hPSCs as building blocks in 3D bioprinting comes from their ability to generate ideally any cell type of interest by in vitro differentiation. Laser-assisted [1] and extrusion-based [2] bioprinting are two layer-by-layer deposition methods recently applied to undifferentiated hPSCs [3–6]. Once embedded in a 3D construct, hPSCs maintain their plurilineage potential [3–5] and could be converted by directed differentiation into neural [4], cartilage [6] or cardiac cells [3]. An alternative approach relies on prior differentiation of hPSCs into cell types of interest, which are then printed to generate tissue-like 3D constructs. Examples of liver [7–9], cardiac [9,10], vascular [11], cornea [12] and spinal cord [13,14] cells, all derived from hPSCs by conventional differentiation and subsequently used for bioprinting, have been recently reported. Notably, to the best of our knowledge, cortical neurons and glial cells derived from hPSCs have never been successfully used for bioprinting. Obtaining cells that cannot be isolated from primary human tissues is one of the major purposes of hPSCs, which have been successfully used to generate a wide variety of derivatives of the nervous system, including neuron subtypes of interest for translational or basic science applications [15].

In this work we took advantage of a custom-made extrusion-based bioprinter, implemented with co-axial wet-spinning microfluidic devices [16], to build 3D constructs made of iPSC-derived cortical neurons and glial cells. Optimization of the printing process and bioink composition resulted in high survival of human neural cells. Bioprinting did not impair further differentiation of the cells within the 3D construct. We also report long term maintenance and acquisition of mature functional properties.

2. Experimental Section

2.1. Cell Culture and Differentiation

Generation and maintenance of iPSCs (WT I line) is described in Lenzi et al. (2015) [17]. In brief, cells were cultured in Nutristem-XF (Biological Industries, Cromwell, CT, USA) supplemented with 0.1% Penicillin-Streptomycin (Thermo Fisher Scientific, Waltham, MA, USA) in hESC-qualified Matrigel (CORNING, New York, NY, USA) coated plates. Medium was changed every day and cells were passaged every 4–5 days using 1 mg/mL Dispase (Gibco, Waltham, MA, USA). The cortical neurons differentiation protocol has been adapted and modified from Shi et al. (2012) [18]. iPSCs were treated with Accutase (Thermo Fisher Scientific) promoting single cell dissociation and plated in Matrigel coated dishes in Nutristem-XF supplemented with 10 µM Rock Inhibitor (Enzo Life Sciences, Farmingdale, NY, USA) and 0.1% Penicillin-Streptomycin with a seeding density of 65,000 cells per cm^2. After three days, medium was changed to N2B27 medium (DMEM-F12, Dulbecco's Modified Eagle's Medium/Nutrient Mixture F-12 Ham, Sigma Aldrich; Neurobasal Medium, Gibco; 1X N2 supplement, Thermo Fisher Scientific; 1X Glutamax, Thermo Fisher Scientific; 1X NEAA, Thermo Fisher Scientific; 1X B27, Miltenyi Biotech; 1X Penicillin-Streptomycin) supplemented with SMAD inhibitors, 10 µM SB431542 and 500 nM LDN-193189 (both from Cayman Chemical, Ann Arbor, MI, USA). This was considered day 0 (D0). Medium was changed every day. After 10 days, cells were passaged with 1 mg/mL Dispase and re-plated into poly-L-ornithine/laminin (Sigma Aldrich, St. Louis, MO, USA) coated dishes in N2B27 medium. Starting from day 10, medium was changed every other day. At day 20, cells were dissociated using Accutase and plated into poly-L-ornithine/laminin coated dishes with a seeding density of 65,000 cells per cm^2 in N2B27 medium supplemented with 10 µM Rock Inhibitor for 24 h. Medium was changed twice a week and 2 µM Cyclopamine (Merck, Kenilworth, NJ, USA) was supplemented to N2B27 medium at day 27 for 4 d. Around day 30, cells were dissociated again with Accutase and re-plated into poly-L-ornithine/laminin coated dishes with a seeding density of 65,000 cells/cm^2 in N2B27 medium supplemented with 10 µM Rock Inhibitor for 24 h. From day 40, N2B27 medium was supplemented with 20 ng/mL BDNF (Sigma Aldrich, St. Louis, MO, USA), 20 ng/mL GDNF (Peprotech, London, UK), 200 ng/mL Ascorbic Acid (Sigma Aldrich), 1 mM cyclic AMP (Sigma Aldrich, St. Louis, MO, USA) and 5 µM DAPT (Adipogen Life Sciences, San Diego, CA, USA).

2.2. Preparation of Gel-Adhesive Glass Substrates and Bioink for 3D Bioprinting

Standard microscopy glass slides were functionalized following a published protocol [19] with minor changes. Briefly, standard glass slides were exposed to air plasma (3 min, 27 W, 600 mTorr) and quickly soaked in a 5% v/v solution of 3-aminopropyl triethoxysilane (Aptes, Sigma Aldrich, St. Louis, MO, USA) in deionized water for 2 h, washed with deionized water and ethanol and then air dried. Afterwards, slides were soaked in 0.2 M solution of 4-morpholineethanesulfonic acid (MES, PH4.5,

Sigma Aldrich, St. Louis, MO, USA) containing 1% w/v alginate (Fmc Biopolymers, Philadelphia, PA, USA), EDC (0.4% w/v; Sigma Aldrich, St. Louis, MO, USA) and NHS (0.3% w/v; Sigma Aldrich, St. Louis, MO, USA) overnight at room temperature. Finally, slides were washed with water and ethanol, air dried, cut into 5 mm × 5 mm squares using a glass cutting pen, UV-sterilized and stored for later use. Alginate solution was prepared by dissolving alginate powder (GP1740, Fmc Biopolymers, Philadelphia, PA, USA) in 25 mM HEPES buffered saline (HBS). A stock solution of alginate was prepared at a concentration of 4% w/v, sterile-filtered, divided in working aliquots and stored at +4 °C for later use. The day of the bioprinting experiment, Matrigel precursor solution was thawed in ice for 2 h and mixed with alginate stock solution at a ratio of 1:1 v/v. Typically, 300 µL of Matrigel/alginate mixture was prepared for each experiment. All solutions were manipulated and kept in ice baths. Differentiating cells were collected from cell culture plates by single cell dissociation mediated by Accutase treatment. Cells were resuspended in the Matrigel/alginate mixture at a 1:1 ratio to obtain the bioink with 2% alginate as final concentration.

2.3. 3D Cell Printing and Post-Processing of Printed Samples

The bioink was loaded in a reservoir consisting of a micro-tube coil of known internal volume, as schematized in Figure 1A. The reservoir was placed in a poly(methyl methacrylate) cylindrical tank (3 cm radius, 15 cm height) covered with a thermal isolating tape (Armaflex L414, Armacell, Munster, DE) and filled with ice in order to prevent the gelation of Matrigel in the reservoir. The total dimension of the system, shown in Figure S1, was rationalized in order to limit the encumbrance of the extruder while ensuring the maintenance of a temperature around 0 °C for the total duration of the printing step (~1 h). The reservoir was connected with the internal needle of a coaxial wet-spinning extruder, while the outer needle was fed with a calcium chloride solution (225 mM $CaCl_2$ in HBS). Two independent microfluidic pumps (Cetoni, Korbussen, DE) controlled the flow of the bioink (5 µL/min) and the crosslinking solution (3.5 µL/min) through the coaxial extruder. The extruder and the ice-bath tank were mounted on a three-axis motorized system (PI-miCos, Eschbach, DE) with a computer-numerical-control (CNC) interface (Twintec, Auburn, WA, USA). Printing instructions were expressed in g-code language, and printing codes were generated using a custom MATLAB algorithm. The geometry described in these codes consisted of two alternating perpendicular layers of microfibers with theoretical diameter of 100 µm, separated by gaps of 200 µm, a layer thickness of 100 µm, deposited at a speed of 240 mm/min, forming a squared fiber mesh of 5 mm × 5 mm × 200 µm. Typically, printing time for generated codes was around 40–50 s, and each sample was constituted of 3 to 5 µL of solution depending on the desired dimension of the construct. Printed samples were collected, washed with sterile saline solution and placed in cell culture incubator for 10 min to trigger the gelation process of Matrigel. Samples were then transferred in 12-well cell culture plates, soaked with cell culture media and incubated for additional 2 h to terminate Matrigel gelation. Afterwards, samples were exposed to alginate-lyase enzyme (Sigma Aldrich, 0.2 µg/mL in cell culture media) overnight, washed with fresh media and maintained in culture for characterization and maturation.

2.4. RNA Analysis

Total RNA was extracted with the Quick RNA MiniPrep (Zymo Research, Freiburg, DE) and retrotranscribed with iScript Reverse Transcription Supermix for RT-qPCR (Bio-Rad, Hercules, CA, USA). Targets were analyzed by PCR with the enzyme MyTaq DNA Polymerase (Bioline, Boston, MA, USA). Thirty cycles of amplification were used for *PAX6* and *GAPDH*, while *FOXG1*, *TBR1*, *TBR2* and *GFAP* were amplified for 34 reaction cycles. The internal control used was the housekeeping gene *GAPDH*. Primer sequences are reported in Table S1.

2.5. Live/Dead Cell Analysis

Cell viability was assessed with the LIVE/DEAD Viability/Cytotoxicity Kit (Thermo Fisher Scientific), which uses green-fluorescent calcein AM and red-fluorescent ethidium homodimer-1 to identify live and dead cells, respectively, according to the manufacturer's instructions. Briefly, bioprinted constructs were incubated with calcein-AM and ethidium homodimer-1 at 37 °C for 30 min, followed by a PBS wash, and a further media change before acquisition. Image acquisition was performed with a custom fluorescent integrated system (Crisel Instruments, Rome, IT) based on an IX73 Olympus inverted microscope equipped with the x-light spinning disk module (Crestoptics, Rome, IT) for confocal acquisition, Lumencor Spectra X LED illumination and a CoolSNAP MYO CCD camera (Photometrics, Tucson, AZ, USA). The widefield images were acquired using Metamorph software version 7.10.2 (Molecular Device, San Jose, CA, USA) with 10×, 20× and 40× air objectives. The construct was sectioned in z with a step size of 5 µm to obtain at least five optical planes per construct to capture the whole structure. For the live/dead cells quantification, the entire image stacks were analyzed in 3D and cells were counted using Spots in Imaris 8.1.2 (Bitplane, Belfast, UK); nine fields were analyzed for each time point. Percentage of viability is reported as the mean value ± standard deviation of the mean, from three independent bioprinted constructs at DPP1 and DPP7 and one bioprinted construct at DPP50.

2.6. Immunostaining

Cells were fixed in 4% paraformaldehyde for 15 min at room temperature and washed twice with PBS. Fixed cells were then permeabilized with PBS containing 0.2% Triton X-100 for 10 min at room temperature and incubated overnight with primary antibodies at 4 °C. The primary antibodies used were anti-PAX6 (1:50, sc-81649, Santa Cruz Biotechnology, Dallas, TX, USA), anti-NCAD (1:100, ab18203, Abcam, Cambridge, UK), anti-TUJ1 (1:1000, T2200, Sigma-Aldrich), anti-MAP2 (1:2000, ab5392, Abcam), anti-NeuN (1:50, MAB377, Merck Millipore), anti-GFAP (1:500, MAB360, Merck Millipore) and anti-TBR1 (1:150, 20932-1-AP, Proteintech, Rosemont, IL, USA). The secondary antibodies used were goat anti-mouse Alexa Fluor 488 (1:250, Immunological Sciences, Rome, IT), goat anti-chicken Alexa Fluor 488 (1:500, Thermo Fisher Scientific), goat anti-rabbit Alexa Fluor 488 (1:250, Immunological Sciences), goat anti-mouse Alexa Fluor 594 (1:500, Thermo Fisher Scientific), goat anti-rabbit Alexa Fluor 594 (1:500, Thermo Fisher Scientific) and goat anti-rabbit Alexa Fluor 647 (1:500, Thermo Fisher Scientific). DAPI (Sigma-Aldrich) was used to label nuclei.

2.7. Microscopy Imaging

Confocal images of panels 1D, 2D and 2D' were acquired at the Olympus iX83 FluoView1200 laser scanning confocal microscope using an air 10× NA0.4 or a silicon oil 30× NA1.05 objective (Olympus, Shinjuku, JP) and 405, 473, 559 and 635 nm lasers. Filter setting for DAPI, Alexa Fluor 488, Alexa Fluor 594 and Alexa Fluor 647 were used when needed. Each stack consisted of individual images with a z-step of 0.5, 5 and 1 µm respectively. Stack images of 1024 × 1024 pixels were stitched together in a mosaic view with the Multi Area Viewer tool of Fluoview 4.2 image software (Olympus). The 3D rendering shown was performed using the Imaris image analysis software v.8.1.2 (Bitplane). Widefield images of panels 2C were acquired with the same system described above with a 20× air objective.

2.8. Patch Clamp Recordings

Whole-cell patch-clamp recordings were used for the functional characterization of 3D bioprinted constructs. Cells in the 3D bioprinted structures were visualized with a BX51WI microscope (OLYMPUS), in a recording chamber continuously perfused with an external solution containing 140 mM NaCl, 2.8 mM KCl, 2 mM $CaCl_2$, 2 mM $MgCl_2$, 10 mM HEPES and 10 mM D-glucose (pH 7.3 with NaOH; 290 mOsm) at room temperature. Borosilicate pipettes were filled with a solution containing 140 mM K-gluconate, 5 mM BAPTA, 2 mM $MgCl_2$, 10 mM HEPES, 2 mM Mg-ATP and 0.3 mM Na-GTP (pH 7.3 with KOH; 280 mOsm). Voltage- and current-clamp recordings were performed using Axon DigiData 1550 (MOLECULAR DEVICES). Signals were filtered at 10 KHz, digitized (25 kHz) and collected using Clampex 10 (MOLECULAR DEVICES). Whole-cell capacitance (Cm), cell membrane resistance (Rm) and resting membrane potential (RMP) were measured on-line by Clampex. Cells were clamped at −70 and 0 mV to measure spontaneous activity. An on-line P4 leak subtraction protocol was used for all recordings of voltage-activated currents. Voltage steps (50 ms duration) from −80 to +40 mV (10 mV increment; holding potential −70 mV) were applied to study voltage-activated sodium currents. Voltage-activated potassium currents were evoked by voltage steps (50 ms duration) from −80 to +40 mV (10 mV increment; holding potential −70 mV). Firing properties were investigated in current-clamp mode, injecting current pulses (1 s duration) of increasing amplitude (from 10 to 80 pA; 10 pA increment), after imposing a membrane potential of −70 mV to each cell (injection of −79 ± 20 pA). Data were analyzed off-line with Clampfit 10 and Origin 7 software.

2.9. Calcium Imaging Recordings

Fluorescence images were acquired at room temperature using a customized digital imaging microscope. Between 5–8 field of views (FOVs) per bioprinted construct were recorded in each experiment session. Excitation of calcium dye was achieved using a 1-nm-bandwidth monocromator (Cairn Optoscan, Faversham, UK) equipped with a 150 W xenon lamp. Fluorescence was visualized using the upright microscope Olympus BX51WI equipped with a 40× water immersion objective and a CoolSnap Myo camera. Image acquisition and processing were obtained using MetaFluor software (Molecular Devices). Changes in the intracellular Ca^{2+} level were monitored using the high-affinity Ca^{2+}-sensitive indicator Fluo4-AM (Invitrogen). 3D bioprinted constructs were loaded by incubating for 30 min at 37 °C in external solution containing the following: 140 mM NaCl, 2.8 mM KCl, 2 mM $CaCl_2$, 2 mM $MgCl_2$, 10 mM HEPES, 10 mM D-glucose (pH 7.3 with NaOH; 290 mOsm) plus 5 µM Fluo4-AM. A custom-made MATLAB guided user interface (GUI) was used to perform calcium imaging data analysis. Fluorescence data collected as a series of images were converted to three-dimensional MATLAB files and the neurons were manually selected from the time-averaged fluorescence recording before running the trace extraction and analysis. Tens of neurons were identified for each field scanned, depending on the confluence and seeding density of the cultures. The calcium traces were acquired with a sampling frequency of 2 Hz and signals were normalized as a function of $\Delta F/F_0 = (F - F_0)/F_0$, where F is the current fluorescence intensity at any time point and F_0 is the basal fluorescence intensity. Single calcium events were detected on the basis of a previously published method [20]. Threshold for peak amplitude, initially set to 3% of the baseline value, was manually adjustable to improve the detection depending on the recording conditions (signal-to-noise ratio, acquisition rate, etc.). Results were visualized, and eventual false or missing detections were manually corrected. Raster plots were created to visualize asynchronous (appearing as sparse vertical lines) and synchronous (appearing as a series of vertically aligned lines) results and the linear dependence between each pair of neurons was calculated by means of Pearson correlation coefficient from binary traces. Neuron firing rate, amplitude of the events and synchrony of the network (evaluated as the relative number of simultaneous events) were exported in Microsoft Excel to perform statistics. Statistical analysis was performed in GraphPad Prism 7 or OriginPro 6.0.

3. Results

3.1. 3D Bioprinting of Differentiating Human iPSC-Derived Neurons and Glia

An outline of the 3D bioprinting method developed in this work is shown in Figure 1A. We used a customized extrusion bioprinter developed in-house (Figure S1). This platform consists of a custom extrusion 3D bioprinter integrating a microfluidic printing head constituted of two independent needles arranged in a coaxial configuration. The deposition strategy is based on the use of calcium-alginate gel as templating agent for the printing of blended extracellular matrices and cells. This provides a precise control on the relative position of cells within the 3D construct, down to the micrometer scale with high reproducibility [16], independently on the 3D embedding matrix of election. Reportedly, bioink composition is crucial to ensure long-term iPSCs viability and maintenance of 3D structures [3,6]. Pilot experiments revealed that Matrigel is the best candidate for in vitro differentiation of neuronal cells in 3D, when compared with transglutaminase/gelatin or photo-crosslinked gelatin methacryloyl gels. For

3D printing experiments, different ratios of Matrigel/alginate and post-printing treatments have been tested. We obtained the best results using a solution containing 2% w/v alginate and 0.5× Matrigel (~50% dilution from stock), printed using 0.33 mM CaCl$_2$ crosslinking solution, and subsequently exposing the printed construct to alginate-lyase enzyme at a concentration of 0.2 μg/mL in cell culture media for 12 h, starting the exposure 3 h after the printing protocol.

The cellular components of the bioink, neuronal and glial precursors, were derived by differentiation of human iPSCs by a multistep protocol in conventional bidimensional (2D) culture conditions (Figure 1B). Efficient induction of a neural cortical fate was obtained by initial dual SMAD inhibition and subsequent block of Hedgehog signaling with cyclopamine [16]. Representative images of differentiating cells are shown in Figure S2. During this standard differentiation process, human iPSCs exited from pluripotency (loss of *NANOG* expression) and gradually acquired a neural character, as shown by the progressive expression of neural progenitor cells (NPCs; *PAX6, NCAD*), neuronal precursors (*TBR2, FOXG1*) and neurons (*TBR1, TUJ1, NeuN, MAP2*) markers (Figure S2A). Further characterization by immunostaining analysis showed progressive acquisition of a neuronal morphology and expression of neurofilament proteins (Figure S2B,C). The astrocyte marker *GFAP* was also expressed at late time points (Figure S2B,C).

3.2. Characterization of 3D Bioprinted Neural Constructs

Neural cells differentiated for about 4 weeks were dissociated, resuspended in the Matrigel/alginate solution and printed. We have performed several experiments in which cells were dissociated in the window of time between day 25 and day 35 of differentiation (indicated in red in the diagram of Figure 1B). During the printing process, the bioink and the crosslinking solution met at the ending tip of the coaxial extruder. Here, Ca^{2+} ions triggered the gelation of alginate in the bioink. This gel adhered to the functionalized glass substrate so that, by moving the extruder, a micrometric cell-embedding gel fiber was spun out and deposited in pre-determined positions. In this work we printed the cells as a reticulum (Figure 1C; Movies S1 and S2). Such architecture was chosen as it allows optimal perfusion of culture medium, which can reach all the cells in the construct. Moreover, areas with lower and higher cell densities are formed along the fibers and at the crossing points, respectively, providing useful information on the behavior of the cells in the 3D construct under different density conditions. Alginate removal by enzymatic treatment 3 h after the printing process promoted the acquisition of neuronal morphology by the first day post printing (Figure S3). Notably, such mild enzymatic treatment did not affect the shape of the printed construct, which was stabilized by Matrigel polymerization. Immunostaining of neurofilaments showed that the structure of the reticulum was maintained over time and that neuronal cells projected their axons and dendrites both within and across the fibers (Figure 1D). Printed cells were then analyzed in terms of viability at different days post printing (DPP). Results shown in Figure 1E indicated that the great majority of the cells were viable at DPP1 (78 ± 3.8% live cells; average ± standard deviation; three constructs, nine fields each) and DPP7 (71 ± 3.5% live cells; average ± standard deviation; three constructs, nine fields each), suggesting that both physical parameters and bioink formulation did not harm neural cells during and immediately after the printing process. Moreover, viability was consistently maintained over time as assessed by live/dead staining up to DPP50 (68 ± 8% live cells; average ± standard deviation; one construct, nine fields). We noticed that the reticulum structure was to some extent maintained at this late time point.

We then assessed possible alterations in neuronal cell fate acquisition caused by either the printing process and/or subsequent cell differentiation within the 3D bioprinted construct. Bioprinted cells were compared with cells maintained in conventional 2D conditions for the same time and cells that were encapsulated in bioink droplets not subjected to printing process (3D bulk). Neuronal morphology was maintained intact in both 3D bulk and 3D bioprinted cells at DPP7 and DPP40 (Figure 2A). In the same samples, marker analysis by RT-PCR showed proper expression of: *PAX6, FOXG1* and *TBR2* as neuronal progenitor markers; *TBR1*, which reveals the presence of mature cortical neurons; and *GFAP*, a common astrocyte marker (Figure 2B and Figure S4). These results were further supported by immunostaining analyses of TBR1 and MAP2 at DPP7 (Figure 2C). Bioprinted neural cells were maintained in neuronal differentiation medium up to DPP70. At this late time point the reticulum structure was, to some extent, maintained and cells properly expressed neuronal and astroglial markers (Figure 2D,D').

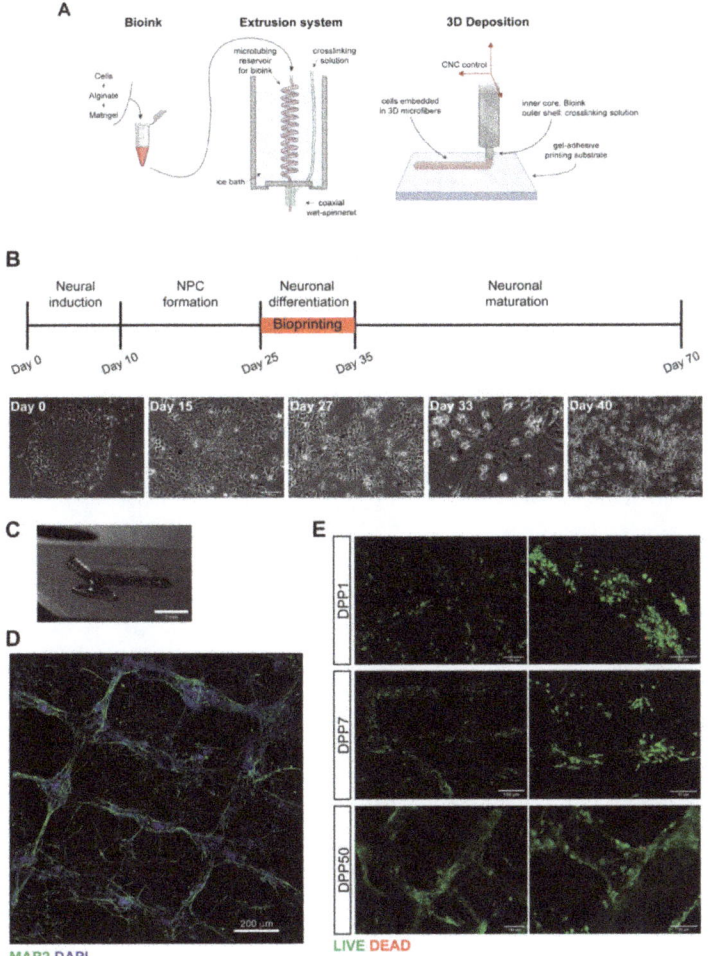

Figure 1. 3D bioprinting method and analysis of viability post printing. (**A**) Schematic representation of the outline of the bioprinting method. (**B**) Outline of the human induced pluripotent stem cell (iPSC) neural differentiation protocol in conventional 2D culture and representative images of differentiating cells in these conditions at the indicated time points. The window of time in which cells have been dissociated for bioprinting experiments in this work is indicated in red. (**C**) Image of the printed 3D construct. Scalebar: 2 mm. (**D**) Mosaic reconstruction of confocal images of bioprinted neural cells at DPP7, stained with a MAP2 antibody (green) and DAPI (blue). Scalebar: 200 μm. (**E**) Live (green) and dead (red) cell staining in the bioprinted construct at the indicated days post printing (DPP). Scalebar: 150 μm (left panels); 50 μm (right panels).

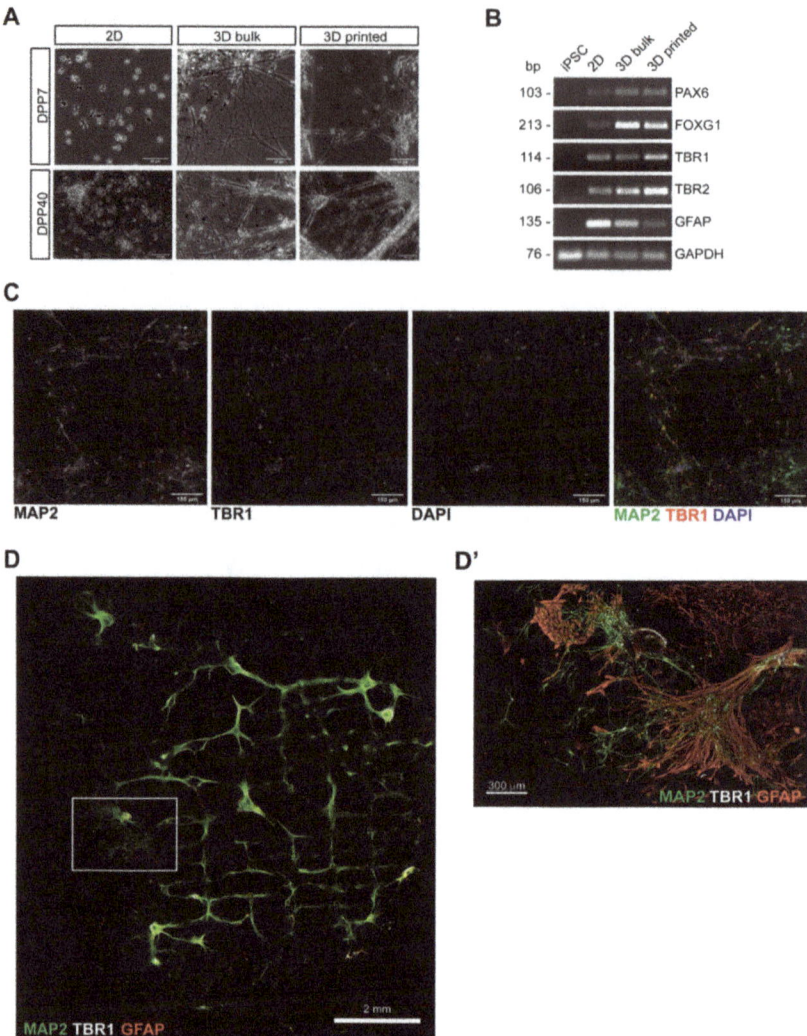

Figure 2. Analysis of neural marker expression in the 3D bioprinted construct. (**A**) Phase contrast images of cells within the 3D bioprinted construct ("3D printed" panels), at the indicated days post printing, and cells in conventional monolayer conditions ("2D" panels) or resuspended in the bioink ("3D bulk" panels) and maintained for the same time of differentiation. (**B**) RT-PCR analysis of neuronal progenitor markers (*PAX6*, *FOXG1*, *TBR2*), a cortical neuron marker (*TBR1*) and an astrocyte marker (*GFAP*). GAPDH was used as a housekeeping control. (**C**) Immunostaining analysis of bioprinted cells at DPP7. MAP2 (green), TBR1 (red) and DAPI (blue) signals are shown. Scalebar: 150 μm. (**D**) Mosaic reconstruction of confocal images of bioprinted neural cells at DPP70, showing the entire sample, stained with MAP2 (green), TBR1 (white) and GFAP (red) antibodies. Scalebar: 2 mm. (**D′**) Mosaic reconstruction of confocal images of the region inside the white box in panel D, acquired at higher resolution. Scalebar: 300 μm.

Collectively, these results demonstrate that iPSC-derived cortical neuronal cells can be bioprinted and further cultured in 3D constructs without causing major survival and differentiation issues.

3.3. Functional Analysis

Single-cell patch-clamp and time-lapse calcium imaging recordings were then performed to assess the degree of maturation achieved by the 3D bioprinted construct. Even though the 3D construct was 300 μm thick, the selected bioink displayed sufficient transparency to visible light and softness to patch pipette insertion (Figure 3A). Using patch clamp recordings, we investigated the expression of the passive and active membrane properties on 3D bioprinted cortical neurons at day 7 after printing. As expected at this experimental point, resting membrane potential (-17.7 ± 1.5 mV; $n = 36$), cell capacitance (14.8 ± 0.89 pF; $n = 45$) and membrane resistance values (1.97 ± 0.23 MΩ; $n = 44$) were typical of neuronal progenitors [21] and similar to those observed in parallel 2D cultures (Figure S5), indicating that the printing process did not impair neuronal viability. We then characterized the ability of cortical neurons to generate action potentials. Neurons in the 3D construct displayed large inward voltage-dependent Na^+ currents (-777.31 ± 73.16 pA at 0 mV; $n = 43$; Figure 3B,C and Figure S5) which activated near -40 mV and peaked at 0 mV, and voltage-dependent K^+ currents (865.75 ± 63.28 pA at $+40$ mV; $n = 43$; Figure 3B,D and Figure S5). Current pulses were able to induce action potentials in almost all tested cells. The mean threshold for first action potential generation was -32.85 ± 2.86 mV ($n = 15$; 20 pA of current injection). However, the minimum current required to elicit firing in some of the tested cells was 10 pA (Figure 3E,F). As expected, no synaptic activity was recorded at 7 days post printing (data not shown).

Given the optical transparency of the 3D bioprinted constructs at DPP7, fluorescence time-lapse recordings lasting 5 min each were performed, thus preserving a good signal-to-noise ratio (Figure 3G). Fluorescence time-lapse analysis of spontaneous calcium oscillation in Fluo4-AM loaded 3D neuronal network indicated the presence of individual calcium activity (mean firing frequency = 0.015 ± 0.001 Hz; FOVs = 38; mean firing amplitude = 0.083 ± 0.002 A.U.) with little synchronized firing (syncro index = 0.223 ± 0.020; FOVs = 38). The small degree of synchronous activity was confirmed by the low correlation coefficient value between each pair of neurons in the field as displayed by the heatmap in Figure 3G (average correlation coefficient value = 0.006; max correlation coefficient value = 0.046 ± 0.005; FOV = 38), thus indicating the establishment of early and immature neuronal networks.

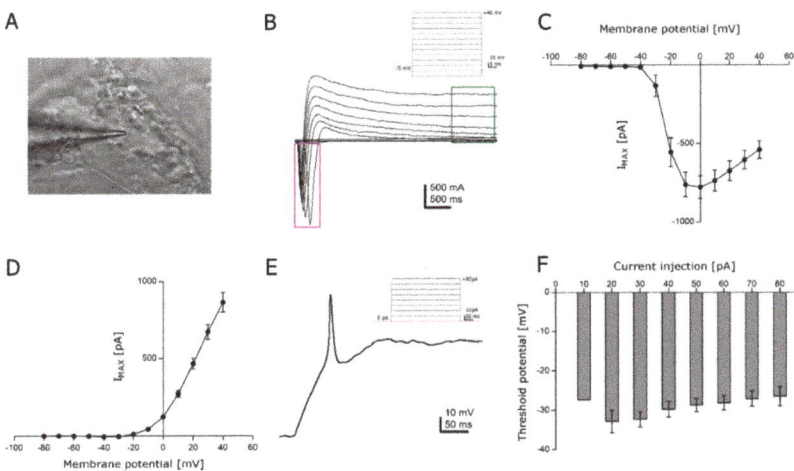

Figure 3. Cont.

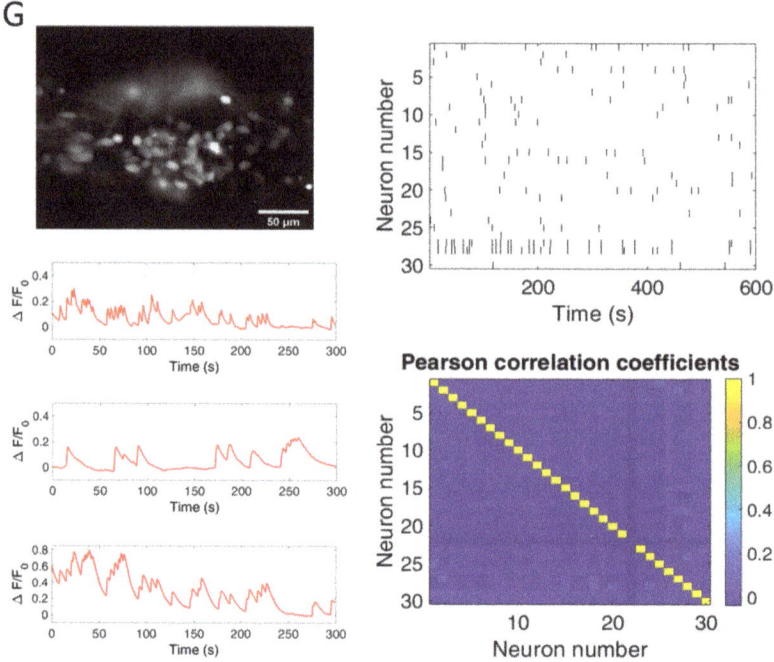

Figure 3. Functional analysis of the 3D bioprinted construct. (**A**) Single-cell patch-clamp recording of an iPSC-derived neuronal cell encapsulated in the 3D bioprinted construct at DPP7. (**B**) Representative scheme of the recording protocol is shown. The inward sodium currents are highlighted in the purple box and the permanent outward potassium currents are highlighted in the green box. (**C**) Average trace of the large inward voltage-dependent Na$^+$ currents. (**D**) Average trace of the outward voltage-dependent K$^+$ currents. (**E**) A single action potential evoked in current clamp recording is shown. The minimum current required to elicit firing was 10 pA, however more of the 50% of tested cells (n = 9 out of 15) responded to 20 pA (**F**). (**G**) Calcium traces as a function of $\Delta F/F_0$ of cortical neurons isolated within the 3D network shown on the left at DPP7. On the right, a representation of the firing pattern and a relative heatmap of the Pearson correlation coefficients within the cells of the same network are shown.

4. Discussion

In this paper we describe a method to obtain 3D cortical constructs in which human cortical neurons and glial cells survive in the long term, holding their cellular characteristics and functional properties. Moving from conventional neuronal cultures, in 2D, to more realistic 3D models is considered a crucial advancement in neurobiology [22]. The recent discovery that differentiating hPSCs have the ability to self-assemble into brain organoids, which recapitulate to some extent the brain structure in 3D [23], has given a twist in the way neurodevelopmental and neurodegenerative diseases are modeled and approached [24]. 3D bioprinting could provide important advantages, in terms of automation and reproducibility, over self-assembled brain organoids [25]. Recent reports showed that undifferentiated human iPSCs and ESCs can be bioprinted and then converted, post-printing, into cell types of interest [4]. This approach will not likely generate useful artificial tissues, as it does not allow control on the position of individual cell types, generated during differentiation, within the construct. The complementary approach, used in this work and in [13,14], and consisting in bioprinting specific cell types obtained by pre-printing hPSCs differentiation, would be more advantageous, allowing better control of the resulting bioprinted construct.

Bioprinting neurons and glial cells represents a challenge. Neurons are vulnerable cells in vitro and environmental stress due to the printing process may affect neural cell viability and influence further differentiation and maturation. Our work is the result of an extensive effort in the optimization of the bioprinting process and bioink composition, with the goal to define proper conditions for generating human artificial 3D cortical neural tissues from hiPSCs. The generation of a bioprinted constructs, by combining hiPSC-derived spinal neuronal progenitor cells and mouse oligodendrocyte progenitor cells, has been recently reported by Joung et al. [13]. Moreover, spinal cord neural progenitors from hiPSCs have been successfully bioprinted by using a commercial lab-on-a-printer platform [14,26]. Here, for the first time, we describe the generation of constructs made of cortical neurons and glial cells by a custom extrusion bioprinter. In this work, we have obtained the best results with a bioink made of Matrigel and alginate. The selection of the bioink most suitable for the viability of the 3D construct remains a controversial issue. Indeed, both fibrin-based and Matrigel-based bioinks have been previously used for bioprinting hiPSC-derived spinal neural cells [13,14]. Matrigel, which is a matrix preparation extracted from the Engelbreth-Holm-Swarm mouse sarcoma, had been successfully used as a bioink component for the generation of hiPSC-derived cardiac and spinal cord bioprinted constructs [3,13]. However, its composition is rather undefined. This could represent an important limitation for basic and translational applications of bioprinted models, including those of the nervous system. Future studies are necessary for identifying more physiological, standardized and defined alternatives to Matrigel. To this direction, promising results have been recently obtained with decellularized extracellular matrix, used for the bioprinting of liver and hearth constructs [9].

Due to the vulnerability of neurons, their viability post printing is a major concern. In this regard, our results (70–80% of live cells) are comparable to previous works using hiPSC-derived neural progenitors [13,14] or an immortalized human neural stem cell line [27]. Moreover, our method allows long term survival of human neurons, up to 70 days post printing. To the best of our knowledge, this is the longest time of maintenance of hiPSC-derived neurons in 3D bioprinted constructs (14 days in [13], 30 days in [14], 40 days in [4] and 41 days in [26]). Further, this work suggests a possible approach to overcome some practical challenges associated with the bioprinting of 3D in vitro models containing cells of limited availability. In order to be able to produce constructs with arbitrary, high cellular density, without affecting the number of samples obtainable from each experiment, we adjusted the amount of bioink necessary for each construct to a few microliters (3 to 5 μL per sample). The dimension, visibility and weight of these samples are very limited, and their handling and maintenance in floating culture condition can be very challenging. To overcome this, we used functionalized micro-slides as receiving substrate during the printing step that guaranteed a prolonged adhesion of the samples to a flat, clear glass surface.

We here report that cortical 3D bioprinted constructs, as well as parallel 2D cultures, display functional properties typical of immature neuronal networks. Indeed, calcium imaging experiments showed sustained calcium spontaneous activity already at DPP7, in line with that reported for 3D bioprinted iPSCs [4,27], and spinal neural progenitors [13], thus suggesting that the printing process does not prevent the development of a functional network. However, passive and active neuronal properties, analyzed at single cell level by means of patch clamp recordings, were typical of immature neurons, and the absence of spontaneous synaptic activity indicated that network activity was mainly not dependent on action potential firing. This result is in line with data on 2D culture at the same time point.

This study opens the possibility for generating more complex human neural 3D constructs, for instance by printing mixed populations with precise ratios of neuronal and glial cells and/or printing iPSCs carrying pathogenic mutations associated to neurological diseases. Notably, the bioprinting approach used herein can be further implemented with more sophisticated microfluidic platforms that might allow the deposition of multiple materials and/or multicellular bioink within a single scaffold, by simultaneously extruding different bioinks or by rapidly switching between one bioink and another, as previously described [16], with the aim of controlling the localization of individual cell types in predetermined positions of the 3D construct. Different specific neuronal subtypes, which can be obtained by iPSC differentiation, might be used as the cellular components of 3D constructs for disease models and drug screening. In the case of complex diseases with clear non-cell autonomous contribution, neural and non-neural cells could be printed together. In the long term, further development of this technology could provide bioprinted cortical neural constructs that can be exploited as customized, standardized and scalable pre-clinical models for drug safety and toxicity studies.

5. Conclusions

In this paper we report the generation of a novel type of bioprinted 3D neuronal construct, based on cortical neurons and glial cells derived from hiPSCs. The cortical construct develops molecular, morphological and functional properties of neuronal networks and can be used for future disease modeling studies as well as for drug screening.

Supplementary Materials: The following are available online at http://www.mdpi.com/2077-0383/8/10/1595/s1, Figure S1: The custom bioprinter used in this work, Figure S2: Neural differentiation of human iPSCs, Figure S3: Effects of the treatment with Alginate-lyase on the bioprinted specimen, Figure S4: Quantitative RT-PCR analysis, Figure S5: Assessment of the 2D conventional cultures functionality, Table S1: Primers used in this study, Video S1 and S2: 3D bioprinting.

Author Contributions: Conceptualization, F.S., C.C., S.D.A. and A.R.; Formal analysis, A.S., V.d.T., S.G. and M.R.; Investigation, F.S., C.C., C.B., A.S., V.d.T and M.C.B.; Methodology, F.S., C.C. and C.B.; Project administration, S.D.A. and A.R.; Supervision, S.D.A. and A.R.; Writing – original draft, S.D.A. and A.R.

Funding: This research received no external funding.

Acknowledgments: The authors wish to thank the Imaging Facility at Center for Life Nano Science (CLNS), Istituto Italiano di Tecnologia, for support and technical advice. We are grateful to Giorgia Belloni for technical help in the qRT-PCR experiments of Figure S2 and Chiara Scognamiglio for advice on 3D bioprinting. We thank Giancarlo Ruocco and the other colleagues of CLNS for helpful discussion.

Conflicts of Interest: The authors declare no conflict of interest.

References

1. Koch, L.; Gruene, M.; Unger, C.; Chichkov, B. Laser assisted cell printing. *Curr. Pharm. Biotechnol.* **2013**, *14*, 91–97. [PubMed]
2. Jiang, T.; Munguia-Lopez, J.G.; Flores-Torres, S.; Kort-Mascort, J.; Kinsella, J.M. Extrusion bioprinting of soft materials: An emerging technique for biological model fabrication. *Appl. Phys. Rev.* **2019**, *6*, 011310. [CrossRef]
3. Koch, L.; Deiwick, A.; Franke, A.; Schwanke, K.; Haverich, A.; Zweigerdt, R.; Chichkov, B. Laser bioprinting of human induced pluripotent stem cells-the effect of printing and biomaterials on cell survival, pluripotency, and differentiation. *Biofabrication* **2018**, *10*, 035005. [CrossRef] [PubMed]
4. Gu, Q.; Tomaskovic-Crook, E.; Wallace, G.G.; Crook, J.M. 3D Bioprinting Human Induced Pluripotent Stem Cell Constructs for In Situ Cell Proliferation and Successive Multilineage Differentiation. *Adv. Healthc. Mater.* **2017**, *6*. [CrossRef]
5. Reid, J.A.; Mollica, P.A.; Johnson, G.D.; Ogle, R.C.; Bruno, R.D.; Sachs, P.C. Accessible bioprinting: Adaptation of a low-cost 3D-printer for precise cell placement and stem cell differentiation. *Biofabrication* **2016**, *8*, 025017. [CrossRef] [PubMed]
6. Nguyen, D.; Hägg, D.A.; Forsman, A.; Ekholm, J.; Nimkingratana, P.; Brantsing, C.; Kalogeropoulos, T.; Zaunz, S.; Concaro, S.; Brittberg, M.; et al. Cartilage Tissue Engineering by the 3D Bioprinting of iPS Cells in a Nanocellulose/Alginate Bioink. *Sci Rep.* **2017**, *7*, 658. [CrossRef]
7. Faulkner-Jones, A.; Fyfe, C.; Cornelissen, D.-J.; Gardner, J.; King, J.; Courtney, A.; Shu, W. Bioprinting of human pluripotent stem cells and their directed differentiation into hepatocyte-like cells for the generation of mini-livers in 3D. *Biofabrication* **2015**, *7*, 044102. [CrossRef]
8. Ma, X.; Qu, X.; Zhu, W.; Li, Y.-S.; Yuan, S.; Zhang, H.; Liu, J.; Wang, P.; Lai, C.S.E.; Zanella, F.; et al. Deterministically patterned biomimetic human iPSC-derived hepatic model via rapid 3D bioprinting. *Proc. Natl. Acad. Sci. USA* **2016**, *113*, 2206–2211. [CrossRef]

9. Yu, C.; Ma, X.; Zhu, W.; Wang, P.; Miller, K.L.; Stupin, J.; Koroleva-Maharajh, A.; Hairabedian, A.; Chen, S. Scanningless and continuous 3D bioprinting of human tissues with decellularized extracellular matrix. *Biomaterials* **2019**, *194*, 1–13. [CrossRef]
10. Ong, C.S.; Fukunishi, T.; Zhang, H.; Huang, C.Y.; Nashed, A.; Blazeski, A.; Di Silvestre, D.; Vricella, L.; Conte, J.; Tung, L.; et al. Biomaterial-Free Three-Dimensional Bioprinting of Cardiac Tissue using Human Induced Pluripotent Stem Cell Derived Cardiomyocytes. *Sci. Rep.* **2017**, *7*, 4566. [CrossRef]
11. Moldovan, L.; Barnard, A.; Gil, C.-H.; Lin, Y.; Grant, M.B.; Yoder, M.C.; Prasain, N.; Moldovan, N.I. iPSC-Derived Vascular Cell Spheroids as Building Blocks for Scaffold-Free Biofabrication. *Biotechnol. J.* **2017**, *12*. [CrossRef] [PubMed]
12. Sorkio, A.; Koch, L.; Koivusalo, L.; Deiwick, A.; Miettinen, S.; Chichkov, B.; Skottman, H. Human stem cell based corneal tissue mimicking structures using laser-assisted 3D bioprinting and functional bioinks. *Biomaterials* **2018**, *171*, 57–71. [CrossRef] [PubMed]
13. Joung, D.; Truong, V.; Neitzke, C.C.; Guo, S.-Z.; Walsh, P.J.; Monat, J.R.; Meng, F.; Park, S.H.; Dutton, J.R.; Parr, A.M.; et al. 3D Printed Stem-Cell Derived Neural Progenitors Generate Spinal Cord Scaffolds. *Adv. Funct. Mater.* **2018**, *28*, 1801850. [CrossRef]
14. De la Vega, L.; Rosas Gómez, A.D.; Abelseth, E.; Abelseth, L.; Allisson da Silva, V.; Willerth, S. 3D Bioprinting Human Induced Pluripotent Stem Cell-Derived Neural Tissues Using a Novel Lab-on-a-Printer Technology. *Appl. Sci.* **2018**, *8*, 2414. [CrossRef]
15. Bellin, M.; Marchetto, M.C.; Gage, F.H.; Mummery, C.L. Induced pluripotent stem cells: The new patient? *Nat. Rev. Mol. Cell Biol.* **2012**, *13*, 713–726. [CrossRef]
16. Colosi, C.; Costantini, M.; Barbetta, A.; Dentini, M. Microfluidic Bioprinting of Heterogeneous 3D Tissue Constructs. *Methods Mol. Biol.* **2017**, *1612*, 369–380.
17. Lenzi, J.; De Santis, R.; de Turris, V.; Morlando, M.; Laneve, P.; Calvo, A.; Caliendo, V.; Chiò, A.; Rosa, A.; Bozzoni, I. ALS mutant FUS proteins are recruited into stress granules in induced Pluripotent Stem Cells (iPSCs) derived motoneurons. *Dis. Model. Mech.* **2015**, *8*, 755–766. [CrossRef]
18. Shi, Y.; Kirwan, P.; Livesey, F.J. Directed differentiation of human pluripotent stem cells to cerebral cortex neurons and neural networks. *Nat. Protoc.* **2012**, *7*, 1836–1846. [CrossRef]
19. Yuk, H.; Zhang, T.; Lin, S.; Parada, G.A.; Zhao, X. Tough bonding of hydrogels to diverse non-porous surfaces. *Nat. Mater.* **2016**, *15*, 190–196. [CrossRef]
20. Palazzolo, G.; Moroni, M.; Soloperto, A.; Aletti, G.; Naldi, G.; Vassalli, M.; Nieus, T.; Difato, F. Fast wide-volume functional imaging of engineered in vitro brain tissues. *Sci Rep.* **2017**, *7*, 8499. [CrossRef]
21. Vitali, I.; Fièvre, S.; Telley, L.; Oberst, P.; Bariselli, S.; Frangeul, L.; Baumann, N.; McMahon, J.J.; Klingler, E.; Bocchi, R.; et al. Progenitor Hyperpolarization Regulates the Sequential Generation of Neuronal Subtypes in the Developing Neocortex. *Cell* **2018**, *174*, 1264–1276. [CrossRef] [PubMed]
22. Centeno, E.G.Z.; Cimarosti, H.; Bithell, A. 2D versus 3D human induced pluripotent stem cell-derived cultures for neurodegenerative disease modelling. *Mol. Neurodegener.* **2018**, *13*, 27. [CrossRef] [PubMed]
23. Lancaster, M.A.; Renner, M.; Martin, C.-A.; Wenzel, D.; Bicknell, L.S.; Hurles, M.E.; Homfray, T.; Penninger, J.M.; Jackson, A.P.; Knoblich, J.A. Cerebral organoids model human brain development and microcephaly. *Nature* **2013**, *501*, 373–379. [CrossRef] [PubMed]
24. Kelava, I.; Lancaster, M.A. Dishing out mini-brains: Current progress and future prospects in brain organoid research. *Dev. Biol.* **2016**, *420*, 199–209. [CrossRef] [PubMed]
25. Salaris, F.; Rosa, A. Construction of 3D in vitro models by bioprinting human pluripotent stem cells: Challenges and opportunities. *Brain Res.* **2019**, *1723*, 146393. [CrossRef] [PubMed]
26. Abelseth, E.; Abelseth, L.; De la Vega, L.; Beyer, S.T.; Wadsworth, S.J.; Willerth, S.M. 3D Printing of Neural Tissues Derived from Human Induced Pluripotent Stem Cells Using a Fibrin-Based Bioink. *ACS Biomater. Sci. Eng.* **2019**, *5*, 234–243. [CrossRef]
27. Gu, Q.; Tomaskovic-Crook, E.; Lozano, R.; Chen, Y.; Kapsa, R.M.; Zhou, Q.; Wallace, G.G.; Crook, J.M. Functional 3D Neural Mini-Tissues from Printed Gel-Based Bioink and Human Neural Stem Cells. *Adv. Healthc. Mater.* **2016**, *5*, 1429–1438. [CrossRef] [PubMed]

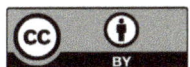

© 2019 by the authors. Licensee MDPI, Basel, Switzerland. This article is an open access article distributed under the terms and conditions of the Creative Commons Attribution (CC BY) license (http://creativecommons.org/licenses/by/4.0/).

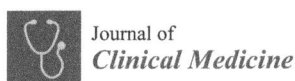

Article

Identification and Expression of Neurotrophin-6 in the Brain of *Nothobranchius furzeri*: One More Piece in Neurotrophin Research

Adele Leggieri [1,†], Chiara Attanasio [1,2,3,†], Antonio Palladino [2], Alessandro Cellerino [4,5], Carla Lucini [1], Marina Paolucci [6], Eva Terzibasi Tozzini [4], Paolo de Girolamo [1] and Livia D'Angelo [1,7,*]

1. Department of Veterinary Medicine and Animal Productions, University of Naples Federico II, I-80137 Naples, Italy; adele.leggieri@unina.it (A.L.); chiara.attanasio@unina.it (C.A.); lucini@unina.it (C.L.); degirola@unina.it (P.d.G.)
2. Interdepartmental Center for Research in Biomaterials (CRIB) University of Naples Federico II, I-80125 Naples, Italy; a.palladino1986@gmail.com
3. Center for Advanced Biomaterials for Healthcare-Istituto Italiano di Tecnologia, I-80125 Naples, Italy
4. Laboratory of Biology Bio@SNS, Scuola Normale Superiore, I-56126 Pisa, Italy; alessandro.cellerino@sns.it (A.C.); eva.terzibasi@sns.it (E.T.T.)
5. Laboratory of Biology of Aging, Leibniz Institute on Aging-Fritz Lipmann Institute, D-0445 Jena, Germany
6. Department of Sciences and Technologies, University of Sannio, I-82100 Benevento, Italy; paolucci@unisannio.it
7. Department of Biology and Evolution of Marine Organisms, Stazione Zoologica Anton Dohrn, I-80121 Naples, Italy
* Correspondence: livia.dangelo@unina.it; Tel.: +39-0812536131
† These two authors shared the co-authorship.

Received: 13 March 2019; Accepted: 22 April 2019; Published: 30 April 2019

Abstract: Neurotrophins contribute to the complexity of vertebrate nervous system, being involved in cognition and memory. Abnormalities associated with neurotrophin synthesis may lead to neuropathies, neurodegenerative disorders and age-associated cognitive decline. The genome of teleost fishes contains homologs of some mammalian neurotrophins as well as a gene coding for an additional neurotrophin (NT-6). In this study, we characterized this specific neurotrophin in the short-lived fish *Nothobranchius furzeri*, a relatively new model for aging studies. Thus, we report herein for the first time the age-related expression of a neurotrophin in a non-mammalian vertebrate. Interestingly, we found comparable expression levels of NT-6 in the brain of both young and old animals. More in detail, we used a locked nucleic acid probe and a riboprobe to investigate the neuroanatomical distribution of NT-6 mRNA revealing a significant expression of the neurotrophin in neurons of the forebrain (olfactory bulbs, dorsal and ventral telencephalon, and several diencephalic nuclei), midbrain (optic tectum, longitudinal tori, and semicircular tori), and hindbrain (valvula and body of cerebellum, reticular formation and octavolateral area of medulla oblongata). By combining in situ hybridization and immunohistochemistry, we showed that NT-6 mRNA is synthesized in mature neurons. These results contribute to better understanding the evolutionary history of neurotrophins in vertebrates, and their role in the adult brain.

Keywords: neurotrophin-6; phylogeny; LNA probe; riboprobe; neuroanatomy; fish; aging

1. Introduction

Nothobranchius furzeri is a novel model organism for aging research [1–3] being its captive lifespan the shortest ever recorded for a vertebrate [4]. The life cycle of *N. furzeri*, indeed, is characterized by explosive growth [5] and rapid expression of aging phenotypes at behavioral, histological, and molecular levels [6–8]. Concerning the brain, *N. furzeri* displays typical aging hallmarks, including lipofuscin accumulation, age-dependent gliosis and rapid decay of adult neurogenesis [9]. The identification of specific genes under positive selection revealed potential candidates to explain the compressed lifespan of this fish. Several age-related genes, indeed, are under positive selection in *N. furzeri* and long-lived species, including humans, raising the intriguing hypothesis that the same gene could underlie evolution of both compressed and extended lifespan [10]. Remarkably, one of the variants in this fish granulin (W449 in the shorter-lived strain and C449 in the longer-lived strain) is within a motif that plays a key role in protein folding, and is mutated in human frontotemporal dementia [11]. The fish variant is predicted to generate functional consequences and is also found in wild fish, thus excluding its derivation from a spurious mutation arisen in the laboratory or from the bottleneck of a rare allele [10].

The assessment of the neurotrophin family came after the identification of the first two members: the nerve growth factor (NGF) [12] and the brain derived neurotrophic factor (BDNF) [13]. These members share stretches of highly homologous amino acid sequences [13], and both support the survival of cultured dorsal root ganglia neurons [14]. Afterwards, three more neurotrophins have been identified in vertebrate genomes: neurotrophin 3 (NT-3), neurotrophin 4 (NT-4) and the fast evolving neurotrophin-5 (NT-5) [15]. Neurotrophins are produced as pre-pro-peptides and undergo proteolytic cleavage before being secreted [16]. They exert many biological effects by their high affinity binding h to the specific tropomyosin-related kinase (Trk) or by a lower affinity interaction with the receptor p75NTR [17]. Specifically, NGF binds to TrkA, NT-3 to TrkC and, with lower affinity, to TrkA, while BDNF and NT-4 bind to TrkB [18]. In addition, p75 receptor can bind to unprocessed or mature neurotrophin and act as co-receptor of Trks [17]. In general, neurotrophins play a role in distinct, as well as partially overlapping, subsets of peripheral and central neurons. Further, individual neurons may also be responsive to more than one neurotrophin at a given time or at subsequent times during development [19]. According to the differential expression and cellular localization of their receptors, neurotrophins can elicit diverse cellular functions in different types of neurons and at different cellular loci [17,18]. Abnormalities associated with neurotrophins synthesis have been linked with neuropathies and neurodegenerative disorders, as well as age-associated cognitive decline.

The genome of teleost fishes contains homologs of the mammalian neurotrophins NGF, BDNF, NT-3 and NT-4 [20] but also a gene coding for one additional neurotrophin originally isolated and cloned in platyfish [21]: neurotrophin-6 (NT-6). The ortholog of this neurotrophic factor in *Danio rerio* [22] and *Cyprinus carpio* [23] was later described as neurotrophin-7 (NT-7). From the biochemical standpoint, NT-6 is featured by the presence of a 22 amino acid residue inserted between the second and third conserved cysteine containing domain. NT-6 promoted the survival of chick sympathetic and sensory dorsal root ganglion neurons, to the same extent of NGF, despite a lower specific activity [21]. Further molecular and phylogenetic studies have provided evidence that, in teleost fishes, NGF and NT-6 are paralogs and originated from duplication of an ancestral gene as consequence of the whole-genome duplication of teleost fishes [24].

Very few studies have been devoted to the role of this neurotrophin in fish, as well as to its expression and morphological distribution. Götz and coworkers [21] documented that NT-6 transcripts are significantly expressed during the embryonic development and adulthood of *Xiphophorus*, in brain, gill, liver and eye while a weak expression is displayed in heart, skin, spleen and skeletal muscles [21]. A very recent paper described NT-6 mRNA during zebrafish embryogenesis (from 12–96 h post fertilization) by whole-mount in situ hybridization [25]. Nittoli et al. reported that early transcript was detected at 16 hpf in two clusters of cells adjacent to the anterior and posterior of the inner ear primordium, and that its expression was lost from 48 h post fertilization onward [25].

In the present study, we investigated the age-related expression of NT-6 in the short-lived teleost, *N. furzeri*. Our findings contribute to: (i) better understand the evolutionary history of neurotrophins in vertebrates; (ii) elucidate their role in vertebrate brain; (iii) demonstrate that NT-6 is expressed in mature neurons of the adult brain; and (iv) document the stable age-associated changes of NT-6 over time.

2. Experimental Section

2.1. Protocols

The protocols for animal care and use were approved by the appropriate Committee at the University of Naples Federico II (2015/0023947). All animal experimental procedures were carried out in accordance with The European Parliament and The Council of The European Union Directive of 22nd of September 2010 (2010/63/UE) and Italian Law (D.lgs 26/2014).

2.2. Animals and Tissue Preparation

Animals, belonging to the long-lived strain MZM 04/10 were used at the following time points: 5 weeks post hatching (wph) (young-adult, age of the sexual maturity) and 27 wph (old animals). Animal maintenance was performed as previously described [26]. To avoid effects of circadian rhythms and feeding, animals were euthanized at 10:00 in a fasted state, with an overdose of anesthetics. They were placed for approximately 5–10 min in a solution containing 1 mg/mL in buffered ethyl 3-aminobenzoate methanesulfonate without prior sedation and observed until no vital signs (body and operculum movement, righting reflex) were observed.

For RNA extraction, 5 fish for each time point (5 and 27 wph) were decapitated, brains were rapidly dissected, kept in sterile tubes (Eppendorf BioPhotometer, Hamburg, Germany) with 500 μL of RNAlater (Qiagen, Hilden, Germany), and stored at 4 °C until the RNA extraction. For fluorescence in situ hybridization (FISH), 5 adult fish (at 20 wph) were decapitated, brains were rapidly excised and fixed in 4% paraformaldehyde (PFA)/PBS overnight (ON) at 4 °C. Then, brains were incubated in 20% sucrose solution ON at 4 °C and successively in 30% sucrose solution ON at 4 °C. Brains were then embedded in cryomount and frozen at −80 °C. Serial transverse and sagittal sections of 12 μm thickness were cut with a cryostat (Leica, Deerfield, IL, USA).

2.3. RNA Isolation and cDNA Synthesis

Tissues were taken out of RNAlater and cleaned with sterile pipettes. *N. furzeri* (NFu) total RNA was isolated from 10 animals with QIAzol (Qiagen), according to a modified manufacturer's protocol [27]. Homogenization was performed using a TissueLyzer II (Qiagen) at 20 Hz for 2–3 × 1 min. Total RNA was then quantized with Eppendorf BioPhotometer. Then, 500 ng of each sample were retrotranscribed to cDNA in a 20 μL volume, using the QuantiTect® Reverse Transcription Kit (Qiagen), following the supplier's protocol. Newly synthetized cDNAs were then diluted to a final volume of 200 μL with ultra-pure sterile water to an approximate final cDNA's concentration of 40 ng/μL.

2.4. Phylogenetics Analysis

Orthologs of Nfu NT-6 were recovered from Genbank by querying Genbank translated nucleotide sequences with the translated cDNA of NfuNT-6. *D. rerio* glial derived neurotrophic factor (GDNF) sequence was selected as outgroup. All phylogenetic analyses were performed using MEGA X [28]. The analysis involved 17 amino acid sequences of different fish species (differently named as neurotrophin-6/7-like and nerve growth factor-like) and *Homo sapiens* and *Mus musculus*. The most appropriate amino acid substitution model was selected based on Akaike Information Criterion (AIC). Phylogenetic tree was reconstructed by maximum likelihood analysis using a partial deletion (80%) setting, JTT with gamma function and invariant sites as substitution model, and bootstrap analysis.

2.5. Quantitative Real Time-PCR

NfuNT6 primers were designed with Primer3 tool [29]. According to the sequence information, one set of primers was designed to quantize NfuNT-6 cDNA: left 5′-GCATTCGTTGAAGTCTGGCT-3′; right 5′-ATCAGGAAGAGCAGGACCAG-3′. Reactions were performed in 20 μL volume containing 1 μL of diluted cDNA, using BrightGreen 2× qPCR MasterMix kit (abm®, Richmond, VA, Canada) following the manufacturer's instructions. Reactions were performed in triplicate and negative control (water) was always included.

2.6. Statistical Analysis

Expression levels of NfuNT-6 mRNA were analyzed by the ΔΔCt method and normalized to the housekeeping gene TATA box binding protein (*TBP*): left 5'-CGGTTGGAGGGTTTAGTCCT-3'; right 5'-GCAAGACGATTCTGGGTTTG-3'). Fold changes represent the difference in expression levels between young and old age NfuNT-6 cDNAs, respectively, with young and old age TATA-binding protein (TBP) cDNAs. The relative ΔΔ curve threshold was built on fold changes values and p-value was <0.01.

2.7. Probe Design

For the neuroanatomical distribution of NfuNT-6 mRNA, two different DIG-labelled probes were employed: a locked nucleic acid (LNA) probe, and an RNA probe (riboprobe). The LNA probe, unlike the RNA probe, contains an extra bridge which connects the 2' oxygen and 4' carbon locking the ribose in the 3' endo conformation. This conformation significantly increases hybridization properties of the probe.

2.8. Riboprobe Synthesis

mRNA probes to identify NfuNT-6 mRNA were synthetized by in vitro transcription (IVT) using MAXIscript™ SP6/T7 in vitro transcription kit (Invitrogen by Thermo Fisher Scientific–Catalogue number AM1312, Carlsbad, CA, USA) and following the manufacturer's instructions. 1 µg of DNA template was transcribed to RNA in 20 µL volume reaction, using NfuNT6 primer associated with the T7 promoter sequence (left 5'-TGGTCCTGCTCTTCCTGATC-3'; T7 right 5'-GGTAATACGACTCACTATAGG_GTGTGTTTGAAGCTGCTCGA-3') and a DIG RNA Labeling Mix, 10× conc (Roche, Basel, Switzerland) containing digoxigenin labeled uracil. After IVT reaction, product was briefly centrifuged and incubated at 37 °C for 1 h. Then, 1 µL of turbo DNase 1 was added, sample was mixed well and incubated for 15 min at 37 °C. 1 µL of EDTA 0.5 M was added to stop the reaction. Reaction product was analyzed by gel electrophoresis and quantized.

2.9. LNA Probe Synthesis

LNA modified DNA oligonucleotide probe, containing an LNA nucleotide at every third position, and labeled at the 59 end only, or at the 59 and 39 ends, with DIG, were supplied by Exiqon Inc. (Vedbaek, Denmark). NT6 probe was designed using the Primer3 primer design program [28] and checked using the LNA Oligo Optimizer tool on the Exiqon website (www.exiqon.com) (see Table 1). Probe sequence was screened against all known *N. furzeri* sequences using BLAST. LNA probe typically shows single nucleotide specificity [30]. Negative control was mismatch probe, designed and synthesized by Exiqon Inc. (see Table 1).

Table 1. LNA probe and mismatch probe.

Target mRNA	5'-Mod	Synthesis Sequence (5'–3')	3'-Mod
NT-6	DIG	TTGTCTCCTGCTGTCCTGCTCTG	DIG
* mut NT-6	DIG	TTGTCTC**T**CGCTG**CT**CTGCT**T**CG	DIG

* Mutations are shown bolded.

2.10. Fluorescence in Situ Hybridization

FISH experiments were performed on cryostat sections using sterile solutions and materials. Diethylpyrocarbonate (DEPC) was added to phosphate-buffered saline (PBS) and water 1 mL/L to inactivate RNase enzymes; solutions were shaken vigorously and autoclaved.

Sections were dried for 2 h at room temperature (RT), well washed in 1× DEPC/PBS and treated with 10 µg/µL Proteinase K (Sigma-Aldrich, St. Louis, MO, USA) 1:200 in DEPC/PBS for 10 min. Proteinase K action was then inactivated by two washes in 2 mg/mL glycine, 5 min each. Sections were post fixed in 4% PFA for 20 min and well washed in 1× DEPC/PBS at RT. Thereafter, the prehybridization was carried out in a hybridization solution (HB) containing 50% formamide, 25% 20× SSC, 50 µg/mL Heparin, 10 µg/mL yeast RNA, 0.1% Tween 20, and 0.92% citric acid at 55 °C (riboprobes) and 42 °C (LNA probes) for 1 h. All probes were denatured for 10 min at 80 °C and sections were then incubated, in HB containing riboprobes concentration of 500 pg/µL, ON at 55 °C and LNA probes concentration of 2 ng/µg, ON at 42 °C. Post-hybridization washes were carried out at 55 °C as follows: 2 × 20 min in 1× SSC, 2 × 10 min in 0.5× SSC, and then in 1× DEPC/PBS at RT. Sections were blocked in blocking solution (BS) containing 10% normal sheep serum heat inactivated and 0.5% blocking reagent (Roche, Hamburg, Germany) for 1 h at RT. After, sections were incubated in a 1:2000 dilution of anti-digoxigenin Fab fragments conjugated with alkaline phosphatase (Roche) in BS, 2 h at RT. Sections were well washed in 1× DEPC/PBS. The chromogenic reaction was carried out by using Fast Red tablets (Sigma-Aldrich) in Tris buffer and incubating the slides at RT in the dark and were observed every 20 min until the signal detection (1–10 h depending on the probe used). After the signal was developed, sections were washed in 1× DEPC/PBS at RT and mounted with Fluoreshield Mounting Medium with DAPI as counterstaining for the nuclei.

2.11. Combined In Situ Hybridization and Immunohistochemistry

After the detection of the FISH chromogenic reaction, sections were well washed in DEPC/PBS and incubated at RT for 1 h with blocking serum (normal goat serum 1:5 in PBS containing 0.1% Triton X-100, Sigma) and subsequently with primary antiserum ON at 4 °C. Primary antisera employed were: rabbit polyclonal anti-S100 (1:200, Agilent Dako, Santa Clara, CA, USA, Ref. Z 0311); mouse IgG2b, biotin-XX conjugate anti-HuC/D (1:50, Invitrogen by Thermo Fisher Scientific, Carlsbad, CA, USA, Ref. A21272); mouse monoclonal anti-MAP-2 (1:50, Santa Cruz Biotechnology, Ref. Sc-74422, Dallas, TX, USA), rabbit polyclonal anti-Parvalbumin (1:100 Anti-Parvalbumin Rabbit pAB PC255L-100UL, EMD Millipore, Burlington, MA, USA). DEPC/PBS washes preceded the incubation with the secondary antibodies: goat anti-rabbit IgG (H+L) Alexa fluor™ Plus 488 (1:1000, Invitrogen by Thermo Fisher Scientific, Ref. A32731, Carlsbad, CA, USA) for anti-S100β, anti-Parvalbumin; Alexa Fluor® 488 Streptavidin conjugated (1:800, Jackson Immuno Research Labs, West Grove, PA, USA, Ref. 016540084) for HuC/D; goat anti-mouse IgG (H+L) Alexa fluor™ Plus 488 (1:1000, Invitrogen by Thermo Fisher Scientific, Carlsbad, CA, USA, Ref. A32723) for MAP-2.

2.12. Microscopy

FISH images were analyzed with a Zeiss AxioScope AX 1.0 microscope (Carl Zeiss, Jena, Germany) with AxioCam MC5 and AxioVision software. Combined FISH/Immunohistochemistry images were analyzed by Leica–DM6B (Leica, Wetzlar, Germany) and processed with LasX software. The digital raw images were optimized for image resolution, contrast, evenness of illumination, and background using Adobe Photoshop CC 2018 (Adobe Systems, San Jose, CA, USA). Anatomical structures were identified according to the adult *N. furzeri* brain atlas [31].

3. Results

3.1. Molecular Characterization of NfuNT-6

A putative NT-6 coding sequence was retrieved from the *N. furzeri* transcriptome browser [32]: the sequence is deposited under the Genebank accession number GAIB01193979.1. NfuNT-6 was aligned with the predicted NT-6/7 sequences available in some actinopterygians species (*Xiphophorus*, *Cyprinus carpio* and *Danio rerio*), as well as mammalian and *D. rerio* neurotrophins. NT-4/5 of *D. rerio* was not included in the alignment because it is not still annotated on GenBank. GDNF of *D. rerio* was used as outgroup. The evolutionary history was inferred using the Minimum Evolution method, having selected long nucleotides sequences. The evolutionary distances were computed using the *p*-distance method and are in the units of the number of base differences per site. The analysis involved 17 nucleotides sequences (Figure 1). The ME tree was searched using the Close-Neighbor-Interchange (CNI) algorithm at a search level of 1. The Neighbor-joining algorithm was used to generate the initial tree. All positions containing gaps and missing data were eliminated. The resulting phylogram clearly shows that the *N. furzeri* sequence is nested within a clade of Actinopterygian sequences, and high percentage of conservation with fish neurotrophin-3.

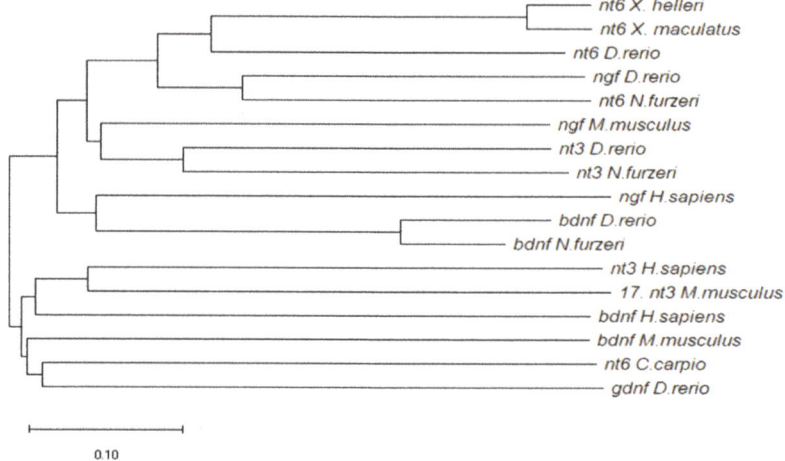

Figure 1. Evolutionary relationships of taxa. The evolutionary history was inferred using the Minimum Evolution method. The optimal tree with the sum of branch length = 4.92138622 is shown. The tree is drawn to scale, with branch lengths in the same units as those of the evolutionary distances used to infer the phylogenetic tree. This analysis involved 17 nucleotide sequences. Codon positions included were 1st+2nd+3rd+Noncoding. All ambiguous positions were removed for each sequence pair (pairwise deletion option). There were 3752 positions in the final dataset.

3.2. Expression Studies

3.2.1. NfuNT-6 mRNA Expression in Young versus Old Animals

We analyzed NfuNT-6 mRNA levels, by qPCR analysis, in brain homogenates of 5 and 27 wph animals. Comparable levels of NfuNT-6 mRNA were found in the brains of young and old animals (*p*-value: 0.70344) (Figure 2). For each time point, NfuNT-6 mRNA was normalized to the reference gene (TBP) and expression levels were compared using the relative delta curve threshold ($\Delta\Delta CT$) method (*p*-value$_{5wph}$ = 0.00387; *p*-value$_{27wph}$ = 0.001085).

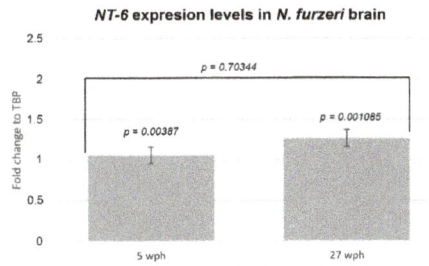

Figure 2. Expression levels of NfuNT-6 mRNA in the brain of young and old *N. furzeri*. Comparable expression levels of NfuNT-6 mRNA in the whole brain of young and old animals (*p*-value: 0.70344). For 5 and 27 wph, NfuNT-6 mRNA was normalized to TBP and expression levels were compared using ΔΔCT method (*p*-value$_{5wph}$ = 0.00387; *p*-value$_{27wph}$ = 0.001085).

3.2.2. Neuroanatomical Expression of NT-6 mRNA

LNA and riboprobes (Figure 3a,b) were used to localize the expression of NT-6 mRNA and revealed overlapping distribution patterns. No specific hybridization signal was observed in sections hybridized with the mismatch probe (Figure 3c). Due to overlapping pattern of expression of riboprobe and LNA, the results refer to NT-6 mRNA. The nomenclature follows the *N. furzeri* brain atlas [30]. Recognition of labeled neurons and/or glial cells was based on morphological criteria and by means of different markers: S100β [9,33], HuC/HuD [34] and MAP2 [35]. Purkinje neurons were identified by using parvalbumin as marker.

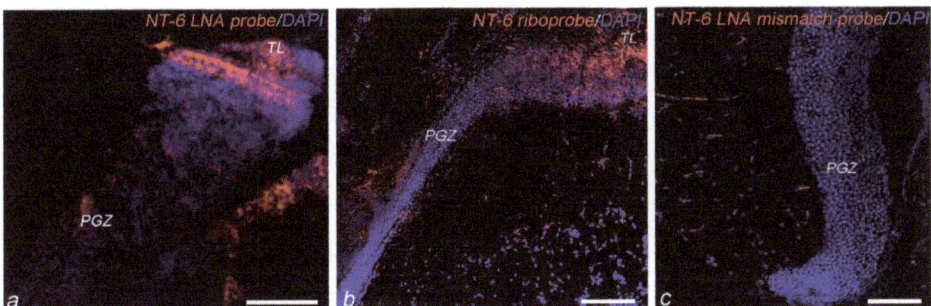

Figure 3. Comparison of riboprobe and LNA and negative control: (**a**) LNA probe and (**b**) Riboprobe to detect NT-6 mRNA expression (red) in the OT, at the margin with TL; and (**c**) mismatch LNA probe in the OT not revealing staining. Scale bar: (**a,c**) 25 µm; and (**b**) 12 µm. Abbreviations: PGZ, periventricular grey zone.

3.2.3. NT-6 mRNA Expression in Mature Neurons

Before analyzing the pattern of expression of NT-6 over different brain areas, we combined in situ hybridization with immunohistochemistry to identify the phenotype of NT-6 mRNA expressing cells. We conducted the experiment on serial sections of the optic tectum, and we employed markers to identify glial and neuronal populations. S100β was used as marker of glial cells [9,33], HuC/HuD as marker of early-differentiated neurons [34,35], and MAP2 as marker of mature neurons [36,37]. NT-6 mRNA was not expressed in S100β immunoreactive cells (Figure 4a,a1,a2) or in HuC/HuD cells (Figure 4b,b1,b2). NT-6 mRNA signal probe was observed in MAP2 immunoreactive cells in the most posterior part of periventricular grey zone of the optic tectum and in some scarce cells in the most superficial layers of the same brain area (Figure 4c,c1,c2).

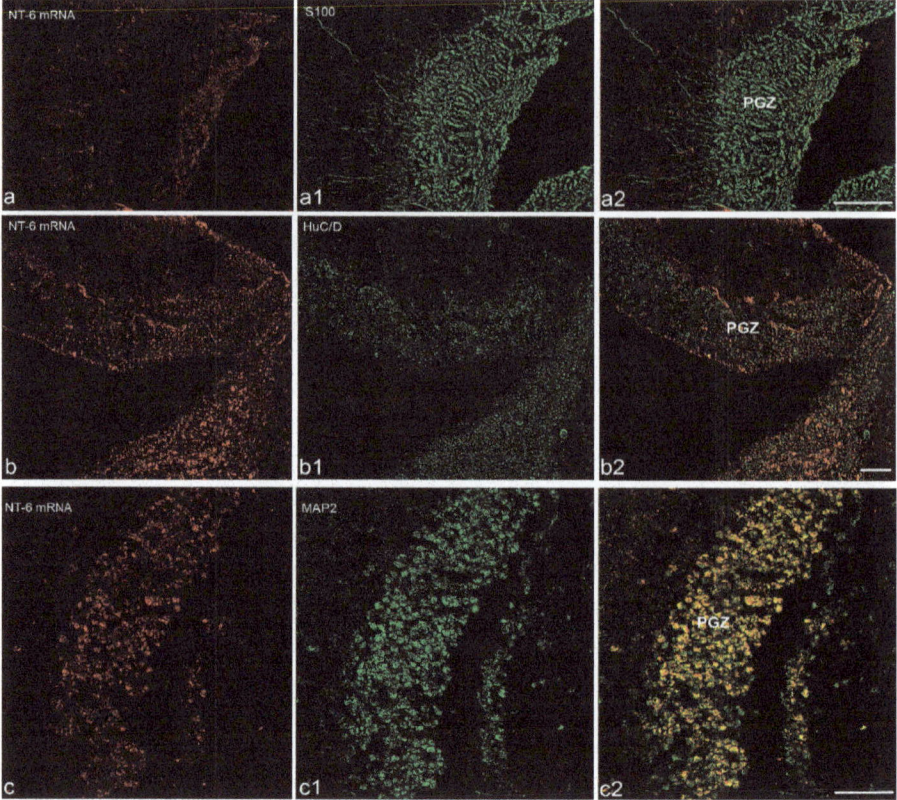

Figure 4. Immunohistochemical characterization of NT-6 mRNA expressing cells in transverse section of optic tectum: (**a,a1,a2**) single images and merge of NT-6 mRNA and S100β positive cells, showing any co-staining in the rostral part of optic tectum; (**b,b1,b2**) single images and merge of NT-6 mRNA and HuC/HuD showing any co-staining in the rostral part of optic tectum; and (**c,c1,c2**) single images and merge of NT-6 mRNA and MAP2 showing that NT-6 is expressed in numerous MAP2 immunopositive. Scale bar: (**a,c**) 50 µm; and (**b**) 25 µm. Abbreviations: PGZ, periventricular grey zone.

3.2.4. Neuroanatomical Distribution of NfuNT-6 mRNA in the Adult *N. furzeri*

Forebrain

In the olfactory bulb, numerous moderately labeled cells were found in the internal and external cellular layers, as well as in the glomerular layer (Figure 5a). In the dorsal telencephalon, the expression pattern of NT-6 mRNA was characterized by weak labeling in few scattered neurons of the central nucleus, whereas intense signal probe was observed in dorso-dorsal, medial (Figure 5b) and lateral nuclei. In the ventral telencephalon, NT-6 mRNA weakly labeled few neurons of dorsal and lateral nuclei. In the preoptic area, NT-6 mRNA expression was detected in the anterior (Figure 5c), parvo- and magnocellular nuclei, and in the suprachiasmatic nucleus. Intense staining was seen in neurons along third ventricle (Figure 5d). In the pretectal area, strong labeling was observed in numerous neurons of cortical nucleus (Figure 5e,f), as well as in neurons of parvocellular superficial pretectal nucleus. Intense staining was observed in few neurons of supraglomerular nucleus. NT-6 mRNA was observed in several weakly positive neurons of dorsal hypothalamus.

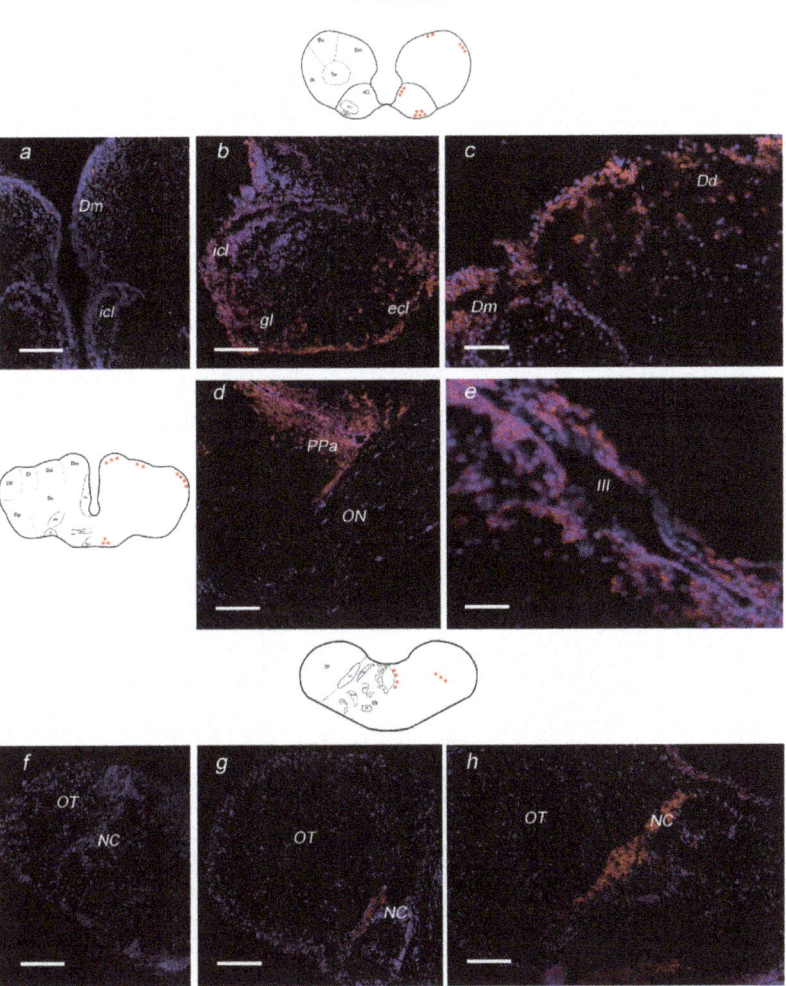

Figure 5. Expression of neurotrophin-6 (NT-6) mRNA in transverse section of forebrain of adult *N. furzeri*. On the left side, schematic drawings of *N. furzeri* brain, with red dots indicating NT-6 mRNA distribution over the different brain areas. Forebrain: (**a**) sense probe staining in the Dm and OB; (**b**) positive cells in icl, ecl and gl of olfactory bulbs; (**c**) positive neurons in the dorso-medial and dorso-dorsal zone of dorsal telencephalon; (**d**) numerous and intensely stained neurons in the anterior part of preoptic area; (**e**) intensely stained neurons scattered along the third ventricle; (**f**) sense probe staining in the NC and anterior part of OT; (**g**) overview of pretectal area and anterior part of optic tectum, with strong positive labeling in the neurons of NC; and (**h**) high magnification of positive neurons of NC. Scale bars: (**a–c,f**) 50 µm; (**d**) 25 µm; and (**e**) 100 µm. Abbreviations: Dd, dorsal zone of dorsal telencephalon; Dm, medial zone of dorsal telencephalon; ecl, external cellular layer; gl, glomerular layer; icl, internal cellular layer; NC, cortical nucleus; OB, olphactory bulb; ON, optic nerve; OT, optic tectum; PPa, anterior preoptic area; III, third ventricle.

Midbrain

The sense probe staining is shown in Figure 6a,b. Between forebrain and midbrain, moderate labeling was observed in neurons of the anterior glomerular nucleus, in neurons bordering the margins of the glomerular nucleus and in few large neurons in its inner part (Figure 6c,d). In the longitudinal tori, NT-6 mRNA was intensely expressed in numerous positive neurons located mainly in the most ventral part (Figure 6e), and along the margin with the optic tectum (Figure 6f). In the optic tectum, positive neurons were observed in the periventricular grey zone (Figures 6g and 7a). However, NT-6 mRNA expressing neurons were few in the most rostral part of the periventricular grey zone (Figure 6f) while became more numerous caudally (Figures 6g and 7a). Furthermore, the neurons lining the margin between the optic tectum and tegmentum were intensely labeled (Figure 6g). In the tegmentum, a positive signal was detected in neurons of Layers 1, 3 and 4 of semicircular tori (TS-1, TS-3, and TS-4) (Figure 6c).

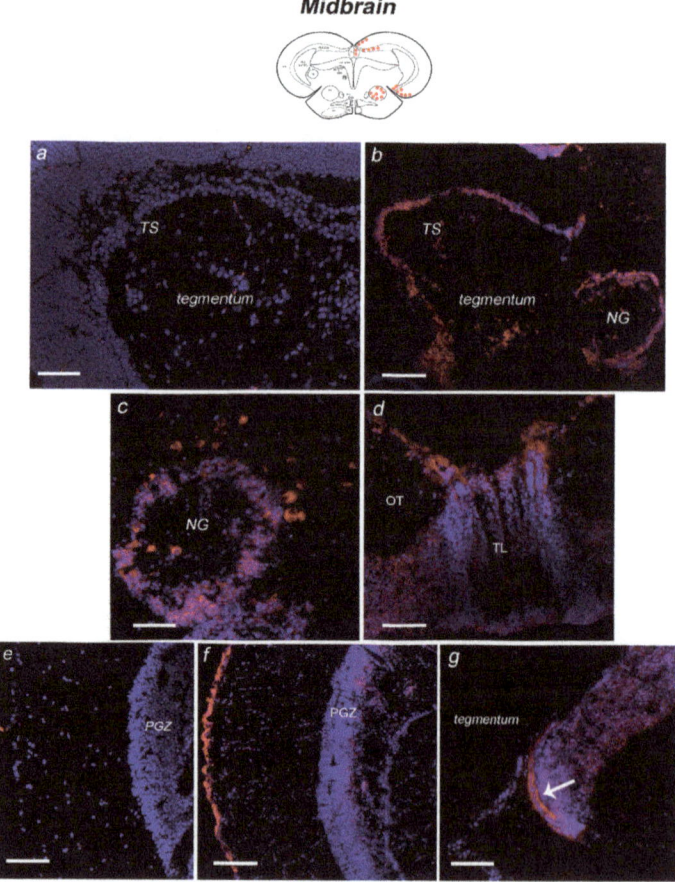

Figure 6. Expression of NT-6 mRNA in transverse section of caudal diencephalon/midbrain of adult *N. furzeri*. On the top, schematic drawings of *N. furzeri* brain, with red dots indicating NT-6 mRNA distribution over the different brain areas. Caudal diencephalon/midbrain: (**a**) sense probe staining in the anterior midbrain tegmentum; (**b**) high magnification of sense probe staining in the NG; (**c**) overview of tegmentum, with probe signal in neurons of TS and NG; (**d**) high magnification of positive neurons, scattered along the margin of NG; (**e**) probe signal in the dorsal and ventral part of TL and along the margin with OT; (**f**) few positive cells of PGZ in the anterior part of OT; and (**g**) numerous positive cells in the most caudal part of OT and intense staining at the margin between OT and the midbrain tegmentum (arrow). Scale bars: (**a,c**) 50 µm; and (**b,d–g**) 25 µm. Abbreviations: NG, glomerular nucleus; OT, optic tectum; PGZ, periventricular grey zone; TL, longitudinal tori; TS, semicircular tori.

Hindbrain

Strong labeling was observed in the most rostral region of cerebellum, with scattered neurons largely diffused in the lateral nucleus of cerebellar valvula (Figure 7a). In the most caudal part of the inferior lobe of hypothalamus, probe signal was seen in numerous small neurons of the diffuse nucleus and in large neurons of the central nucleus (Figure 7b).

NT-6 mRNA was moderately localized in neurons of Purkinje layer of the lateral region of the cerebellar valvula (Figure 7a). Positive neurons in the Purkinje layer were also observed in the ventro-lateral and ventro-ventral subdivisions of cerebellar body (Figure 7c,d). The positive neurons were identified as Purkinje cells by double labeling with Parvalbumin (Figure 8a–b$_2$). Strong labeling was seen also in elongated cells of the dorsal cerebellar subdivision (Figure 7c,d). Few positive neurons were labeled in the cerebellar crista (Figure 7c). In medulla oblongata, the expression pattern was seen in scattered neurons of octavolateral area, and in neurons of superior (Figure 7c) and intermediate reticular formation. Sense probe staining is shown in Figure 7e,f.

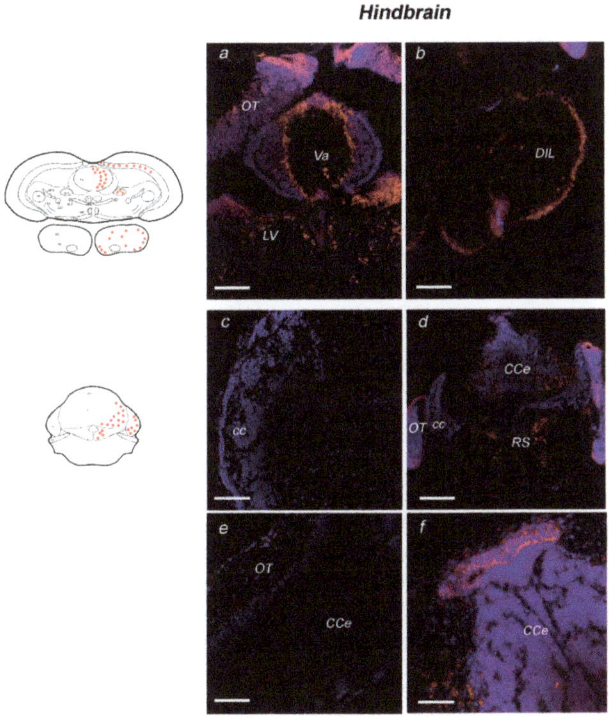

Hindbrain

Figure 7. Expression of NT-6 mRNA in transverse section of hindbrain of adult *N. furzeri*. On the left side, schematic drawings of *N. furzeri* brain, with red dots indicating NT-6 mRNA distribution over the different brain areas. (**a**) Intense staining in the cells of caudal part of PGZ, and along the margin between OT and TL. Positivity in neurons of Purkinje layer of Va and in neurons of LV. (**b**) Positive neurons widespread over the central nucleus and dorsal hypothalamus of the most caudal part of DIL. (**c**) Sense probe staining in the cerebellar crista. (**d**) Intense staining in neurons of Purkinje, in neurons of RS. (**e**) Sense probe staining in the OT and CCe. (**f**) Intense staining labeling in the most upper portion of CCe (arrow) and in neurons of Purkinje layer of CCe. Scale bars: (**a,b,d**) 50 μm; and (**c,e,f**) 100 μm. Abbreviations: CCe, corpus of cerebellum; cc, cerebellar crista, DIL, diffuse inferior lobe of hypothalamus; LV, nucleus of lateral valvula; OT, optic tectum; PGZ, periventricular grey zone; RS, superior reticular formation; TL, longitudinal tori; Va, valvula of cerebellum.

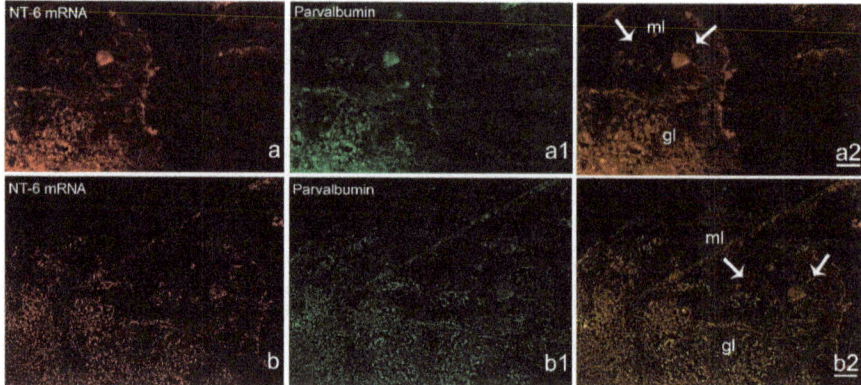

Figure 8. Immunohistochemical characterization of NT-6 mRNA expression in Purkinje cells in sagittal section of cerebellum. (**a,a1,a2**) single images and merge of NT-6 mRNA and Parvalbumin positive cells, showing co-staining in the gl and in Purkinje cells (arrow). (**b,b1,b2**) higher magnification of single images and merge of NT-6 mRNA and Parvalbumin positive cells showing co-staining in the gl and in Purkinje cells (arrow). Scale bar: a = 50 µm; b = 25 µm. Abbreviation: gl, granular layer; ml, molecular layer.

4. Discussion

The accumulated evidence documents an age-associated dysregulation of neurotrophins in the brain of mammals [38,39]. This is the first study reporting both the age-related expression of a neurotrophin in a non-mammalian vertebrate, and a comprehensive description of NT-6 mRNA in the adult brain of a fish species.

NT-6 has been identified in very few fish species: *Xiphophorus maculatus* [21], *Danio rerio* (zebrafish) [22], and *Cyprinus carpio* [23]. Phylogenetic analysis on neurotrophins, carried out on mature amino acid sequences [40,41], supports the hypothesis that during chordate/vertebrate lineage two rounds of duplication events of an ancestral neurotrophin gene occurred. Studies have shown that the genomic organization and transcript structure of NGF and NT-6 in the teleost zebrafish share a high similarity with the mouse NGF [24] and suggest that teleost NT-6 has evolved from a common ancestor after a single "fish specific" duplication of NGF [40,41]. Our phylogenetic studies on nucleotides sequences further confirm the hypothesis of NT-6 originated from NGF/NT-3 ancestors. However, the role of NT-6 needs to be clarified in teleosts fish: despite the degree of functional overlapping among the different neurotrophins, individual neurotrophins display a specific activity [42,43].

According to the few data available in literature, we hypothesize that this fish-specific neurotrophin might have a peculiar function among different fish species. Indeed, NT-6 persists in the brain of *N. furzeri* and the closest relative *Xiphophorus* [21] beyond early stages, whereas in zebrafish its expression is strictly linked to the embryonic stages [25]. The observation that NT-6 mRNA expression displayed comparable levels in the brain of young and old animals suggests us that, in our model species, this molecule plays a role in brain development as well as in its maintenance in adults. However, we cannot exclude that the expression levels, despite appearing very similar, can derive from a modulation of the NT-6 neuronal synthesis. For instance, it could be possible that few neurons express high levels of NT-6, or at the same time, that a high number of neurons express low levels of NT-6, in an age-dependent manner. Most interestingly, the synthesis of NT-6 in the aged brain could be a consequence of microglia activation, as compensatory mechanism of physiological aging process [44]. Further experiments are necessary to test these hypotheses and thus to better understand the role of neurotrophins in aging process. This is the first time we explored the age regulation of a neurotrophin in the brain of *N. furzeri*, while our previous studies had been addressed to investigate the morphological distribution of neurotrophins and their receptors in the adult brain.

Herein, we also provide a complete neuroanatomical description of NT-6 mRNA in the brain of *N. furzeri*. In this respect, we employed two different digoxigenin modified probes: an LNA probe and a riboprobe. LNA probes are generally used to detect short DNA oligonucleotides for microRNA and mRNA detection [30,45–48]. LNA containing DNA probes have been previously employed for in situ hybridization detection of mRNAs [45–48] in whole mount embryos of chicken and on tissue sections in *N. furzeri* [2]. The LNA probes revealed an enhanced hybridization efficiency, hybridization specificity and duplex stability [49]. Remarkably, our in situ experiments showed an overlapping neuroanatomical distribution for both probes.

Briefly, our results demonstrate that NT-6 mRNA is expressed in the forebrain (dorsal and ventral telencephalon, and in several diencephalic nuclei), in the midbrain (optic tectum, longitudinal tori, semicircular tori), and in the hindbrain (valvula and body of cerebellum, reticular formation and octavolateral area of medulla oblongata). NT-6 mRNA has been documented during the developing stages of *Xiphophorus* [21] and zebrafish [25], respectively, expressed in the valvula cerebelli and optic vescicle. In adult *Xiphophorus*, although NT-6 is expressed, a neuroanatomical description has not been reported yet [21]. Overall, our findings document a wide NT-6 mRNA localization throughout the whole brain of *N. furzeri*. In addition, other neurotrophins (NGF, BDNF and NT-4), at either mRNAs or protein level, were observed in the adult brain of *N. furzeri* [48–50]. Remarkably, NT-6 mRNA is expressed in mature neurons, similar to other neurotrophins, such as BDNF, NGF, and NT-4 [50–52], which have been already documented in the brain of this model species. Most interestingly, neurotrophins display a peculiar neuronal expression also in zebrafish and the European eel [35,53–55]. These observations reinforce the hypothesis that the expression of neurotrophins in teleost fish is primarily linked to mature neurons. In adult mammalian brain, the neuronal mRNA levels of NGF and BDNF are tightly regulated by neural activity and influence the modulation of several key events such as synthesis, metabolism and release of neurotransmitters, postsynaptic ion channel fluxes, neuronal firing rates as well as long-term synaptic potentiation of neurons [56]. In this context, further studies are mandatory to explore the evolutionary conserved neuronal role of neurotrophins in the brain of fish species.

In conclusion, our findings document: (1) the identification and molecular characterization of NT-6 coding sequence of *N. furzeri* (NfuNT-6) and the nucleotide degree of conservation in *Xiphophorus*, *D. rerio* and mammalian NGF and BDNF; (2) the efficiency of using a sensitive LNA probe to detect NT-6 mRNA; (3) the unchanged expression levels of NT-6 in the brain of young and old animals; and (4) the expression of NT-6 mRNA in mature neurons of forebrain, midbrain and hindbrain in *N. furzeri*. These results provide a basis for future research on evolutionary function of neurotrophins, which are currently perceived as one of the primary factors underlying the complexity of vertebrate nervous systems. Therefore, their involvement in higher brain functions and aging is undoubtedly a relevant topic.

Further experimental work is noticeably needed both to characterize more in-depth NT-6 in this model and to confirm its importance in brain development and architecture. In addition, functional studies are required to explore and feature the potential role played by NT-6 in aging.

Author Contributions: Conceptualization, C.A. and A.C.; Data curation, A.P.; Funding acquisition, P.d.G.; Methodology, A.L.; Software, E.T.T.; Writing—original draft, L.D.A.; and Writing—review and editing, C.L. and M.P.

Funding: The project was supported by University of Naples Federico II (DR/2017/409–Project F.I.A.T.).

Acknowledgments: The authors are thankful to Antonio Calamo for technical assistance.

Conflicts of Interest: The authors declare no conflict of interest.

References

1. Cellerino, A.; Valenzano, D.R.; Reichard, M. From the bush to the bench: The annual Nothobranchius fishes as a new model system in biology. *Biol. Rev. Camb. Philos. Soc.* **2016**, *91*, 511–533. [CrossRef]

2. D'Angelo, L.; Lossi, L.; Merighi, A.; de Girolamo, P. Anatomical features for the adequate choice of experimental animal models in biomedicine: I. Fishes. *Ann. Anat.* **2016**, *205*, 75–84. [CrossRef]
3. Kim, Y.; Nam, H.G.; Valenzano, D.R. The short-lived African turquoise killifish: An emerging experimental model for ageing. *Dis. Model Mech.* **2016**, *2*, 115–129. [CrossRef]
4. Genade, T.; Benedetti, M.; Terzibasi, E.; Roncaglia, P.; Valenzano, D.R.; Cattaneo, A.; Cellerino, A. Annual fishes of the genus *Nothobranchius* as a model system for aging research. *Anat. Soc.* **2005**, *4*, 223–233. [CrossRef]
5. Blazek, R.; Polacik, M.; Reichard, M. Rapid growth, early maturation and short generation time in African annual fishes. *EvoDevo* **2013**, *4*, 24. [CrossRef]
6. Valenzano, D.R.; Terzibasi, E.; Genade, T.; Cattaneo, A.; Domenici, L.; Cellerino, A. Resveratrol prolongs lifespan and retards the onset of age-related markers in a short lived vertebrate. *Curr. Biol* **2006**, *16*, 296–300. [CrossRef]
7. Di Cicco, E.; Terzibasi Tozzini, E.; Rossi, G.; Cellerino, A. The short-lived annual fish *Nothobranchius furzeri* shows a typical teleost aging process reinforced by high incidence of age-dependent neoplasias. *Exp. Gerontol.* **2011**, *46*, 249–256. [CrossRef]
8. Hartmann, N.; Reichwald, K.; Wittig, I.; Dröse, S.; Schmeisser, S.; Lück, C.; Hahn, C.; Graf, M.; Gausmann, U.; Terzibasi, E.; et al. Mitochondrial DNA copy number and function decrease with age in the short-lived fish *Nothobranchius furzeri*. *Anat. Soc.* **2011**, *10*, 824–831.
9. Terzibasi Tozzini, E.; Baumgart, E.; Battistoni, G.; Cellerino, A. Adult neurogenesis in the short-lived teleost *Nothobranchius furzeri*: localization of neurogenic niches, molecular characterization and effects of aging. *Anat. Soc.* **2012**, *11*, 241–251.
10. Valenzano, D.R.; Benayoun, B.A.; Singh, P.P.; Zhang, E.; Etter, P.D.; Hu, C.K.; Clément-Ziza, M.; Wilemesen, D.; Cui, R.; Harel, I.; et al. The African Turquoise Killifish Genome Provides Insights into Evolution and Genetic Architecture of Lifespan. *Cell Press* **2015**, *163*, 1539–1554. [CrossRef]
11. Wang, W.X.; Wilfred, B.R.; Madathil, S.K.; Tang, G.; Hu, Y.; Dimajuga, J.; Stromberg, A.J.; Huang, Q.; Saatman, K.E.; Nelson, P.T. miR-107 Regulates Granulin/Progranulin with Implications for Traumatic Brain Injury and Neurodegenerative Disease. *Am. J. Pathol.* **2010**, *177*, 334–345. [CrossRef]
12. Cohen, S.; Levi-Montalcini, R.; Hamburger, V. A nerve growth-stimulating factor isolated from sarcom as 37 and 180. *Proc. Natl. Acad. Sci. USA* **1954**, *40*, 1014–1018. [CrossRef]
13. Barde, Y.A.; Edgar, D.; Thoenen, H. Purification of a new neurotrophic factor from mammalian brain. *EMBO J.* **1982**, *1*, 549–553. [CrossRef]
14. Leibrock, J.; Lottspeich, F.; Hohn, A.; Hofer, M.; Hengerer, B.; Masiakowski, P.; Thoenen, H.; Barde, Y.A. Molecular cloning and expression of brain-derived neurotrophic factor. *Nature* **1989**, *341*, 149–152. [CrossRef]
15. Lewin, G.R.; Barde, Y.A. Physiology of the neurotrophins. *Annu. Rev. Neurosci.* **1996**, *19*, 289–317. [CrossRef]
16. Lanave, C.; Colangelo, A.M.; Saccone, C.; Alberghina, L. Molecular evolution of the neurotrophin family members and their Trk receptors. *Gene* **2009**, *394*, 1–12. [CrossRef]
17. Chao, M.V. Neurotrophins and their receptors: A convergence point for many signalling pathways. *Nat. Rev. Neurosci.* **2003**, *4*, 299–309. [CrossRef]
18. Reichardt, L.F. Neurotrophin-regulated signalling pathways. *Philos. Trans. R. Soc. Lond. B Biol. Sci.* **2006**, *361*, 1545–1564. [CrossRef]
19. Skaper, S.D. Compartmented chambers for studying neurotrophic factor action. *Methods Mol. Biol.* **2006**, *846*, 213–222.
20. Heinrich, G.; Lum, T. Fish neurotrophins and Trk receptors. *Int. J. Dev. Neurosci.* **2000**, *18*, 1–27. [CrossRef]
21. Götz, R.; Köster, R.; Winkler, C.; Raulf, F.; Lottspeich, F.; Schartl, M.; Thoenen, H. Neurotrophin-6 is a new member of the nerve growth factor family. *Nature* **1994**, *372*, 266–269. [CrossRef]
22. Nilsson, A.S.; Fainzilber, M.; Falck, P.; Ibáñez, C.F. Neurotrophin-7: A novel member of the neurotrophin family from the zebrafish. *FEBS Lett.* **1998**, *424*, 285–290. [CrossRef]
23. Lai, K.O.; Fu, W.Y.; Ip, F.C.; Ip, N.Y. Cloning and expression of a novel neurotrophin, NT-7, from carp. *Mol. Cell Neurosci.* **1998**, *11*, 64–76. [CrossRef]
24. Dethleffsen, K.; Heinrich, G.; Lauth, M.; Knapik, E.W.; Meyer, M. Insert-containing neurotrophins in teleost fish and their relationship to nerve growth factor. *Mol. Cell Neurosci.* **2003**, *24*, 380–394. [CrossRef]
25. Nittoli, V.; Sepe, R.M.; Coppola, U.; D'Agostino, Y.; De Felice, E.; Palladino, A.; Vassalli, Q.A.; Locascio, A.; Ristoratore, F.; Spagnuolo, A.; et al. A comprehensive analysis of neurotrophins and neurotrophin tyrosine kinase receptors expression during development of zebrafish. *J. Comp. Neurol.* **2018**, *526*, 1057–1072. [CrossRef]

26. Terzibasi, E.; Valenzano, D.R.; Benedetti, M.; Roncaglia, P.; Cattaneo, A.; Domenici, L.; Cellerino, A. Large differences in aging phenotype between strains of the short-lived annual fish Nothobranchius furzeri. *PLoS ONE* **2008**, *3*, e3866. [CrossRef]
27. Baumgart, M.; Groth, M.; Priebe, S.; Appelt, J.; Guthke, R.; Platzer, M.; Cellerino, A. Age-dependent regulation of tumor-related microRNA in the brain of the annual fish Nothobranchius furzeri. *Mech. Ageing Dev.* **2012**, *133*, 226–233. [CrossRef]
28. Kumar, S.; Stecher, G.; Li, M.; Knyaz, C.; Tamura, K. MEGA X: Molecular Evolutionary Genetics Analysis across computing platforms. *Mol. Biol. Evol.* **2018**, *35*, 1547–1549. [CrossRef]
29. Untergasser, A.; Nijveen, H.; Rao, X.; Bisseling, T.; Geurts, R.; Leunissen, J.A. Primer3Plus, an enhanced web interface to Primer3. *Nucleic Acids Res.* **2007**, *35*, W71–W74. [CrossRef]
30. Thomsen, R.; Nielsen, P.S.; Jensen, T.H. Dramatically improved RNA in situ hybridization signals using LNA-modified probes. *RNA* **2005**, *11*, 1745–1748. [CrossRef]
31. D'Angelo, L. Brain atlas of an emerging teleostean model: Nothobranchius furzeri. *Anat. Rec. (Hoboken)* **2013**, *296*, 681–691.
32. Petzold, A.; Reichwald, K.; Groth, M.; Taudien, S.; Hartmann, N.; Priebe, S. The transcript catalogue of the short-lived fish Nothobranchius furzeri provides insights into age-dependent changes of mRNA levels. *BMC Genom.* **2013**, *14*, 185. [CrossRef]
33. D'Angelo, L.; de Girolamo, P.; Cellerino, A.; Tozzini, E.T.; Varricchio, E.; Castaldo, L.; Lucini, C. Immunolocalization of S100-like protein in the brain of an emerging model organism: Nothobranchius furzeri. *Microsc. Res Tech.* **2012**, *75*, 441–447. [CrossRef]
34. Zupanc, G.K.; Hinsch, K.; Gage, F.H. Proliferation, migration, neuronal differentiation, and long-term survival of new cells in the adult zebrafish brain. *J. Comp. Neurol.* **2005**, *488*, 290–319. [CrossRef]
35. Pellegrini, E.; Mouriec, K.; Anglade, I.; Menuet, A.; Le Page, Y.; Gueguen, M.M.; Marmignon, M.H.; Brion, F.; Pakdel, F.; Kah, O. Identification of aromatase-positive radial glial cells as progenitor cells in the ventricular layer of the forebrain in zebrafish. *J. Comp. Neurol.* **2007**, *501*, 150–167. [CrossRef]
36. Kroehne, V.; Freudenreich, D.; Hans, S.; Kaslin, J.; Brand, M. Regeneration of the adult zebrafish brain from neurogenic radial glia-type progenitors. *Development* **2011**, *138*, 4831–4841. [CrossRef]
37. Wohl, S.G.; Reh, T.A. miR-124-9-9* potentiates Ascl1-induced reprogramming of cultured Müller glia. *Glia* **2016**, *64*, 743–762. [CrossRef]
38. Olivera-Pasilio, V.; Lasserre, M.; Castellò, M.E. Cell Proliferation, Migration, and Neurogenesis in the Adult Brain of the Pulse Type Weakly Electric Fish, Gymnotus omarorum. *Front. Neurosci.* **2017**, *11*, 437. [CrossRef]
39. Cacialli, P.; D'angelo, L.; Kah, O.; Coumailleau, P.; Gueguen, M.M.; Pellegrini, E.; Lucini, C. Neuronal expression of brain derived neurotrophic factor in the injured telencephalon of adult zebrafish. *J. Comp. Neurol.* **2018**, *526*, 569–582. [CrossRef]
40. Iulita, F.M.; Cuello, C.A. The NGF Metabolic Pathway in the CNS and its Dysregulation in Down Syndrome and Alzheimer's Disease. *Curr. Alzheimer Res.* **2016**, *13*, 53–67. [CrossRef]
41. Peng, S.; Wuu, J.; Mufson, E.J.; Fahnestock, M. Precursor form of brain-derived neurotrophic factor and mature brain-derived neurotrophic factor are decreased in the pre-clinical stages of Alzheimer's disease. *J. Neurochem.* **2005**, *93*, 1412–1421. [CrossRef]
42. Hallböök, F.; Lundin, L.G.; Kullander, K. Lampetra fluviatilis neurotrophin homolog, descendant of a neurotrophin ancestor, discloses the early molecular evolution of neurotrophins in the vertebrate subphylum. *J. Neurosci.* **1999**, *18*, 8700–8711. [CrossRef]
43. Hallböök, F.; Wilson, K.; Thorndyke, M.; Olinski, R.P. Formation and evolution of the chordate neurotrophin and Trk receptor genes. *Brain Behav. Evol.* **2006**, *68*, 133–144. [CrossRef]
44. Huang, E.J.; Reichardt, L.F. Neurotrophins: Roles in neuronal development and function. *Annu. Rev. Neurosci.* **2001**, *24*, 677–736. [CrossRef]
45. Válóczi, A.; Hornyik, C.; Varga, N.; Burgyán, J.; Kauppinen, S.; Havelda, Z. Sensitive and specific detection of microRNAs by northern blot analysis using LNA-modified oligonucleotide probes. *Nucleic Acids Res.* **2004**, *32*, e175. [CrossRef]
46. Kloosterman, W.P.; Wienhold, E.; de Bruijn, E.; Kauppinen, S.; Plasterk, R.H. In situ detection of miRNAs in animal embryos using LNA-modified oligonucleotide probes. *Nat. Methods* **2006**, *3*, 27–29. [CrossRef]
47. Darnell, D.K.; Stanislaw, S.; Kaur, S.; Antin, P.B. Whole mount in situ hybridization detection of mRNAs using short LNA containing DNA oligonucleotide probes. *RNA* **2010**, *16*, 632–637. [CrossRef]

48. Darnell, D.K.; Antin, P.B. LNA-based in situ hybridization detection of mRNAs in embryos. *Methods Mol. Biol.* **2014**, *1211*, 69–76.
49. McTigue, P.M.; Peterson, R.J.; Kahn, J.D. Sequence-dependent thermodynamic parameters for locked nucleic acid (LNA)-DNA duplex formation. *Biochem* **2004**, *43*, 5388–5405. [CrossRef]
50. D'Angelo, L.; de Girolamo, P.; Lucini, C.; Terzibasi, E.T.; Baumgart, M.; Castaldo, L.; Cellerino, A. Brain-derived neurotrophic factor: mRNA expression and protein distribution in the brain of the teleost Nothobranchius furzeri. *J. Comp. Neurol.* **2014**, *522*, 100–430.
51. D'Angelo, L.; Castaldo, L.; Cellerino, A.; de Girolamo, P.; Lucini, C. Nerve growth factor in the adult brain of a teleostean model for aging research: Nothobranchius furzeri. *Ann. Anat.* **2014**, *196*, 183–191. [CrossRef]
52. D'Angelo, L.; Avallone, L.; Cellerino, A.; de Girolamo, P.; Paolucci, M.; Varricchio, E.; Lucini, C. Neurotrophin-4 in the brain of adult Nothobranchius furzeri. *Ann. Anat.* **2016**, *207*, 47–54. [CrossRef] [PubMed]
53. Dalton, V.S.; Borich, S.M.; Murphy, P.; Roberts, B.L. Brain-derived neurotrophic factor mRNA expression in the brain of the teleost fish, Anguilla anguilla, the European Eel. *Brain Behav. Evol.* **2009**, *73*, 43–58. [CrossRef] [PubMed]
54. Cacialli, P.; Gueguen, M.M.; Coumailleau, P.; D'Angelo, L.; Kah, O.; Lucini, C.; Pellegrini, E. BDNF Expression in Larval and Adult Zebrafish Brain: Distribution and Cell Identification. *PLoS ONE* **2016**, *11*, e0158057. [CrossRef]
55. Cacialli, P.; Gatta, C.; D'Angelo, L.; Leggieri, A.; Palladino, A.; de Girolamo, P.; Pellegrini, E.; Lucini, C. Nerve growth factor is expressed and stored in central neurons of adult zebrafish. *J. Anat.* **2019**. [CrossRef]
56. Park, H.; Poo, M.M. Neurotrophin regulation of neural circuit development and function. *Nat. Rev. Neurosci.* **2013**, *14*, 7–23. [CrossRef] [PubMed]

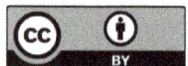

© 2019 by the authors. Licensee MDPI, Basel, Switzerland. This article is an open access article distributed under the terms and conditions of the Creative Commons Attribution (CC BY) license (http://creativecommons.org/licenses/by/4.0/).

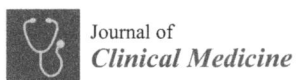

Article

Ontogenetic Pattern Changes of Nucleobindin-2/Nesfatin-1 in the Brain and Intestinal Bulb of the Short Lived African Turquoise Killifish

Alessia Montesano [1,2,3,†], Elena De Felice [4,†], Adele Leggieri [1], Antonio Palladino [5], Carla Lucini [1], Paola Scocco [4], Paolo de Girolamo [1], Mario Baumgart [2,‡] and Livia D'Angelo [1,6,*,‡]

1. Department of Veterinary Medicine and Animal Production, University of Naples Federico II, 80137 Naples, Italy; alessia.montesano@leibniz-hki.de (A.M.); adele.leggieri@unina.it (A.L.); lucini@unina.it (C.L.); degirola@unina.it (P.d.G.)
2. Leibniz Institute on Aging–Fritz Lipmann Institute, 07745 Jena, Germany; mario.baumgart@leibniz-fli.de
3. Leibniz Institute for Natural Product Research and Infection Biology–Hans Knöll Institute, 07745 Jena, Germany
4. School of Bioscience and Veterinary Medicine, University of Camerino, 62032 Camerino, Italy; elena.defelice@unicam.it (E.D.F.); paola.scocco@unicam.it (P.S.)
5. Center for Advanced Biomaterials for Health Care, IIT@CRIB, Istituto Italiano di Tecnologia, 80125 Naples, Italy; a.palladino1986@gmail.com
6. Stazione Zoologica Anton Dohrn, 80122 Naples, Italy
* Correspondence: livia.dangelo@unina.it; Tel.: +39-081-253-6131; Fax: +39-081-253-6097
† Alessia Montesano and Elena De Felice shared first co-autorship.
‡ Mario Baugmart and Livia D'Angelo shared senior co-autorship.

Received: 21 November 2019; Accepted: 24 December 2019; Published: 31 December 2019

Abstract: Nesfatin-1 (Nesf-1) was identified as an anorexigenic and well conserved molecule in rodents and fish. While tissue distribution of NUCB2 (Nucleobindin 2)/Nesf-1 is discretely known in vertebrates, reports on ontogenetic expression are scarce. Here, we examine the age-related central and peripheral expression of NUCB2/Nesf-1 in the teleost African turquoise killifish *Nothobranchius furzeri*, a consolidated model organism for aging research. We focused our analysis on brain areas responsible for the regulation of food intake and the rostral intestinal bulb, which is analogous of the mammalian stomach. We hypothesize that in our model, the stomach equivalent structure is the main source of NUCB2 mRNA, displaying higher expression levels than those observed in the brain, mainly during aging. Remarkably, its expression significantly increased in the rostral intestinal bulb compared to the brain, which is likely due to the typical anorexia of aging. When analyzing the pattern of expression, we confirmed the distribution in diencephalic areas involved in food intake regulation at all age stages. Interestingly, in the rostral bulb, NUCB2 mRNA was localized in the lining epithelium of young and old animals, while Nesf-1 immunoreactive cells were distributed in the submucosae. Taken together, our results represent a useful basis for gaining deeper knowledge regarding the mechanisms that regulate food intake during vertebrate aging.

Keywords: Nesf-1; vertebrate; *Nothobranchius furzeri*; aging; brain-gut axis

1. Introduction

Nucleobindin (NUCB) belongs to the family of calcium and DNA binding proteins and comprises two members, NUCB1 and NUCB2. In mammals, NUCB1 is expressed within the pituitary, liver, and kidney, where it regulates calcium homeostasis and G protein signaling [1,2], while NUCB2 is expressed in the appetite-controlling hypothalamic nuclei, such as the lateral area of the hypothalamus (LHA), paraventricular nucleus (PV), arcuate nucleus (ARC), supraoptic nucleus (SON), tractus solitarius nucleus (NTS), and dorsal nucleus of the vagus [3]. NUCB2 is post-translationally cleaved by prohormone convertases into one N-terminal fragment, Nesfatin-1 (residues 1–82), and two C-terminal peptides, Nesfatin-2 (residues 85–163) and Nesfatin-3 (residues 166–396) [4]. Only the mid-segment of Nesfatin-1 (Nesf-1) is considered the bioactive core, exercising anorexigenic effects [3–5]. In fact, Kohno and colleagues [6] showed that in PV and SON nuclei, which are immunoreactive (ir) to oxytocin and vasopressin, Nesf-1 positive neurons play a key role in the post-prandial regulation of food intake and peripheral metabolism. Hypothalamic neurons which co-expressed Nesf-1, antidiuretic hormone (ADH), corticotropin (CRH), and thyrotropin-releasing hormone (TRH) constitute an important network which regulates food intake. This network acts through the anorexigenic system of the melanocortin above all. It has been shown that the intracerebro-ventricular administration of both NUCB2 and Nesf-1 reduces food intake and body weight as well as increases sympathetic nerve activity and blood pressure in rats [3]. However, the use of anti-Nesf-1 antibodies is not enough to inhibit the sense of satiety induced by leptin: therefore, Nesf-1 is an anorexigenic molecule with a leptin-independent action in mammals [7]. As with many other central appetite regulators, NUCB2/Nesf-1 was also detected in peripheral tissues in different vertebrate models that had an important role in energy homeostasis, such as adipose tissue [8], pancreas [9,10], and in middle and lower segments of gastric mucosal glands [11], as well as in the submucosal layer of the duodenum [9]. Stengel and colleagues described NUCB2/Nesf-1 in the gastric X/A-like endocrine cells of the stomach and showed co-localization with the orexigenic hormone ghrelin in mammals. Moreover, expression levels of NUCB2/Nesf-1 in purified small endocrine cells of gastric mucosa have been reported to be 10-fold higher compared to brain levels [11]. Based on these indications, the stomach is considered one of the main sources of circulating NUCB2/Nesf-1 [12], supporting the hypothesis that NUCB2 is cleaved and Nesf-1 is produced at the gastric level [13].

In the last few years, several studies have described the distribution pattern of NUCB2/Nesf-1, also reporting the appetite regulatory effect in non-mammalian vertebrates. Particularly, in teleost fish, NUCB2 mRNA is widely expressed in central and peripheral tissues, mostly in the brain and gut. Similarly to mammals, the highest NUCB2/Nesf-1 mRNA expression was found in the gastrointestinal tract [14–16]. Nesf-1 ir-cells were found in the feeding regulatory nuclei of the hypothalamus and anterior intestine of the goldfish [14] and in the mucosal cellular layer of the anterior gastrointestinal tract in zebrafish [16]. NUCB2/Nesf-1 and ghrelin co-localize in the enteroendocrine cells of the anterior intestine [17] and in the hepatopancreas of goldfish [18], in the gut mucosal cells of zebrafish [16], and in intestinal enteroendocrine cells of pejerry [19]. Furthermore, the anorexigenic role of Nesf-1 seems to also be conserved in goldfish and Ya-fish, where central or peripheral administration of Nesf-1 induces feeding behavior suppression [14,15,17] as well as in Siberian sturgeon, where it acts through the cholecystokinin signal pathway [20,21].

Despite the fact that tissue distribution patterns are well described in vertebrates, few studies are dedicated to the determination of the expression of NUCB2 mRNA and Nesf-1 immunoreactivity during ontogenesis and postnatal development. Mohan and Unniappan [22] demonstrated that NUCB2/Nesf-1 immunoreactivity in the pancreas and gastrointestinal tract of rats increased from embryonic day 21 through to postnatal day 27, which is likely related to weaning. Senin and colleagues [23] confirmed and expanded previous data on gastroenteropancreatic tissues of rats by analyzing NUCB2/Nesf-1 expression from 2 until 8 weeks of age, corresponding to adulthood. However, there are no reports regarding age-related changes of NUCB2/Nesf-1 in the brain and stomach of any vertebrate. Here, we investigate the expression of Nesf-1 in the African turquoise killifish *Nothobranchius furzeri*, a well consolidated model organism for aging research. *N. furzeri* is the shortest-lived vertebrate that can be kept in captivity, with a lifespan of certain strains of 4 to 6 months in optimal laboratory conditions (6–10 times shorter than the lifespan of mice and zebrafish, respectively) [24]. In fact, *N. furzeri* is characterized by rapid growth, early sexual maturation [25,26], and the development of several biomarkers of aging during the short lifespan [27].

Thus, the aim of the present study is to investigate for the first time the age-related central and peripheral expression of NUCB2/Nesf-1 in *N. furzeri*, achieving deeper knowledge in food intake regulation during aging. Additionally, this study contributes to widely characterize the food intake regulation of the African turquoise killifish [28] and enrich data on neuropeptides that regulate food intake in fish [29–32].

2. Materials and Methods

2.1. Protocols and Ethics Statement

All experiments were performed on group-housed *N. furzeri* belonging to the long-lived strain MZM 04/10 (Leibniz Institute on Aging Friz-Lipmann Institute, Germany, Jena) at the following time points: 5 weeks post hatching (wph) (young-adult) and 27 wph (onset of aging-related features). Animal maintenance was performed as described [24]. Animals were bred and kept in FLI's fish facility according to paragraph 11 of the German Animal Welfare Act. The protocols of animal maintenance were approved by the local authority in the State of Thuringia (Veterinaer- und Lebensmittelueberwachungsamt) with license number J-003798. Euthanasia and organ harvesting was performed according to paragraph 4 (3) of the German Animal Welfare Act and The Council of The European Union Directive of 22nd of September 2010 (2010/63/UE).

2.2. Animals and Tissue Preparation

Fish at the selected time point were euthanized at 10 a.m. with an overdose of anesthetics. Fish, without prior sedation, were placed in a buffered Tricaine methanesulfonate solution (MS-222, TricanePharmaq, Pharmaq) at a concentration of 1 mg/mL for approximately 5–10 min until no vital signs were observed (body and operculum movement, righting reflex), followed by decapitation. The whole heads, brains, and intestines were dissected and processed according to the experimental protocols. For RNA extraction, brains were immediately processed as described in Baumgart et al. 2014 [33]. For morphological analysis, the whole heads were opened by a small incision to allow penetration of a fixative and were fixed in paraformaldehyde (PFA, 4% in diethylpyrocarbonate treated phosphate saline buffer (PBS)) overnight (ON) at 4 °C and the brains were prepared the next day to maintain structural integrity. For cryostatic embedding, tissues were successively incubated in 20% and 30% sucrose solution ON at 4 °C, embedded in cryomount (Tissue-Tek® O.C.T.™, Sakura Finetek USA Inc., Torrance, CA, USA), and frozen at −80 °C. Serial coronal sections of 14 µm thickness for the brain and sagittal sections of 16 µm for the intestine were cut with a Leica cryostat (Deerfield, IL, USA). For paraffin embedding, tissues were dehydrated in a graded ethanol series, embedded in paraffin, and serial coronal 7 µm thick sections were cut at the microtome.

2.3. Sequence Analysis

N. furzeri NUCB2 gene structure was recovered from the *Nothobranchius furzeri* Genome Browser–NFINgb [34], while human, mouse, and zebrafish sequences were recovered from the Ensembl Genome Browser [35]. The gene structure analysis was based on sequences retrieved by the Ensembl Genome Browser (Table S1). The evolutionary history was inferred using the Minimum Evolution method [36]. The optimal tree with the sum of branch length = 3.06014219 is shown. The tree is drawn to scale, with branch lengths in the same units as those of the evolutionary distances used to infer the phylogenetic tree. The evolutionary distances were computed using the Poisson correction method [37] and are in the units of the number of amino acid substitutions per site. The ME tree was searched using the Close-Neighbor-Interchange (CNI) algorithm [38] at a search level of 1. The Neighbor-joining algorithm [39] was used to generate the initial tree. This analysis involved 5 amino acid sequences. All ambiguous positions were removed for each sequence pair (pairwise deletion option). There were a total of 496 positions in the final dataset. Evolutionary analyses were conducted in MEGA X [40]. NUCB2 aminoacidic sequences were recovered from the National Center for Biotechnology Information–NCBI [41] and the alignment was performed using Clustal

Omega [42]. Identity percentage among sequences was calculated with the Basic local alignment search tool—Blast [43].

2.4. RNA Extraction and Reverse Transcription of cDNA Synthesis

Homogenization of tissues was performed using a Tissue Lyzer II (Qiagen, Hilden, Germany) at 20 Hz for 2 to 3 rounds × 1 min [44]. Total RNA was quantized with a NanoDrop 1000 (PeqLab, Erlangen, Germany). Then, 500 ng of each sample was retro-transcribed in a total reaction volume of 20 µL using the QuantiTect® Reverse Transcription Kit (Qiagen), following the supplier's protocol. The cDNAs were diluted to a final volume of 200 µL with nuclease-free water (Qiagen) and stored at −20° C.

2.5. Quantitative Real Time PCR

Primers were designed with Primer3 tool [45]: forward and reverse primers were always located in two different exons. The primers that were used were summarized in Table S2. The correct amplicon size was verified by 1% agarose-gel electrophoresis. Real-time PCR reactions were performed in 20 µL volume with 1 µL diluted cDNA using the Quantitect® SYBR Green PCR kit (Qiagen) following the manufacturer's instructions. A cDNA pool was serially diluted (from 80 to 2.5 ng per reaction) and used to create standard as well as melting curves and to calculate amplification efficiencies for the primer pair prior to use for quantification. All reactions were performed in triplicates and negative (water) as well as genomic (without reverse transcriptase) controls were always included.

2.6. Statistical Analysis

We analyzed the expression levels NUCB2 mRNA in the whole brain and stomach of 22 animals in total at 5 wph ($n = 12$) and 27 wph ($n = 10$). Expression levels were analyzed by the $\Delta\Delta Ct$ method and normalized to the housekeeping gene TATA box binding protein (TBP) (Table S2). Fold changes represent the normalized fold difference in expression levels relative to 5 weeks-old brain. T-test and p-value were calculated with Graphpad Prism among young and old brains and young and old rostral intestinal bulbs. Furthermore, T-test and p-value were also calculated for young brains versus young intestinal bulbs and old brains versus old intestinal bulbs.

2.7. Riboprobes Synthesis

mRNA probes to identify NUCB2B were synthesized by *in vitro* transcription (IVT). Oligonucleotide primers were designed using Primer3 software [45]. Reverse primer contained a T7-promotor sequence to allow direct IVT and the experiment was carried out by means of a DIG RNA labeling mix containing digoxigenin-11-dUTP (Roche, cat. 11277073910). Primers sequences that were used for this study are summarized in Table S2. Primers were diluted to a final concentration of 10 pM. A standard PCR was run to amplify the target region prior to IVT and the amplicon was checked by agarose electrophoresis. Alignment of the obtained sequences was performed by MEGA X software (Molecular Evolutionary Genetics Analysis from www.megasoftware.net) to validate the expected sequence of the amplicon. The concentration of the mRNA probe was measured using the Nanodrop® (Thermo Scientific, Waltham, MA, USA) system.

2.8. In Situ Hybridization

In situ hybridization (ISH) experiments have been conducted on brain and intestine sections and by means of sterile solutions and materials. Dyethilpyrocarbonate (DEPC) was added to millipore water (1 mL/L) to inactivate RNases, shaken and autoclaved. All solutions that were used in the steps until probe revelation were made with RNase free water and RNAse free conditions were kept during all prehybridization and hybridization steps.

Sections were dried for 2 h at room temperature (RT), washed well in 1× DEPC/PBS, and treated with 10 μg/μL Proteinase K (Sigma–Aldrich) 1:200 in 1× DEPC/PBS for 10 min. Proteinase K was inactivated by two washes in 2 mg/mL glycine, 5 min each. Sections were post fixed in 4% PFA for 20 min and well washed in 1× DEPC/PBS at RT. Prehybridization was carried out in a hybridization solution containing 50% formamide, 0.5% SSC (Saline-Sodium Citrate), 500 μg. Heparin, 50 μg/mL yeast RNA, and 0.1% Tween 20 at 55 °C for 1 h. Probes were denatured for 10 min at −80 °C and sections were then incubated ON at 55 °C in hybridization solution containing antisense NUCB2B probe at a concentration of 2 ng/μL. Post hybridization washes were carried out at 55 °C as follows: 2 × 20 min in 1× SSC, 2 × 10 min in 0.5× SSC and then in PBS added with tween20 (PBT) at RT. The sections were blocked with a blocking solution (BS) containing 10% normal sheep serum heat inactivated and 0.5% blocking reagent (Roche, Basel, Switzerland, cat. 11096176001) for 1 h at RT. Sections were incubated ON at 4 °C in fresh blocking buffer containing a 1:2000 dilution of anti-digoxigenin Fab fragments conjugated with alkaline phosphatase (Roche, cat. 11093274910). After washing in PBS and levamisole (Vector Labs., Burlingame, CA, USA, SP-5000), the reaction was developed using Fast Red substrate (Roche, cat. 11496549001) under periodic inspection with an epifluorescence microscope. To stop the reaction, the sections were washed repeatedly in PBT and mounted with Fluoroshield Mounting Medium with DAPI (IBSC, Hermon, ME, USA, cat. AR-6501-0) as counterstaining for the nuclei.

2.9. Western Blot

Brain samples of young and old fish were extracted in RIPA buffer (Radio Immuno Precipitation Assay) with Lysis buffer (50 mM Tris–HCl pH 7.4, 1% Triton X-100, 0.25% Na-deoxycholate, 150 mM NaCl, 1 mM EDTA), containing protease inhibitors 2 mM phenylmethylsulfonyl fluoride (PMSF) and protease inhibitor cocktail (P8340; Sigma-Aldrich, St. Louis, MO, USA). Samples were homogenized with an Ultra-Turrax T25 (IKA Labortechnik, Staufer, Germany) at 13,500 rpm. Homogenates were centrifuged 15,000 rpm for 30 min at 4 °C; supernatants were collected separately and the protein concentration was determined with Bio-Rad dye protein assay (Bio-Rad Laboratories Inc., Hemel Hempstead, UK). For each sample, 20 μL of protein were boiled at 100 °C for 10 min in 20 μL of 2× loading buffer (50 mM Tris–HCl pH 6.8, 100 mM b-mercaptoethanol, 4% SDS, 0.1% blue bromophenol, 10% glycerol). Proteins were separated on a 12% SDS–polyacrylamide gel electrophoresis with 4% stacking gel in 1% Tris–glycine buffer (0.025 M Tris, 0.190 M glycine, and 0.1%SDS [pH 8.3]) in a miniprotean cell (Bio-Rad) at 100 V for 2 h. The separated proteins were electro-transferred on a nitrocellulose membrane with transfer buffer (48 mM Tris base, 39 mM glycine, 0.04% SDS, and 20% methanol [pH 8.5]) in a minitransfer cell (Bio-Rad) at 100 V at 4 °C for 1 h. Membranes were incubated at 4 °C for 1 h in blocking buffer containing 1% PBS and 0.05% Tween 20 with 5% dry non-fat milk and probed with polyclonal antibody raised in rabbit against Nesf-1 (H-003-24; Phoenix Pharmaceuticals; Belmont, CA, USA) and β-actin (A5060, Sigma, St. Louis, MO, USA) used as an internal marker. Primary antibody was diluted 1:2000 and incubated overnight at 4 °C, followed by incubation with the secondary goat anti-rabbit IgG (Sigma 1:3000) antibody for 1 h at RT. Signals were detected by chemoluminescence with the Pico Enhanced Chemiluminescence Kit (Pierce Chemical) with Chemidoc (Bio-Rad, Hercules, CA, USA). A pre-stained molecular-weight ladder (Novex Sharp Pre-Stained Protein Standard, Life Technologies, Monza, Italy) was used to determine protein size. Specificity was determined by pre-absorption of primary antibodies with their relative control peptides before western blotting.

2.10. Immunohistochemistry

Immunohistochemistry (IHC) was conducted on both paraffin and cryosections of brain and intestine. Paraffin slides were deparaffinized in xylene and rehydrated in progressively diluted alcohols, while cryosections were dried for 2 h at RT, placed in a bath of acetone 100% for 10 min at 4 °C, air-dried for a few minutes, and washed once in water and twice in 1× PBS. Then, both slides were treated for 30 min with 3% H_2O_2 and, after washing with 1× PBS, were incubated in normal goat serum (1:5 in 1×

PBS) at RT for 30 min. Incubation with primary polyclonal antibody raised in rabbit against Nesf-1 (1:1000, H-003-24; Phoenix Pharmaceuticals; Belmont, CA, USA) was performed at 4 °C ON. Sections were rinsed in 1× PBS for 15 min and incubated with EnVision reagent (DAKO, K406511) for 30 min at RT. Immunoreactive sites were visualized using a fresh solution of 10 µg of 3,3′-diaminobenzidine tetrahydrochloride (DAB, Sigma-Aldrich, #D5905) in 15 mL of a 0.5 M Tris buffer.

2.11. Controls of Specificity

The specificity of each in situ hybridization reaction was checked in repeated trials using sense NUCB probe at a concentration of 2 ng/µL.

The specificity of each immunohistochemical reaction was checked in repeated trials via pre-absorption of primary antibody Nesf-1 (H-003-24; Phoenix Pharmaceuticals) with homologous antigen Nesf-1 (1–45)/Nesf-1, N-terminal (Human) (003-24; Phoenix pharmaceuticals) (up to 50 mg/mL antiserum in the final dilution). Positive controls were made by sections of rat testis [10]. Internal reaction controls were carried out by substituting primary antisera or secondary antisera with 1× PBS or normal serum in the specific step.

2.12. Image Acquisition

Fluorescent and light images were observed and analyzed with Zeiss Apotome and processed with Zeiss blue software. Digital raw images were optimized for image resolution, contrast, evenness of illumination, and background using Adobe Photoshop CC 2018 (Adobe Systems, San Jose, CA, USA). Anatomical structures were identified according to the adult *N. furzeri* brain atlas [46]. The immunoreactive cells in the rostral intestinal bulb have been counted. The cell count was carried out manually by using an open source image-processing program (ImageJ). Cells were identified on the basis of their morphological aspect.

3. Results

3.1. Sequence Analysis and Antibody Specificity

The structure of the gene consisted of 13 exons and 12 introns (Figure 1A). Due to the third round of whole-genome duplication in teleost, two paralogues are present in the genome of *N. furzeri*: NUCB2A and NUCB2B. Sequences were obtained from the *Nothobranchius furzeri* Genome Browser–NFINgb (https://nfingb.leibniz-fli.de/): accession number was Nfu_g_1_003870 for NUCB2A and Nfu_g_1_018131 for NUCB2B [34]. Even if the differences between NUCB2A and NUCB2B are very slight, we designed primers to detect only NUCB2B, since it has a higher evolutionary conservation towards mice or humans (Figure 1B). As a result, the primers for generating the ISH probe as well as the qPCR primer bound only to the NUCB2B transcript and the synthetized probe showed 100% identity to NUCB2B (in total 417 nucleotides, transcript position 210 to 626), whereas the identity to NUCB2A was only 36% (in total, 154 nucleotides: transcript position 247 to 341 with 16 mismatches, position 358 to 402 with 6 mismatches, and position 535 to 575 with 5 mismatches).

In *N. furzeri*, like in other fish, Nesf-1 is an 81 amino acid anorexigenic peptide (82 in mammals) encoded in the N-terminal of its translated precursor, nucleobindin-2 (NUCB2). *N. furzeri* Nesf-1 protein sequence showed an overall identity of 78% with Nesf-1 of medaka, 73% with zebrafish, 60% with mouse, and 58% with human (Figure 1C). The antibody specificity was tested by western blot. Currently, there are no commercially available antibodies raised against fish sequences and thus, we employed a polyclonal antibody raised against human Nesf-1 (1–45), recognizing a region highly conserved and corresponding to the bioactive segment of the neuropeptides [47]. The western blot revealed a defined band of ~40 kDa in *N. furzeri* brain homogenates of young and old fish (Figure 1D). β-actin, used as an internal marker, showed a band of about 42 kDa.

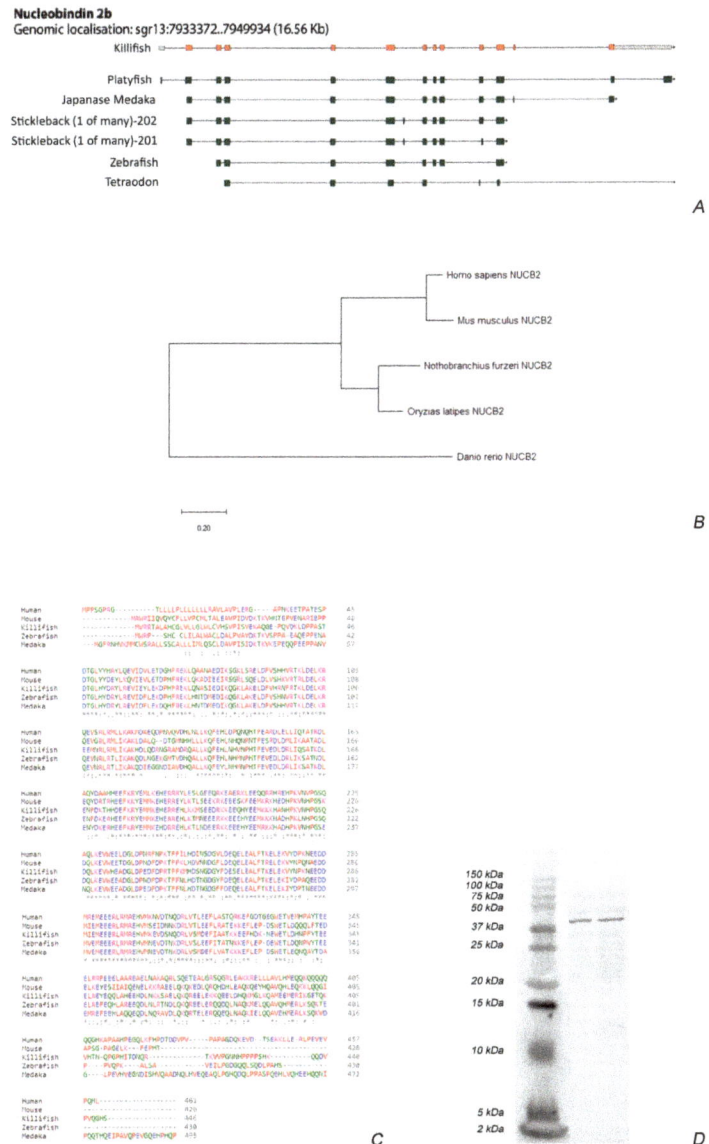

Figure 1. NUCB2B gene structure and Nesfatin–1 peptide analysis: (**A**) NUCB2B intron/exon gene structure of *N. furzeri* and alignment of transcripts from other fish species (downloaded and modified from http://nfingb.leibniz-fli.de/, transcript information for the other fish species can be found at http://www.ensembl.org/). The structure of the two paralogues NUCB2A and NUCB2B were highly similar. In the image, NUCB2B is shown as a template. (**B**) The evolutionary history of NUCB2B peptide sequences was inferred by using the Minimum Evolution method. The phylogenetic tree of amino acid sequences was reconstructed by MEGA X. (**C**) NUCB2B peptide sequence alignments in different species: *Nothobranchus furzeri* (killifish), *Oryzias latipes* (medaka), *Carassius auratus* (goldfish), *Homo sapiens* (human), and *Mus musculus* (mouse). Asterisks mark conserved amino acids (alignment was done with Clustal Omega http://www.ebi.ac.uk/Tools/msa/clustalo/). (**D**) Western blot in the brain of young and old killifish showing an immunoreactive band of about 40 kDa.

3.2. Expression Levels of NUCB2B mRNA in the Whole Brain and in the Rostral Intestinal Bulb of Young and Old Animals

The levels of NUCB2B mRNA varied between the two organs and over age. In the brain, we observed a slight augment of NUCB2B levels in old compared to young animals ($p = 0.0169$). In the rostral intestinal bulb, we did not detect a significant variation in the expression levels of NUCB2B in old animals (Figure 2) compared to young ($p = 0.0591$). Furthermore, we questioned which organ could represent the main source of NUCB2B. At sexual maturity, expression levels of NUCB2B were comparable between the rostral intestinal bulb and brain ($p = 0.5899$), although there was a slight increase in the intestinal bulb; whereas at the old stage, NUCB2B mRNA levels were significantly higher in the rostral intestinal bulb than in the brain ($p = 0.0001$) (Figure 2).

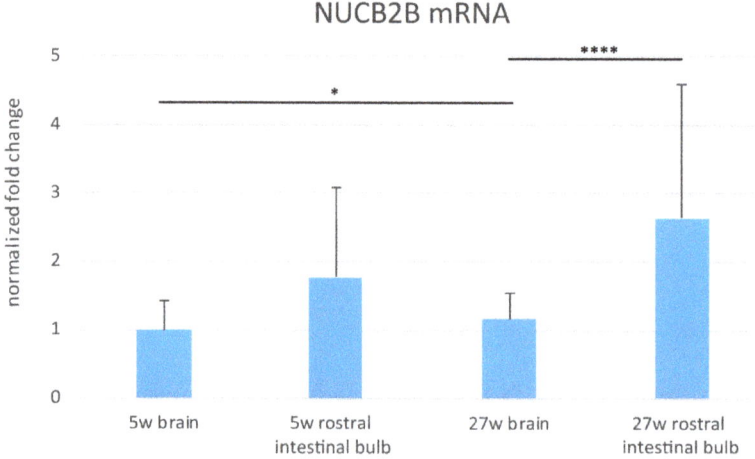

Figure 2. Expression levels of mRNA encoding NUCB2B in the brain and rostral intestinal bulb of young and old *N. furzeri*. The graphic was built on ΔΔCT method and data were normalized to the young brain. T-test and p-value were calculated among young ($n = 12$) and old ($n = 10$) brains and young ($n = 12$) and old ($n = 10$) rostral intestinal bulbs. Furthermore, T-test and *p*-value were also calculated for young brains versus young intestinal bulbs and old brains versus old intestinal bulbs. (p brain old versus young = 0.0169; p rostral intestine bulb old versus young = 0.0591; p young rostral intestinal bulb versus brain = 0.5899; p old rostral intestinal bulb versus brain = 0.0001). (*) indicates the level of significance.

3.3. Morphological Studies of the Whole Brain of Young and Old Animals

In the present study, the attention was focused on the expression and distribution of either mRNA (ISH) and protein (IHC) onto the areas responsible for the regulation of food intake: the ventral part of the telencephalon and the diencephalon in toto. However, positive labeling was also detected outside the above-mentioned areas, such as olfactory bulbs and dorsal telencephalon in the forebrain, optic tectum, and semicircular tori in the midbrain, which are known to mediate food appetite behavior [32]. Table 1 summarizes positive neurons and fibers localization of NUCB2B mRNA/Nesf-1 protein in young and old brains of *N. furzeri*. The neuroanatomical terminology followed the *N. furzeri* brain atlas [46].

Table 1. Summary of positive perikarya and fibers localization of NUCB2B mRNA and Nesf-1 protein in the forebrain of young and old *N. furzeri*.

	Young Brain			Old Brain		
	mRNA	Protein		mRNA	Protein	
	Perikarya	Perikarya	Fibers	Perikarya	Perikarya	Fibers
Telencephalon						
Dorsal Telencephalon						
Sopracommissural Zone of the Ventral Telencephalon (Vs)			+			+
Central Part of the Ventral Telencephalon (Vc)			+			+
Preoptic area						
Preoptic Nucleus, Parvocellular Part (PPp)		+			+	
Cortical Nucleus (CN)	+	+			+	
Lateral Preglomerular Nucleus (PGl)		+			+	
Medial Preglomerular Nucleus (PGm)		+			+	
Tuberal hypothalamus						
Dorsal Hypothalamus (Hd)	+	+	+	+	+	+
Ventral Hypothalamus (Hv)	+	+	+	+	+	+
Caudal Hypothalamus (Hc)	+	+		+	+	
Periventricular Nucleus of Posterior Tuberculum (TPp)			+	+		+
Glomerular Nucleus (NG)		+	+		+	+
Nucleus of Posterior Recess (NRP)	+		+	+		+
Diffuse Inferior Lobe of Hypothalamus (DIL)	+	+	+		+	+
Posterior tubercle						
Paraventricular Organ (PVO)	+	+	+	+	+	+
Thalamus						
Dorsal Posterior Talamic Nucleus (DP)		+			+	
Ventro-Medial Talamic Nucleus (VM)	+	+			+	

3.3.1. In Situ Hybridization

In the diencephalon of young fish, NUCB2B mRNA was detected in neurons of the cortical nucleus (Figure 3E–G). Positive neurons were displayed in the ventro-medial thalamic nucleus (Figures 3E–H and 4C), in the paraventricular organ (Figure 3G–J), and in the periventricular nucleus of the posterior tubercle (Figures 3G–J and 5C–E) along the ventricle. Labelled neurons were found in the dorsal (Figures 3I,J and 4C), central, and ventral part of the hypothalamus (Figure 3G–J), close to the ventricle. Small and intensely positive neurons were detected in the diffuse inferior lobe of the hypothalamus (Figures 3L,M and 4E). In the diencephalon of old fish, some positive neurons were detected in the periventricular nucleus of the posterior tuberculum. Many packed positive neurons were observed in the hypothalamic region, particularly in the dorsal, ventral, lateral, and caudal parts (Figure 5A). Moreover, many neurons were positively stained in the nucleus of posterior recess (Figure 5C–E), unlike in the young subjects.

In addition, in young fish, positive neurons were detected in non-diencephalic areas: along the margin of the dorsal telencephalon (Figures 3A–C and 4A) and in the periventricular grey zone of the optic tectum (Figures 3G and 6A). Conversely, in old fish, only scarcely positive neurons were detected along the margin of the dorsal telencephalon (Figures 5E and 6C).

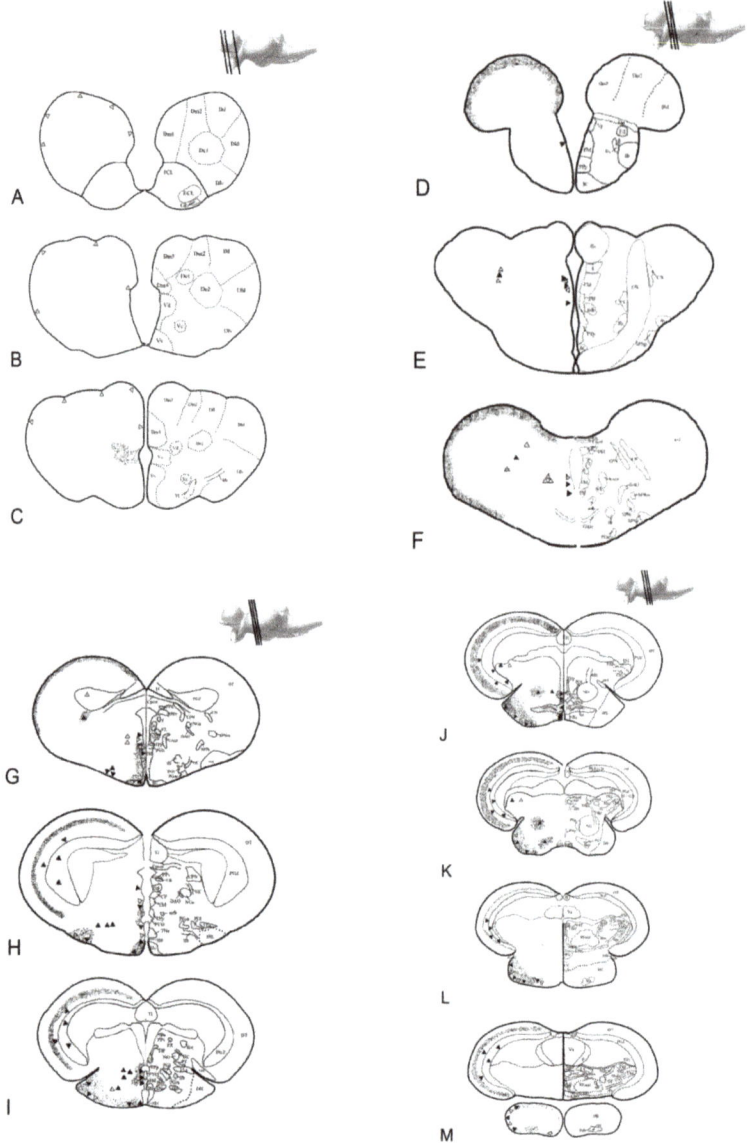

Figure 3. Atlas of NUCB2B gene and Nesf-1 protein distribution: schematic drawings of transversal sections of *N. furzeri* brain [46], specifically referred to (**A–F**) forebrain; (**G–M**) midbrain. White triangles indicate sites of mRNA positive neurons (ISH); black triangles indicate sites of immunopositive neurons (IHC); small dots indicate immunoreactive fibres (IHC). Scale bar: 200 µm.

3.3.2. Immunohistochemistry

In young fish, immunoreactivity to Nesf-1 protein was found in the ventral telencephalon and diencephalon. In the telencephalic ventral areas, especially in the supracommissural zone, abundant positive ir-fibers were observed (Figures 3C and 4B). In the diencephalon, positive neurons were detected in the magno- and parvo-cellular parts of the preoptic nucleus (Figure 3D–F). Also, ir-neurons enveloped in a tight net of projections were visible in the cortical nucleus (Figure 3E–G), preglomerular nucleus, mainly in its medial part (Figure 3G), pretectal nucleus, as well as in the paraventricular organ (Figure 3G–J). Numerous immune-labelled neurons, with a notable quantity of fibers surrounding, was identified in the ventral, dorsal, and caudal parts of the tuberal hypothalamus. Several stained neurons and fibers were recognized in the thalamic nucleus, both dorsal posterior and ventro-medial parts (Figures 3G–J and 4D). Ir-perikarya were located around the margin of the periventricular nucleus of the posterior tuberculum (Figure 3E–G). Many ir-projections were found in the medial part of the glomerular nucleus (Figure 3J,K). Positive ir-neurons were disseminated in the diffuse inferior lobe of the hypothalamus, especially on the external margin (Figures 3K–M and 4F), with some fibers spread in the medial zone. In non-diencephalic regions, several ir-positive neurons were detected in the optic tectum (Figure 6B), especially packed in the periglomerular grey zone (Figure 6B), with projections towards the external margin (Figure 3G–M). Moreover, weakly ir-neuronal cells were widespread in the different layers of semicircular tori (Figure 3J,K).

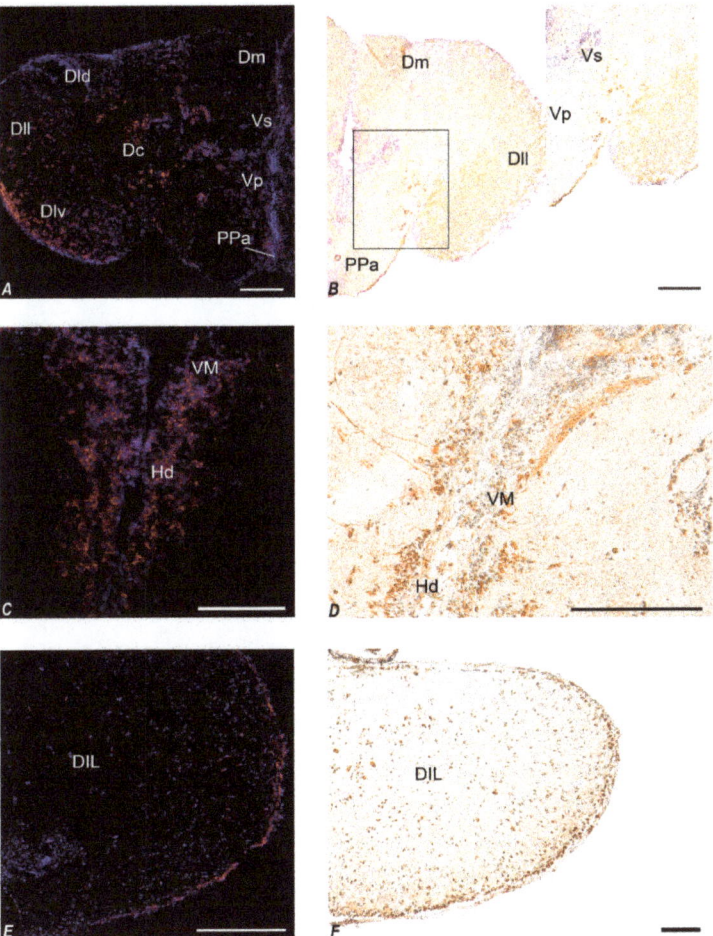

Figure 4. Transversal section showing localization of NUCB2B mRNA and Nesf-1 protein in the young brain of *N. furzeri*. (**A**) NUCB2B expressing neurons in Dc, Dld, Dll, Dlv, Dm, PPa, Vp, and Vs; (**B**) Nesf-1 immunoreactivity (ir) in neurons of Dm, DIL, PPa, Vp, and Vs; (**C**) NUCB2B expressing neurons in VM and Hd; (**D**) Nesf-1 ir in neurons of VM and Hd; (**E**) NUCB2B expressing neurons in DIL; (**F**) Nesf-1 ir in neurons of DIL. Scale bars: A-B-F 100 µm; C-E 200 µm; D 300 µm.

Nesf-1 protein distribution did not show notable differences between the young and elderly subjects (Figures 5B,D,F and 6D).

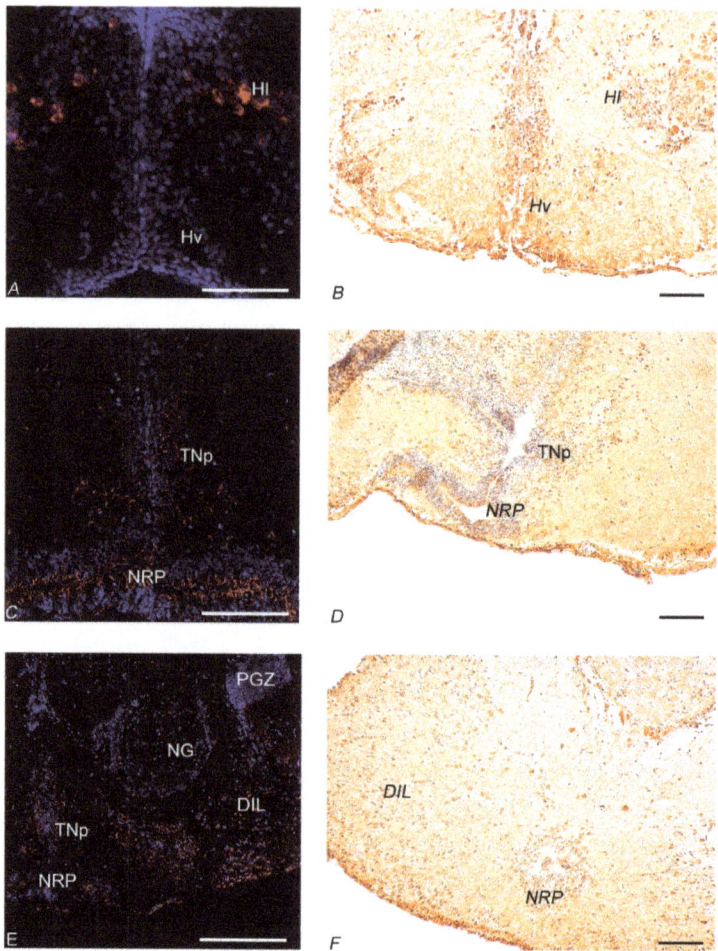

Figure 5. Transversal section showing localization of NUCB2B mRNA and Nesf-1 protein in the brain of old *N. furzeri*. (**A**) NUCB2B expressing neurons in HI and Hv; (**B**) Nesf-1 immunoreactivity (ir) in neurons of HI and Hv; (**C**) NUCB2B expressing neurons in TNp and NRP; (**D**) Nesf-1 ir in neurons of NRP and TNp; (**E**) NUCB2B expressing neurons in DIL, NG, NRP, PGZ, and TNp; (**F**) Nesf-1 ir-neurons of DIL and NRP. Scale bars: A-C-E 200 µm, B-D-F 100 µm.

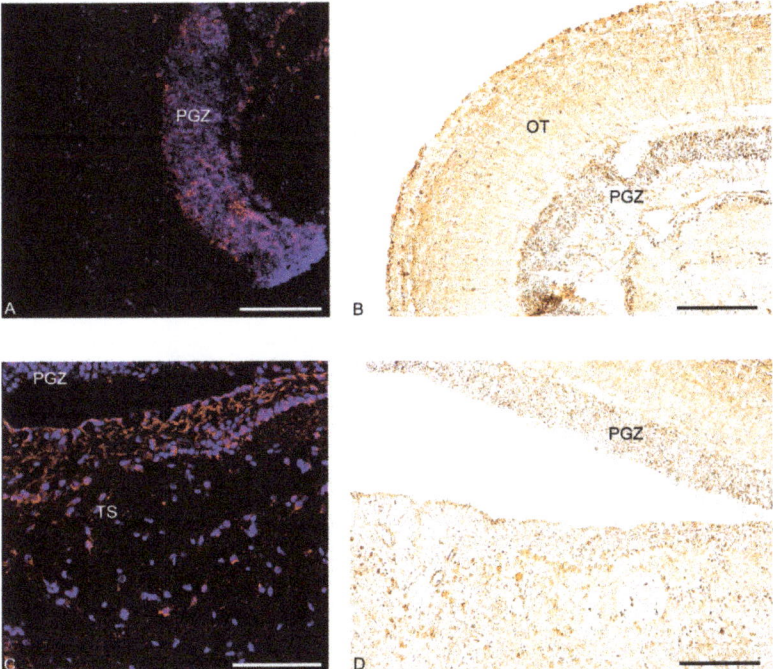

Figure 6. Transversal section showing localization of NUCB2B mRNA and Nesf-1 protein in non-diencephalic regions of *N. furzeri* brain. (**A,B**) young fish: (**A**) NUCB2B expressing neurons in PGZ; (**B**) Nesf-1 immunoreactivity (ir) in neurons of PGZ and OT; (**C,D**) old fish: (**C**) NUCB2B expressing neurons in PGZ and TS; (**D**) Nesf-1 ir-neurons of PGZ. Scale bars: 200 µm.

3.4. Morphological Studies of the Intestine of Young and Old Animals

N. furzeri, as a Cyprinodontiformes species, belongs to the group of agastric fish in which the intestine transits directly from the esophagus [48]. In adults, the intestine is folded into three sections: the rostral intestinal bulb, mid-intestine, and caudal intestine. We focused our analysis on the rostral intestinal bulb, which is known to likely serve a similar function to the mammalian stomach [49]. Sagittal sections of the rostral intestinal bulb reveal a simple architecture of a mucosa, submucosa, muscularis externa, and serosa layer (Figure 7A,B). The intestinal mucosa consists of columnar shaped enterocytes (Figure 7B). We observed that the intestine surface is covered by ridges that are oriented circumferentially across the intestine axis (Figure 7A,B). These ridges in the cross-section resemble the spatially separate villi in the mouse or human small intestine.

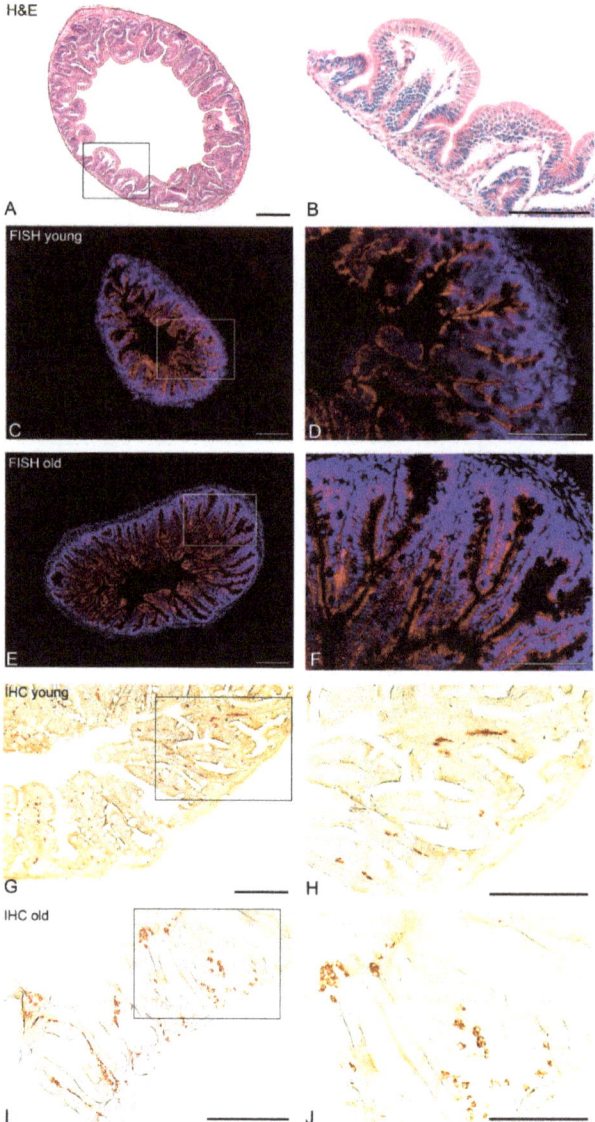

Figure 7. Transversal section showing localization of NUCB2B mRNA and Nesf-1 protein in the rostral intestinal bulb of *N. furzeri*. (**A**) Hematoxylin/eosin staining reveals a simple architecture of a mucosa, submucosa, muscularis externa, and serosa layer; (**B**) Higher magnification of A; (**C**) in young fish NUCB2B mRNA was detected in the lining epithelium; (**D**) Higher magnification of C; (**E**) in old fish, NUCB2B mRNA was detected in the lining epithelium; (**F**) Higher magnification of E; (**G**) in young subjects, Nesf-1-immuonoreactivity (ir) was detected within rounded or flask-shaped cells in submucosa, most of them scattered deep within the folds of the ridges; (**H**) Higher magnification of G; (**I**) in old fish, Nesf-1-ir cells were more abundant in the submucosa and in addition, some of the cells were dispersed along the apical regions of the ridges; (**J**) Higher magnification of I. Scale bars: A-C-E 100 μm, B-D-F-H-I-J 300 μm, G 200 μm.

3.4.1. In Situ Hybridization

In the rostral intestinal bulb of young fish, NUCB2B mRNA was detected in the lining epithelium. Signal was restricted to the columnar shaped enterocytes of the apical regions of the ridges (Figure 7C,D). NUC2B mRNA distribution did not show notable differences between young and old subjects (Figure 7E,F).

3.4.2. Immunohistochemistry

Cross sections of the rostral intestinal bulb of young fish showed Nesf-1 positive rounded or flask-shaped cells in submucosa, mainly scattered deep within the folds of the ridges (Figure 7G,H). In old fish, Nesf-1 ir-cells were more abundant in the submucosa and, in addition, some of the cells were dispersed along the apical regions of the ridges (Figure 7I,J). The number of positive cells did not reveal differences between the young and old animals (Figure S1).

4. Discussion

In the present survey, we characterized NUCB2B/Nesf-1 in the brain and in the mammalian stomach equivalent structure of *N. furzeri* and reported, for the first time, its regulation upon aging in a teleost species.

In fish, two isoforms of NUCB2 (NUCB2A and NUCB2B) exist, which presumably arose due to the teleosts-specific whole genome duplication known as 3R (third round of genome duplication) [50]. Also, in *N. furzeri* [34], two paralogues exist: NUCB2A and NUCB2B. Here, we determined that NUCB2A and NUCB2B gene sequences in killifish are highly similar to NUCB2 from other fish and mammals. This suggests that NUCB2 and its paralogues are highly conserved genes; therefore, Nesf-1 (a product of proteolytic processing of NUCB2 protein) has a similar aminoacid sequence among vertebrates. In fish, the proposed prohormone convertase cleavage site (Lys-Arg) is ubiquitously conserved in both NUCB2A and NUCB2B genes, suggesting that the putative Nesf-1 peptide can be cleaved from the larger NUCB2 precursor [14,15]. We analyzed the distribution of NUCB2B mRNA in the whole brain and the transcript was mainly detected in the hypothalamic nuclei, as previously reported in mammals [3,6,51–54], as well as in other vertebrate species such as frogs [55] and goldfish [14]. In young animals, neurons expressing NUCB2B mRNA were localized in the cortical nucleus, ventro-medial thalamic nucleus, paraventricular organ, and diffuse inferior lobe of the hypothalamus. We also studied Nesf-1 protein distribution by a commercial antibody, detecting the precursor Nesf-1 (1–82). Western blot analysis on the whole brain of *N. furzeri* reveals that the protein is expressed with the expected molecular weight of about 40 kDa, as also reported in goldfish [14] and mammals [51]. In *N. furzeri*, immunoreactivity to Nesf-1 was detected in the hypothalamic area, both in neuronal perikarya and fibers of young and old animals. Some areas, i.e., paraventricular organ and the diffuse inferior lobe of the hypothalamus, displayed positive neurons in ISH and IHC. Interestingly, mRNA expression and protein distribution were also detected in non-diencephalic areas, specifically in the telencephalon, optic tectum, and semicircular tori of both young and old animals. In mammals, Nesf-1 immunoreactivity was observed in non-diencephalic areas as well, including the nucleus of tractus solitarius, another brain region implicated in the regulation of feeding [6,51,52]. Our results in the brain of *N. furzeri* agree with previous observations in goldfish, where immunohistochemical studies showed the presence of Nesf-1-like ir within the hypothalamus and preoptic areas [14]. In teleost fish, both telencephalon and optic tectum are known to be involved in the control of appetite [56]. For example, electrical stimulation of either the ventral telencephalon, secondary gustatory nucleus, or optic tectum induces enhanced feeding behavior [57], whereas feeding behavior is depressed by olfactory tract lesions [57,58]. It might be possible that the presence of NUC2B/Nesf-1 in non-diencephalic areas of *N. furzeri* brain implicates that these areas could also be involved in the regulation of feeding in this species and/or several other homeostatic systems [59].

The primary source of NUCB2/Nesf-1 is currently unknown in vertebrates. In mammals, the expression level of NUCB2 in the stomach was found to be 10-fold higher than the levels of the brain [11], suggesting a prominent role for this organ in the synthesis and secretion of NUCB2/Nesf-1. As the most common teleost fish used as an animal model, such as zebrafish [60], medaka [48], or goldfish [14], *N. furzeri* also has no proper stomach, which is different from what has been reported in a previous paper [31]. According to Smith [61], a true stomach always has mucosal glands producing hydrochloric acid juice and can be closed by a sphincter at its caudal end. In addition, the loss of the stomach phenotype is accompanied by the loss of pepsinogen and gastric proton pump genes [48]. In agastric fish, the intestine transits directly from the esophagus and usually it can be divided into three sections (anterior, mid-intestine, and caudal intestine), where the dilatation of the first section of the intestine (named the rostral intestinal bulb or J-loop) is considered homologous to the mammalian stomach [48]. For the first time, we described the rostral intestinal bulb of *N. furzeri*. The wall of the intestine showed the superposition of four tunicae, which is typical of vertebrates. Genome analysis indicates the absence of pepsinogen gene in *N. furzeri*. In the rostral intestinal bulb, NUCB2B mRNA was detected in the epithelial cells lining while Nesf-1 immunoreactivity was mainly observed in the submucosa. The morphological pattern observed in the intestine of *N. furzeri* agree with previous observations in zebrafish, where NUCB2/nesfatin-1-like ir was detected in most of the cells scattered deep within the folds of the villi of J-loop [16], and disagree with a previous study of goldfish, where Nesf-1-like ir was only detected in enteroendocrine like cells of the intestinal villi [14]. It is likely that NUCB2 concurs to regulate the high turnover of epithelial intestinal cells. Future studies are mandatory to explore the peripheral role of NUCB2B/Nesf-1in *N. furzeri*, taking into consideration that currently the receptor(s) mediating the regulatory mechanisms of actions of Nesf-1 remain unknown [47].

Up to now, this is the first study reporting the regulation of NUCB2/Nesf-1 during aging in a vertebrate model. Interestingly, we document the increase of NUCB2B during aging, with the highest expression at the peripheral level. This could be related to an energy drive failure leading to anorexic phenotype, which indeed is well described and typically occurs during aging [62]. There are enough demonstrations available to indicate that nucleobindin and its encoded peptides have a pleiotropic role in cell biology, such as inhibition of proliferation and enhancing apoptosis [63]. In this context, it is relevant to specify that in the current genome annotation of *N. furzeri*, neither ghrelin nor leptin b were annotated, which are highly conserved during vertebrate evolution. With the exclusion of any annotation error, it is likely that that they are evolutionarily lost. This will be in line with the presence of an anorexic phenotype in old *N. furzeri* and it would elucidate a new role of nesfatin as an independent anorexigenic player in this short-living species.

These results, obtained in a phylogenetically distant vertebrate, highlight the growing evidence in support of a role for Nesf-1 as a novel brain-gut regulatory peptide. The communication between the central nervous system and the gastrointestinal tract plays a fundamental role in the regulation of food intake and energy balance, modulating short-term satiety and hunger responses. This axis also has a role in the regulation of blood glucose levels and adipocyte function [64]. The gut-brain axis has both neuronal and humoral components that convey information to the key brain regions involved in the homeostatic regulation of feeding, located mainly in the hypothalamus (including the arcuate nucleus) and brainstem (including the nucleus tractus solitarius) [65]. A number of gut hormones have been identified in the gastrointestinal system, including Nesf-1 [66], which are released from enteroendocrine cells. In addition to the coordination of the digestive process, they also relay information regarding the current state of energy balance, exerting endocrine effects on other organ systems, particularly the brain, where some have also been found to exist as neurotransmitters [67].

5. Conclusions

In conclusion, the present work provides the first evidence for the occurrence of NUCB2B/Nesf-1 in *N. furzeri* and to the best of our knowledge, it is the first description of aging regulation reported in any vertebrate. We consider that the experimental modulation could contribute to validate the

African turquoise killifish in clinical and preclinical studies. Indeed, in previous work [28], we used 96 h of fasting as a paradigm to better evaluate the regulation of neuropeptides involved in food intake. In that experimental design, 96 h of fasting represents a metabolic stimulus in this species, since we have demonstrated that it is able to activate neurons (pS6 marker), although in the brain of old animals, very few neurons were activated, suggesting that the metabolic stimulus needs to be more intense in old organisms with physiologically low metabolic rates. Based on these evidences, we are planning a similar experiment with a longer starvation period to evaluate the activated metabolic pathways at central and peripheral levels.

Supplementary Materials: The following are available online at http://www.mdpi.com/2077-0383/9/1/103/s1, Figure S1: NESF-1 positive cells in the submucosa of the rostral intestinal bulb of young and old animals. Cell count was carried out manually on 7 consecutive sections by using an open source image-processing program (ImageJ). Cells were identified on the basis of their morphological aspect. The graphical analysis was produced by Excel and did not reveal any significance difference between the two age points studied, Table S1: Ensemble Species Code, Table S2: Summary of primer pair sequences used for Real Time PCR (RT- PCR) and in situ hybridization (ISH).

Author Contributions: Conceptualization, A.M., M.B., and L.D.; Data curation, A.P.; Formal analysis, A.M., A.L., and L.D.; Funding acquisition, P.d.G.; Investigation, A.M., E.D.F., and A.L.; Project administration, M.B. and L.D.; Supervision, P.d.G. and M.B.; Validation, A.M. and E.D.F.; Visualization, E.D.F. and L.D.; Writing—original draft, E.D.F.; Writing—review & editing, C.L., P.S., and M.B. All authors have read and agreed to the published version of the manuscript.

Funding: This work was supported by a grant from the University of Naples Federico II (DR/2017/409-Project F.I.A.T.).

Acknowledgments: We are grateful to Alessandro Cellerino for their critical revision of the work. We thank Sabine Matz for their technical work and Antonio Calamo for their imaging assistance.

Conflicts of Interest: The authors declare no conflict of interest.

Abbreviations

Dc	central zone of dorsal telencephalon
Dld	dorso-lateral zone of dorsal telencephalon
Dll	latero-lateral zone of dorsal telencephalon
Dlv	ventro-lateral zone of dorsal telencephalon
Dm	medial zone of dorsal telencephalon
DIL	inferior lobe of hypothalamus
Hd	dorsal hypothalamus
Hl	lateral hypothalamus
Hv	ventral hypothalamus
NG	glomerular nucleus
NRP	nucleus of posterior recess
OT	optic tectum
PGZ	periventricular grey zone of Optic Tectum
PPa	anterior preoptic nucleus
TNp	posterior tuberal nucleus
TS	semicircular tori
VM	ventro-medial thalamic nucleus
Vp	posterior zone of ventral telencephalon
Vs	supracommisural zone of ventral telencephalon

References

1. Gonzalez, R.; Mohan, H.; Unniappan, S. Nucleobindins: Bioactive precursor proteins encoding putative endocrine factors? *Gen. Com. Endocrin.* **2012**, *176*, 341–346. [CrossRef] [PubMed]
2. Brailoiu, G.C.; Deliu, E.; Tica, A.A.; Rabinowitz, J.E.; Tilley, D.G.; Benamar, K.; Koch, W.J.; Brailoiu, E. Nesfatin-1 activates cardiac vagal neurons of nucleus ambiguus and elicits bradycardia in conscious rats. *J. Neurochem.* **2013**, *126*, 739–748. [CrossRef] [PubMed]

3. Oh-I, S.; Shimizu, H.; Satoh, T.; Okada, S.; Adachi, S.; Inoue, K.; Eguchi, H.; Yamamoto, M.; Imaki, T.; Hashimoto, K.; et al. Identification of nesfatin-1 as a satiety molecule in the hypothalamus. *Nature* **2006**, *443*, 709–712. [CrossRef] [PubMed]
4. Mohan, H.; Unniappan, S. Phylogenetic aspects of nucleobindin-2/nesfatin-1. *Curr. Pharm. Des.* **2013**, *19*, 6929–6934. [CrossRef] [PubMed]
5. Palasz, A.; Krzystanek, M.; Worthington, J.; Czajkowska, B.; Kostro, K.; Wiaderkiewicz, R.; Bajor, G. Nesfatin-1, a unique regulatory neuropeptide of the brain. *Neuropeptides* **2012**, *46*, 105–112. [CrossRef]
6. Kohno, D.; Nakata, M.; Maejima, Y.; Shimizu, H.; Sedbazar, U.; Yoshida, N.; Dezaki, K.; Onaka, T.; Mori, M.; Yada, T. Nesfatin-1 neurons in paraventricular and supraoptic nuclei of the rat hypothalamus coexpress oxytocin and vasopressin and are activated by refeeding. *Endocrinology* **2008**, *149*, 1295–1301. [CrossRef]
7. Brunner, L.; Nick, H.P.; Cumin, F.; Chiesi, M.; Baum, H.P.; Whitebread, S.; Stricker-Krongrad, A.; Levens, N. Leptin is a physiologically important regulator of food intake. *Int. J. Obes. Relat. Metab. Disord.* **1997**, *21*, 1152–1160. [CrossRef]
8. Ramanjaneya, M.; Chen, J.; Brown, J.E.; Tripathi, G.; Hallschmid, M.; Patel, S.; Kern, W.; Hillhouse, E.W.; Lehnert, H.; Tan, B.K.; et al. Identification of nesfatin-1 in human and murine adipose tissue: A novel depot-specific adipokine with increased levels in obesity. *Endocrinology* **2010**, *151*, 3169–3180. [CrossRef]
9. Zhang, A.Q.; Li, X.L.; Jiang, C.Y.; Lin, L.; Shi, R.H.; Chen, J.D.; Oomura, Y. Expression of nesfatin-1/NUCB2 in rodent digestive system. *World J. Gastroenterol.* **2010**, *6*, 1735–1741. [CrossRef]
10. Gatta, C.; De Felice, E.; D'Angelo, L.; Maruccio, L.; Leggieri, A.; Lucini, C.; Palladino, A.; Paolucci, M.; Scocco, P.; Varricchio, E.; et al. The case study of Nesfatin-1 in the pancreas of *Tursiops truncatus*. *Front. Physiol.* **2018**, *9*, 1845. [CrossRef]
11. Stengel, A.; Goebel, M.; Yakubov, I.; Wang, L.; Witcher, D.; Coskun, T.; Taché, Y.; Sachs, G.; Lambrecht, N.W. Identification and characterization of nesfatin-1immunoreactivity in endocrine cell types of the rat gastric oxyntic mucosa. *Endocrinology* **2009**, *150*, 232–238. [CrossRef] [PubMed]
12. Stengel, A.; Goebel-Stengel, M.; Jawien, J.; Kobelt, P.; Taché, Y.; Lambrecht, N.W. Lipopolysaccharide increases gastric and circulating NUCB2/nesfatin-1 concentrations in rats. *Peptides* **2011**, *32*, 1942–1947. [CrossRef]
13. Li, Z.; Mulholland, M.; Zhang, W. Regulation of gastric nesfatin-1/NUCB2. *Curr. Pharm. Des.* **2013**, *19*, 6981–6985. [CrossRef] [PubMed]
14. Gonzalez, R.; Kerbel, B.; Chun, A.; Unniappan, S. Molecular, cellular and physiological evidences for the anorexigenic actions of nesfatin-1 in goldfish. *PLoS ONE* **2010**, *5*, e15201. [CrossRef] [PubMed]
15. Lin, F.; Zhou, C.; Chen, H.; Wu, H.; Xin, Z.; Liu, J.; Gao, Y.; Yuan, D.; Wang, T.; Wei, R.; et al. Molecular characterization, tissue distribution and feeding related changes of NUCB2A/nesfatin-1 in Ya-fish (*Schizothoraxprenanti*). *Gene* **2014**, *536*, 238–246. [CrossRef] [PubMed]
16. Hatef, A.; Shajan, S.; Unniappan, S. Nutrient status modulates the expression of nesfatin-1 encoding nucleobindin 2A and 2B mRNAs in zebrafish gut, liver and brain. *Gen. Comp. Endocrin.* **2015**, *215*, 51–60. [CrossRef] [PubMed]
17. Kerbel, B.; Unniappan, S. Nesfatin-1 suppresses energy intake, co-localises ghrelin in the brain and gut, and alters ghrelin, cholecystokinin and orexin mRNA expression in goldfish. *J. Neuroendocr.* **2011**, *24*, 366–377. [CrossRef]
18. Bertucci, J.I.; Blanco, A.M.; Canosa, L.F.; Unniappan, S. Glucose, amino acids and fatty acids directly regulate ghrelin and NUCB2/nesfatin-1 in the intestine and hepatopancreas of goldfish (*Cariassus auratus*) in vitro. *Comp. Biochem. Physiol. Part A* **2017**, *206*, 24–35. [CrossRef]
19. Bertucci, J.I.; Blanco, A.M.; Sanchez-Bretano, A.; Unniappan, S.; Canosa, L.F. Ghrelin and NUCB2/Nesfatin-1 co-localization with digestive enzymes in the intestine of Pejerrey (*Odontesthes bonariensis*). *Anat. Rec.* **2019**, *302*, 973–982. [CrossRef]
20. Zhang, X.; Qi, J.; Tang, N.; Wang, S.; Wu, Y.; Chen, H.; Tian, Z.; Wang, B.; Chen, D.; Li, Z. Intraperitoneal injection of nesfatin-1 primarily through the CCK-CCK1R signal pathway affects expression of appetite factors to inhibit the food intake of Siberian sturgeon (*Acipenser baerii*). *Peptides* **2018**, *109*, 14–22. [CrossRef]
21. Zhang, X.; Wang, S.; Chen, H.; Tang, N.; Qi, J.; Wu, Y.; Hao, J.; Tian, Z.; Wang, B.; Chen, D.; et al. The inhibitory effect of NUCB2/nesfatin-1 on appetite regulation of Siberian sturgeon (*Acipenser baerii* Brandt). *Hormon. Behav.* **2018**, *103*, 111–120. [CrossRef] [PubMed]
22. Mohan, H.; Unniappan, S. Ontogenic pattern of nucleobindin-2/nesfatin-1 expression in the gastroenteropancreatic tissues and serum of Sprague Dawley rats. *Reg. Pept.* **2012**, *175*, 61–69. [CrossRef] [PubMed]

23. Senin, L.; Al-Massadi, O.; Barja-Fernandez, S.; Folgueira, C.; Castelao, C.; Tovar, S.A.; Leis, R.; Lago, F.; Baltar, J.; Baamonde, I.; et al. Regulation of NUCB2/nesfatin-1production in rat'stomach and adipose tissue is dependent on age, testosterone levels and lactating status. *Mol. Cell. Endocrinol.* **2015**, *411*, 105–112. [CrossRef] [PubMed]
24. Terzibasi, E.; Valenzano, D.R.; Benedetti, M.; Roncaglia, P.; Cattaneo, A.; Domenici, L.; Cellerino, A. Large differences in aging phenotype between strains of the short-lived annual fish *Nothobranchius furzeri*. *PLoS ONE* **2008**, *3*, e3866. [CrossRef]
25. Cellerino, A.; Valenzano, D.R.; Reichard, M. From the bush to the bench: The annual Nothobranchius fishes as a new model system in biology. *Biol. Rev. Camb. Philos. Soc.* **2016**, *91*, 511–533. [CrossRef]
26. D'Angelo, L.; Lossi, L.; Merighi, A.; de Girolamo, P. Anatomical features for the adequate choice of experimental animal models in biomedicine: I. Fishes. *Ann. Anat. Anat. Anz.* **2016**, *205*, 75–84. [CrossRef]
27. Genade, T.; Benedetti, M.; Terzibasi, E.; Roncaglia, P.; Valenzano, D.R.; Cattaneo, A.; Cellerino, A. Annual fishes of the genus Nothobranchius as a model system for aging research. *Aging Cell* **2005**, *4*, 223–233. [CrossRef]
28. Montesano, A.; Baumgart, M.; Avallone, L.; Castaldo, L.; Lucini, C.; Tozzini, E.T.; Cellerino, A.; D'Angelo, L.; de Girolamo, P. Age-related central regulation of orexin and NPY in the short lived African killifish Notobranchius furzeri. *J. Comp. Neurol.* **2019**, *527*, 1508–1526. [CrossRef]
29. Arcamone, N.; Neglia, S.; Gargiulo, G.; Esposito, V.; Varricchio, E.; Battaglini, P.; de Girolamo, P.; Russo, F. Distribution of ghrelin peptide in the gastrointestinal tract of stomachless and stomach-containing teleosts. *Microsc. Res. Tech.* **2009**, *72*, 525–533. [CrossRef]
30. Russo, F.; de Girolamo, P.; Neglia, S.; Gargiulo, A.; Arcamone, N.; Gargiulo, G.; Varricchio, E. Immunohistochemical and immunochemical characterization of the distribution of leptin-like proteins in the gastroenteric tract of two teleosts (*Dicentrarchus labrax* and *Carassius auratus* L.) with different feeding habits. *Microsc. Res. Tech.* **2011**, *74*, 714–719. [CrossRef]
31. D'Angelo, L.; Castaldo, L.; de Girolamo, P.; Lucini, C.; Paolucci, M.; Pelagalli, A.; Varricchio, E.; Arcamone, N. Orexins and receptor OX2R in the gastroenteric apparatus of two teleostean species: *Dicentrarchu sLabrax* and *Carassius Auratus*. *Anat. Rec.* **2016**, *299*, 1121–1129. [CrossRef] [PubMed]
32. Volkoff, H. Fish as models for understanding the vertebrate endocrine regulation of feeding and weight. *Mol. Cell. Endocrinol.* **2019**. [CrossRef] [PubMed]
33. Baumgart, M.; Groth, M.; Priebe, S.; Savino, A.; Testa, G.; Dix, A.; Ripa, R.; Spallotta, F.; Gaetano, C.; Ori, M.; et al. RNA-seq of the aging brain in the short-lived fish N. furzeri—conserved pathways and novel genes associated with neurogenesis. *Aging Cell* **2014**, *13*, 965–974. [CrossRef] [PubMed]
34. Reichwald, K.; Petzold, A.; Koch, P.; Downie, B.R.; Hartmann, N.; Pietsch, S.; Baumgart, M.; Chalopin, D.; Felder, M.; Bens, M.; et al. Insights into sex chromosome evolution and aging from the genome of a short-lived fish. *Cell* **2015**, *163*, 1527–1538. [CrossRef]
35. Hunt, S.E.; McLaren, W.; Laurent, G.; Thormann, A.; Schuilenburg, H.; Sheppard, D.; Parton, A.; Armean, I.M.; Trevanion, S.J.; Flicek, P.; et al. Ensembl variation resources. *Database* **2018**, *2018*. [CrossRef] [PubMed]
36. Rzhetsky, A.; Nei, M. A simple method for estimating and testing minimum evolution trees. *Mol. Biol. Evol.* **1992**, *9*, 945–967.
37. Zuckerkandl, E.; Pauling, L. Evolutionary divergence and convergence in proteins. In *Evolving Genes and Proteins*; Bryson, V., Vogel, H.J., Eds.; Academic Press: New York, NY, USA, 1965; pp. 97–166.
38. Nei, M.; Kumar, S. *Molecular Evolution and Phylogenetics*; Oxford University Press: New York, NY, USA, 2000.
39. Saitou, N.; Nei, M. The neighbor-joining method: A new method for reconstructing phylogenetic trees. *Mol. Biol. Evol.* **1987**, *4*, 406–425. [CrossRef]
40. Kumar, S.; Stecher, G.; Li, M.; Knyaz, C.; Tamura, K. MEGA X: Molecular Evolutionary Genetics Analysis across computing platforms. *Mol. Biol. Evol.* **2018**, *35*, 1547–1549. [CrossRef]
41. Geer, L.Y.; Marchler-Bauer, A.; Geer, R.C.; Han, L.; He, J.; He, S.; Liu, C.; Shi, W.; Bryant, S.H. The NCBI BioSystems database. *Nucleic Acids Res.* **2010**, *38*, D492–D496. [CrossRef]
42. Sievers, F.; Higgins, D.G. Clustal Omega for making accurate alignments of many protein sequences. *Protein Sci.* **2018**, *27*, 135–145. [CrossRef]

43. Altschul, S.F.; Gish, W.; Miller, W.; Myers, E.W.; Lipman, D.J. Basic local alignment search tool. *J. Mol. Biol.* **1990**, *215*, 403–410. [CrossRef]
44. Baumgart, M.; Groth, M.; Priebe, S.; Appelt, J.; Guthke, R.; Platzer, M.; Cellerino, A. Age-dependent regulation of tumor-related microRNA in the brain of the annual fish Nothobranchius furzeri. *Mech. Ageing Dev.* **2012**, *133*, 226–233. [CrossRef] [PubMed]
45. Untergasser, A.; Nijveen, H.; Rao, X.; Bisseling, T.; Geurts, R.; Leunissen, J.A. Primer3Plus, an enhanced web interface to Primer3. *Nucleic Acids Res.* **2007**, *35*, W71–W74. [CrossRef]
46. D'Angelo, L. Brain atlas of an emerging teleostean model: *Nothobranchiusfurzeri*. *Anat. Rec.* **2013**, *296*, 681–691. [CrossRef] [PubMed]
47. Leung, A.K.; Ramesh, N.; Vogel, C.; Unniappan, S. Nucleobindins and encoded peptides: From cell signaling to physiology. *Adv. Prot. Chem. Struct. Biol.* **2019**, *116*, 91–133. [CrossRef]
48. Wilson, J.M.; Castro, L.F.C. Morphological diversity of the gastrointestinal tract in fishes. *Fish Physiol.* **2010**, *30*, 1–55.
49. Kapoor, B.G.; Smit, H.; Verighina, I.A. The alimentary canal and digestion in teleosts. *Adv. Mar. Biol.* **1976**, *13*, 109–239.
50. Taylor, J.S.; Braasch, I.; Frickey, T.; Meyer, A.; Van de Peer, Y. Genome duplication, a trait shared by 22000 species of ray-finned fish. *Genome Res.* **2003**, *13*, 382–390. [CrossRef]
51. Brailoiu, G.C.; Dun, S.L.; Brailoiu, E.; Inan, S.; Yang, J.; Chang, J.K.; Dun, N.J. Nesfatin-1: Distribution and interaction with a G protein-coupled receptor in the rat brain. *Endocrinology* **2007**, *148*, 5088–5094. [CrossRef]
52. Fort, P.; Salvert, D.; Hanriot, L.; Jego, S.; Shimizu, H.; Hashimoto, K.; Mori, M.; Luppi, P.H. The satiety molecule nesfatin-1 is co-expressed with melanin concentrating hormone in tuberal hypothalamic neurons of the rat. *Neuroscience* **2008**, *155*, 174–181. [CrossRef]
53. Nonogaki, K.; Ohba, Y.; Sumii, M.; Oka, Y. Serotonin systems upregulate the expression of hypothalamic NUCB2 via 5-HT2C receptors and induce anorexia via a leptin-independent pathway in mice. *Biochem. Biophys. Res. Commun.* **2008**, *372*, 186–190. [CrossRef] [PubMed]
54. Foo, K.S.; Brismar, H.; Broberger, C. Distribution and neuropeptide coexistence of nucleobindin-2 mRNA/nesfatin-like immunoreactivity in the rat CNS. *Neuroscience* **2008**, *156*, 563–579. [CrossRef] [PubMed]
55. Senejani, A.G.; Gaupale, T.C.; Unniappan, S.; Bhargava, S. Nesfatin-1/nucleobindin-2 like immunoreactivity in the olfactory system, brain and pituitary of frog, *Microhyla ornata*. *Gen. Comp. Endocrin.* **2014**, *202*, 8–14. [CrossRef]
56. Volkoff, H.; Canosa, L.F.; Unniappan, S.; Cerdá-Reverter, J.M.; Bernier, N.J.; Kelly, S.P.; Peter, R.E. Neuropeptides and the control of food intake in fish. *Gen. Comp. Endocrin.* **2005**, *142*, 3–19. [CrossRef]
57. Demski, L.S.; Knigge, K.M. The telencephalon and hypothalamus of the bluegill (*Lepomis macrochirus*): Evoked feeding, aggressive and reproductive behavior with representative frontal sections. *J. Comp. Neur.* **1971**, *143*, 1–16. [CrossRef]
58. Stacey, N.E.; Kyle, A.L. Effects of olfactory tract lesions on sexual and feeding behavior in the goldfish. *Physiol. Behav.* **1983**, *30*, 621–628. [CrossRef]
59. Stengel, A. Nesfatin-1- More than a food intake regulatory peptide. *Peptides* **2015**, *72*, 175–183. [CrossRef] [PubMed]
60. Cheng, D.; Shami, G.J.; Morsch, M.; Chung, R.S.; Braet, F. Ultrastructural mapping of the zebrafish gastrointestinal system as a basis for experimental drug studies. *BioMed Res. Int.* **2016**, *2016*. [CrossRef]
61. Smit, H. Gastric secretion in the lower vertebrates and birds. In *Handbook of Physiology Section 6 Alimentary Canal Vol. V Bile, Digestion, Ruminal Physiology*; Code, C.F., Ed.; American Physiological Society: Washington, DC, USA, 1968; pp. 2791–2805.
62. Morley, J.E.; Silver, A.J. Anorexia in the elderly. *Neurobiol. Aging* **1988**, *9*, 9–16. [CrossRef]
63. Ramanjaneya, M.; Tan, B.K.; Rucinski, M.; Kawan, M.; Hu, J.; Kaur, J.; Patel, V.H.; Malendowicz, L.K.; Komarowska, H.; Lehnert, H.; et al. Nesfatin-1 inhibits proliferation and enhances apoptosis of human adrenocortical H295R cells. *J. Endocrinol.* **2015**, *226*, 1–11. [CrossRef]
64. Murphy, K.G.; Bloom, S.R. Gut hormones and the regulation of energy homeostasis. *Nature* **2006**, *444*, 854–859. [CrossRef] [PubMed]
65. Ahima, R.S.; Antwi, D.A. Brain regulation of appetite and satiety. *Endocrinol. Metab. Clin. N. Am.* **2008**, *37*, 811–823. [CrossRef] [PubMed]

66. Štimac, D.; Klobučar Majanović, S.; Franjić, N. Stomach—keyplayer in the regulation of metabolism. *Dig. Dis.* **2014**, *32*, 192–201. [CrossRef]
67. Hussain, S.S.; Bloom, S.R. Theregulation of food intake by the gut-brain axis: Implications for obesity. *Int. J. Obes.* **2013**, *37*, 625–633. [CrossRef] [PubMed]

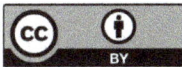

© 2019 by the authors. Licensee MDPI, Basel, Switzerland. This article is an open access article distributed under the terms and conditions of the Creative Commons Attribution (CC BY) license (http://creativecommons.org/licenses/by/4.0/).

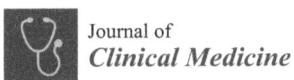

Article

New Chondrosarcoma Cell Lines with Preserved Stem Cell Properties to Study the Genomic Drift During In Vitro/In Vivo Growth

Veronica Rey [1,2,†], Sofia T. Menendez [1,2,3,†], Oscar Estupiñan [1,2,3], Aida Rodriguez [1], Laura Santos [1], Juan Tornin [1], Lucia Martinez-Cruzado [1], David Castillo [4], Gonzalo R. Ordoñez [4], Serafin Costilla [5], Carlos Alvarez-Fernandez [6], Aurora Astudillo [7], Alejandro Braña [8] and Rene Rodriguez [1,2,3,*]

- [1] University Central Hospital of Asturias—Health and Research Institute of Asturias (ISPA), 33011 Oviedo, Spain; reyvazquezvero@gmail.com (V.R.); sofiatirados@gmail.com (S.T.M.); o_r_e_s_@hotmail.com (O.E.); aidarp.finba@gmail.com (A.R.); laurasd.finba@gmail.com (L.S.); juantornin@gmail.com (J.T.); lucialmc24@gmail.com (L.M.-C.)
- [2] University Institute of Oncology of Asturias, 33011 Oviedo, Spain
- [3] CIBER in Oncology (CIBERONC), 28029 Madrid, Spain
- [4] Disease Research and Medicine (DREAMgenics) S.L., 33011 Oviedo, Spain; david.castillo@dreamgenics.com (D.C.); gonzalo.ordonez@dreamgenics.com (G.R.O.)
- [5] Department of Radiology of the Servicio de Radiología of the University Central Hospital of Asturias, 33011 Oviedo, Spain; costillaserafin@uniovi.es
- [6] Department of Medical Oncology of the Servicio de Radiología of the University Central Hospital of Asturias, 33011 Oviedo, Spain; carlos.alvfer@gmail.com
- [7] Department of Pathology of the Servicio de Radiología of the University Central Hospital of Asturias, 33011 Oviedo, Spain; astudillo@hca.es
- [8] Department of Traumatology of the University Central Hospital of Asturias, 33011 Oviedo, Spain; albravigil@gmail.com
- * Correspondence: renerg.finba@gmail.com; Tel.: +34-98510-7956
- † These authors contributed equally to the manuscript.

Received: 4 March 2019; Accepted: 1 April 2019; Published: 4 April 2019

Abstract: For the cancer genomics era, there is a need for clinically annotated close-to-patient cell lines suitable to investigate altered pathways and serve as high-throughput drug-screening platforms. This is particularly important for drug-resistant tumors like chondrosarcoma which has few models available. Here we established and characterized new cell lines derived from two secondary (CDS06 and CDS11) and one dedifferentiated (CDS-17) chondrosarcomas as well as another line derived from a CDS-17-generated xenograft (T-CDS17). These lines displayed cancer stem cell-related and invasive features and were able to initiate subcutaneous and/or orthotopic animal models. Different mutations in Isocitrate Dehydrogenase-1 (*IDH1*), Isocitrate Dehydrogenase-2 (*IDH2*), and Tumor Supressor P53 (*TP53*) and deletion of Cyclin Dependent Kinase Inhibitor 2A (*CDKN2A*) were detected both in cell lines and tumor samples. In addition, other mutations in *TP53* and the amplification of Mouse Double Minute 2 homolog (*MDM2*) arose during cell culture in CDS17 cells. Whole exome sequencing analysis of CDS17, T-CDS17, and matched patient samples confirmed that cell lines kept the most relevant mutations of the tumor, uncovered new mutations and revealed structural variants that emerged during in vitro/in vivo growth. Altogether, this work expanded the panel of clinically and genetically-annotated chondrosarcoma lines amenable for in vivo studies and cancer stem cell (CSC) characterization. Moreover, it provided clues of the genetic drift of chondrosarcoma cells during the adaptation to grow conditions.

Keywords: chondrosarcoma; primary cell lines; cancer stem cells; whole exome sequencing; genomic drift; animal model; cancer preclinical model

1. Introduction

Chondrosarcoma is a malignant cartilage-forming tumor that represents, with approximately 25% of the cases, the second most common bone sarcoma. The most common subtype, representing 80% of the total, is the primary or conventional central chondrosarcoma which is characterized by the pathological formation of hyaline cartilage within the medullar cavity [1]. Other less common subtypes include the periosteal chondrosarcoma, which occurs in the surface of the bone, and secondary chondrosarcoma, which arises in benign lesions such as enchondroma, frequently associated to Ollier disease or Maffucci syndrome, or osteochondroma [1]. The dedifferentiated chondrosarcoma is a distinct variety of chondrosarcoma, accounting for approximately a 10% of the cases. This subtype is characterized by the presence of a low-grade well-differentiated cartilaginous tumor juxtaposed to a high-grade anaplastic sarcoma [1].

Within the complex cytogenetic scenario characteristic of chondrosarcomas, a few chromosomal alterations and gene mutations are frequently found. Thus, mutations in Isocitrate Dehydrogenase-1 (*IDH1*) and -2 (*IDH2*) are found in 87% of enchondromas, up to 70% of conventional central chondrosarcomas and 54% of dedifferentiated chondrosarcomas and may drive sarcomagenic processes [2–4]. In addition, mutations in the major cartilage collagen (*COL2A1*) or Tumor Supressor P53 (*TP53*) genes have been found in approximately 35% and 20% of the chondrosarcomas respectively [5,6]. Other frequent copy number variations, such as the amplification of the 12q13 region, containing Mouse Double Minute 2 homolog (*MDM2*) and the cyclin-dependent kinase 4 genes, and the deletion of the 9p21 region, which includes the Cyclin Dependent Kinase Inhibitor 2A (*CDKN2A*) locus, contribute to the deregulation of the p53 and Retinoblastoma (RB) pathways [5,7].

Wide surgical resection is the mainstay therapeutic option for localized chondrosarcomas. However, these tumors often show high local recurrence and metastatic potential. Furthermore, chondrosarcomas are inherently resistant to conventional chemo and radiotherapy and nowadays there are no effective treatments available for metastatic or inoperable tumors [8–12]. Proposed mechanisms of chemoresistance include the role of the cartilaginous extracellular matrix as a barrier for drug diffusion, the overexpression of members of the adenosine triphosphate (ATP) binding cassette transmembrane family of efflux pumps and antiapoptotic proteins, and the presence of a high percentage of low proliferating/quiescent cells [9,11,12]. Interestingly, some of these features are related to those described for tumor cell subsets presenting stem cell properties (cancer stem cells, CSC). These CSC subpopulations have been characterized in several subtypes of sarcomas and associated to the expression/activity of pluripotency factors, like Sex Determining Region Y-Box 2 (SOX2), stem cell markers, like Aldehyde Dehydrogenase 1 Family Member A1 (ALDH1), or to the ability to grow as floating clonal spheres (tumorspheres) [13,14]. CSC subpopulations have been barely characterized in chondrosarcoma and therefore new models amenable for the study of these subpopulations are needed to find vulnerabilities against these drug-resistant subpopulations.

Despite their failure to completely reproduce the genetic and microenvironmental conditions of tumors, cell lines are still indispensable models to investigate altered mechanisms in cancer, to study CSC subpopulations, and to serve as drug-screening platforms in a high-throughput and logistically simple and rapid way [15–17]. To our knowledge, 14 tumor-derived chondrosarcoma lines, corresponding to seven conventional, five dedifferentiated, and two secondary chondrosarcomas, have been reported so far [18–27]. In this work, we succeeded in establishing three cell lines from two secondary (CDS06 and CDS11) and one dedifferentiated (CDS-17) chondrosarcoma as well as another cell line derived from a CDS-17 xenograft (T-CDS17). We studied their tumorigenic and invasive potential, characterized the present CSC subpopulations, and analyzed the most relevant chondrosarcoma-related genetic alterations both in the cell lines and their original tumors. Furthermore, using a whole exome sequencing (WES) approach in CDS17 and T-CDS17 cells and their matched patient samples we were able to track the genomic adaptation of tumor cells to in vitro and in vivo growth.

2. Experimental Section

2.1. Establishment of Cell Lines

Human samples and data from donors included in this study were provided by the Principado de Asturias BioBank (PT17/0015/0023) integrated in the Spanish National Biobanks Network upon obtaining of written informed consent from patients. All experimental protocols have been performed in accordance with institutional review board guidelines and were approved by the Institutional Ethics Committee of the University Central Hospital of Asturias (approval number: 45/16). This study was performed in accordance with the Declaration of Helsinki.

Tumor samples were subjected to mechanical disaggregation followed by an enzymatic dissociation using MACS® Tissue Dissociation Kit and the GentleMACS Dissociator system (Miltenyi Biotec, Bergisch Gladbach, Germany). At the end of the incubation, culture medium (DMEM-Dulbecco's Modified Eagle Medium supplemented with 10% FBS, 2 mM L-glutamine, 100 U/mL penicillin and 100 µg/mL streptomicin) was added and the cell suspension was filtered to remove clusters. Tumor cells were collected by centrifugation, resuspended in fresh culture medium and seeded in culture flasks. As an alternative protocol to derived cell lines, some fresh tumor specimens were cut into several small fragments, transferred to dry 25 cm^2 culture flasks, covered with a drop of medium and incubated until outgrowth of tumor cells was observed. Cell cultures derived by both methods were subcultured when they reached 80–90% confluence. As a procedure to select tumoral cells and rid of stromal cells, we performed soft agar colony formation assays using the CytoSelect^{TM} 96-Well Cell Transformation Assay Kit (Cell Biolabs Inc, San Francisco, CA, USA). Cells able to form colonies under these anchorage-independent growth conditions are supposed to be transformed. These colonies were recovered, left to attach to plastic substrate and grow in culture medium as normal adherent cultures. Short Tandem Repeat (STR) analyses were performed to compare the identity of cell lines with matched tumor sample (Supplemental Information).

2.2. Tumorsphere Culture

The tumorsphere formation protocol was previously described [28].

2.3. Western Blotting

Whole cell protein extraction and western blotting analysis were performed as previously described [29]. Antibodies used are described in Supplementary Materials.

2.4. Aldefluor Assay and Cell Sorting

Cells with high Aldehyde Dehydrogenase (ALDH) activity was detected and isolated using the Aldefluor^{TM} reagent (Stem Cells Technologies, Grenoble, France) as previously described [13].

2.5. Three-Dimensional Spheroid Invasion Assay

Invasion assays using 3D spheroids in the presence or not of dasatinib or PF-573228 (Selleckchem, Houston, TX, USA) were performed as previously described [30] (see Supplementary Materials information for details).

2.6. In Vivo Tumor Growth

All animal research protocols were carried out in accordance with the institutional guidelines of the University of Oviedo and were approved by the Animal Research Ethical Committee of the University of Oviedo prior to the study (approval code: PROAE 11/2014; date of approval: 9 December 2014). Experiments were done using female NOD.CB17/Prkdcscid/scid/Rj inbreed mice (Janvier Labs,

St. Berthevin, France). For subcutaneous (s.c.) inoculations in the flanks of the mice, 5×10^5 cells mixed 1:1 with BD Matrigel Matrix High Concentration (Becton Dickinson-BD Biosciences, Erembodegem, Belgium) previously diluted 1:1 in culture medium were injected. Tumor volume was determined using a caliper as previously described [31]. One month after inoculation, mice were sacrificed by CO_2 asphyxiation and tumors were extracted and processed for histological analysis. Limited dilution assays (LDA) and calculation of tumor-initiating frequencies (TIF) was performed as described in Supplemental Information. For the intra-bone (i.b.) inoculation, mice were anesthetized with isoflurane and the leg was bent 90° in order to drill the tip of the tibia with a 25G needle before cell inoculation (2×10^5 cells in 5 µl of culture media per mouse) using a 27G needle [32]. In these experiments, tumor growth was evaluated in the preclinical image laboratory of the University of Oviedo using a computed tomography (CT) system (Argus CT, Sedecal, Madrid, Spain) at week 8 after cell inoculation and a µCT system (SkyScan 1174, Bruker, Antwerp, Belgium) following mice sacrifice at week 12 (see Supplementary Materials for analysis conditions).

2.7. Histological Analysis

Human and xenograft samples were fixed in formol, decalcified using solutions with nitric acid (10%) or formic acid (4%)/chlorhydric acid (4%) and embedded in paraffin. Sections of 4-µm were stained with hematoxylin and eosin (H&E) as previously described [29].

2.8. MDM2 and CDKN2A Gene Copy Number Analysis

Genomic DNA was extracted using the QIAmp DNA Mini Kit (Qiagen, Hilden, Germany) and gene amplification was evaluated by real-time PCR. Reactions were carried out using the following primers: for MDM2 gene, Fw 5′-TGGCTGTGTTCAAGTGGTTC-3′ and Rv 5′-GTGGTGACAGGGTGCTCTAAC-3′; for CDKN2A gene, Fw 5′-CACATTCATGTGGGCATTTC-3′ and Rv 5′-TGCTTGTCATGAAGTCGACAG-3′ (Exon 3, recognizing both $p14^{ARF}$ and $p16^{INK4}$ sequences); and for the reference gene RPPH1 (ribonuclease P RNA component H1), Fw 5′-GAGGGAAGCTCATCAGTGG-3′ and Rv 5′-ACATGGGAGTGGAGTGACAG-3′. Dissociation curve analysis of all PCR products showed a single sharp peak and the relative gene copy number was calculated using the $2^{-\Delta\Delta CT}$ method. For each set of samples, DNA from the corresponding healthy tissue was used as a calibrator.

2.9. Mutational Analysis of TP53, IDH1, IDH2, PI3KCA

Genomic DNA were amplified by PCR (Taq PCR Master Mix (2x), EURx Ltd. (Gdańsk, Poland)). The fragments analyzed include: exon 4 of *IDH1* and *IDH2* genes, identified as mutation hot spots in chondrosarcoma; exon 20 of the *PI3KCA* gene; and exons 4 and 6 of the *TP53* gene. Reactions were carried out using the forward and reverse primers detailed in Supplemental Information and the different PCR products were detected by gel electrophoresis in 1.5% agarose, showing a single band. Samples were purified and sequenced by Macrogen Ltd. (Madrid, Spain) and were aligned with the reference sequences of the genes using SnapGene® 4.2.11 (GSL Biotech; available at snapgene.com).

2.10. Library Construction and WES

WES was performed by Macrogen (Seoul, Korea) using 1 µg of genomic DNA from each sample. DNAs were sheared with a Covaris S2 instrument and used for the construction of a paired-end sequencing library as described in the paired-end sequencing sample preparation protocol provided by Illumina. Enrichment of exonic sequences was then performed for each library using the Sure Select All Exon V6 kits following the manufacturer's instructions (Agilent Technologies, Santa Clara, CA, USA). Exon-enriched DNA was pulled down by magnetic beads coated with streptavidin (Invitrogen, Carlsbad, CA, USA), followed by washing, elution, and additional cycles of amplification of the captured library. Enriched libraries were sequenced (2×101 bp) in an Illumina HiSeq4000 sequencer. WES results were processed using the bioinformatics software HD Genome One (DREAMgenics, Oviedo, Spain), certified with IVD/CE-marking (see Supplementary Materials for a comprehensive description of the exome analysis, [33–47]). The datasets generated during the study are available in the European Nucleotide Archive repository [48].

3. Results

3.1. Establishment of Patient-Derived Chondrosarcoma Cell Lines and Analysis of In Vivo Tumorigenic Potential

Surgically resected tumor samples from 11 patients diagnosed of chondrosarcoma at the Hospital Universitario Central de Asturias (Spain) were processed to establish primary cultures. Cultures from two secondary chondrosarcoma, CDS06 (associated with a previous osteochondroma) and CDS11 (presenting Ollier disease), and one from a dedifferentiated chondrosarcoma (CDS-17), were able to growth long term in vitro (Table S1 show an overview of patient and tumor characteristics). These cell lines were able to form colonies in soft agar, an in vitro transformation assay to test the ability of the cells to grow in anchorage independent conditions (Table 1). In order to select the more tumorigenic populations within the cultures, the colonies able to grow in soft agar were recovered and placed back in adherent culture to continue with the corresponding cell line development. Recovered cell lines could be passaged at least 20 times (Table 1) and their identity with the original tumor was confirmed by STR genotyping (Table S2).

Table 1. Functional characterization of chondrosarcoma cell lines.

| Cell Line | Chondrosar. Subtype | Anchorage Independ. Growth § | Passage * | Tumorsphere Growth (% Frequency ± SD) | | In Vivo Tumor Growth ** | | | Aldefluor Assay (%) | Invasion ‡ |
| | | | | 1st Tumorsph. Passage | 2nd Tumorsph. Passage | Subcutaneous | | Intra-Bone | | |
						Tumor Growth (Tumors/Mice)	Mean Volume (mm³ ± SD)	Tumor Growth (Tumors/Mice)		
CDS06	Secondary	Yes	20	Yes (0.24 ± 0.10)	Yes (0.10 ± 0.05)	n/a	n/a	n/a	Yes (4.01)	No
CDS11	Secondary	Yes	25	Yes (0.28 ± 0.11)	Yes (0.16 ± 0.06)	Yes (3/3)	77.00 ± 10.91	n/a	Yes (5.05)	Yes
CDS17	Different.	Yes	<35	Yes (0.20 ± 0.08)	Yes (0.10 ± 0.01)	Yes (3/3)	198.27 ± 5.11	Yes (1/2)	Yes (2.94)	Yes
T-CDS17	Dedifferent.	Yes	<35	Yes (0.26 ± 0.08)	Yes (0.11 ± 0.01)	Yes (3/3)	350.32 ± 39.45 ¶	Yes (2/2)	Yes (14.50)	Yes

(§) Ability to growth forming colonies in embedded in soft agar. (*) number of passages reached so far in adherent cultures. (**) Tumor growth was follow for 1 and 2.5 months in subcutaneous and intra-bone experiments respectively. (‡) Ability of 3D spheroids to invade collagen matrices. (¶) There is a significant difference between the volumes of tumors generated by CDS17 and T-CDS17 cells ($p = 0.043$; two side Student's t-test. SD: Standard Deviation).

Two of the cell lines (CDS11, CDS17) were assayed for their ability to initiate tumor growth in vivo. Both of them were able to form small slow-growing tumors after subcutaneous (s.c.) inoculation in immunodeficient mice after 1 month (Figure 1A and Table 1). Following this, we generated a new cell line derived from a CDS17-xenograft tumor. Subsequent transplantation of this new cell line, T-CDS17, resulted in a more aggressive tumor growth (formation of significantly bigger tumors in similar latency periods), thus indicating that the tumor could be effectively propagated in vivo (Table 1). Histological analysis showed that the original CDS11 tumor was a malignant chondrosarcoma invading intra-trabecular bone matrix and presenting well differentiated and dedifferentiated areas. There was no inflammatory infiltrate and the dedifferentiated subcomponent displayed a mitotic index of 15 mitoses per 10 high power fields (HPF, 40X). The histology of tumors grown from the CDS11 line resembled that of the more undifferentiated/dedifferentiated areas of the original patient.

Tumor, with tumor cells distributed diffusely in a mesenchymal matrix. No well-differentiated component was found in these tumors. Inflammation was also absent and tumors showed 9 mitoses per 10 HPF (Figure 1A). The CDS17 patient sample was a high-grade chondrosarcoma displaying the characteristic chondroid differentiation, with tumor cells presenting pericellular matrix and surrounded by a chondroid extracellular matrix. There was no inflammation present in this tumor and its mitotic index was 18 mitoses per 10 HPF. Tumors derived from CDS17 and T-CDS17 cells lines maintained chondroid differentiation, with tumor cells presenting pericellular halos and embedded in a chondroid basophilic extracellular matrix. There were no inflammatory infiltrates in these tumors and its mitotic index was 17 and 25 mitoses per 10 HPF for CDS17 and T-CDS17 respectively (Figure 1A).

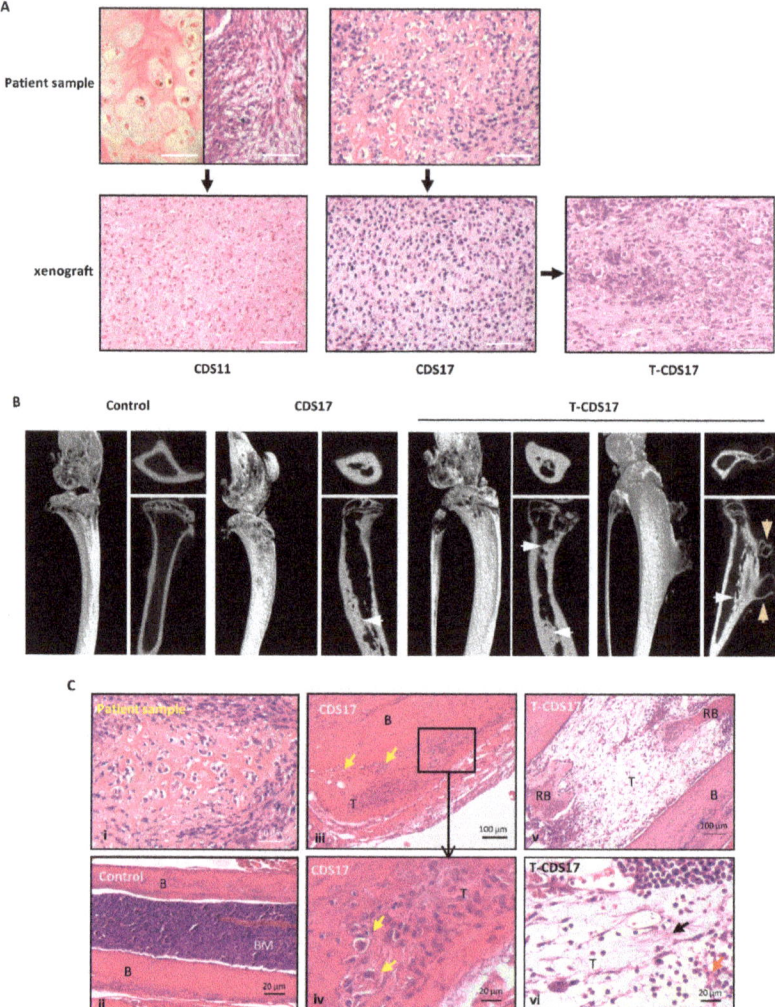

Figure 1. In vivo tumorigenicty of chondrosarcoma cell lines. (**A**) Histological analysis (H&E staining) of original patient tumors and tumors developed 1 month after subcutaneous (s.c.) inoculation of CDS11, CDS17, and T-CDS17 cell lines in immunodeficient mice. Two different areas of the CDS11 patient tumor sample are shown. scale bars = 150 µm. (**B**) Radiologic examination (µCT scan) of tumors developed after intra-bone (i.b.) inoculation of CDS17 and T-CDS17 cells in immunodeficient mice. Coronal, sagittal and axial images are shown. Compared to a control leg, intra-medullar formation of tumor bone/osteoid formation (white arrows) is shown in mice inoculated with both cell lines. In addition, a mouse inoculated with T-CDS17 cells presented an extra-medullar lesion compatible with the radiographic features of osteochondrosarcoma (orange arrows). (**C**) H&E staining of an original patient sample (i), a control leg (ii), and tumors formed after i.b. inoculation of CDS17 (iii and iv) and T-CDS17 (v and vi) cells lines. Chondroid.like cells (yellow arrows) and areas of fibrillar (black arrow) and amorphous (orange arrow) osteo-chondroid matrix are indicated. (B: bone; RB: reactive bone).

In an attempt to create more faithful animal models CDS17 and T-CDS17 cells were inoculated intra-tibia in immunodeficient mice. Both CDS17 (1 out of 2 mice) and T-CDS17 (2 out of 2 mice) cells were able to generate tumor growth in this orthotopic location. Computerized tomography (CT) analysis at day 50 after inoculation (Figure S1) and microCT analysis at the end point of the experiment (day 80) (Figure 1B) revealed the formation of tumors resembling the radiological features of human chondrosarcomas. These tumors showed the presence of a dotted pattern chondroid-like matrix inside the bone marrow cavity. In addition, one of the T-CDS17 generated tumors also displayed extra-medullar tumor growth, forming an osteochondroid exostosis-like lesion (Figure 1B and Figure S1). Histological sections of these orthotopically grown tumors also resembled the main features of the patient sample (Figure 1C(i)), with chondrogenic tumor cells presenting pericellular halos and embedded in cartilaginous matrix (Figure 1C(iii,iv)). In addition, legs inoculated with tumor cells showed bone marrow cavities filled by dedifferentiated mesenchymal cells producing fibrillar and amorphous osteo-chondroid matrix and presenting extensive areas of reactive bone (Figure 1C(v,vi)). None of tumors presented inflammatory component and they showed mitotic indexes between 7 (CDS17) and 10 (T-CDS17) mitoses per 10 HP.

3.2. Genetic Characterization of Chondrosarcoma Cell Lines

Sequencing analysis of common mutations in chondrosarcoma identified point mutations in *IDH1* (p.R132L) in CDS01 cells and *IDH2* (p.R172G) in CDS17 and T-CDS17 cells which were also detected in the corresponding patient tumor samples. Otherwise, CDS06 cells did not show any *IDH1* or *IDH2* mutations. Analysis of *TP53* (exons 4 and 6) revealed the presence of nonsynonymous homozygous in all cell lines. The single nucleotide variants (SNV) p.P72R was found in all cell lines and also in CDS06 and CDS11 patient samples, meanwhile the mutation p.S215R was only found in CDS17 and T-CDS17 cell lines but not in the corresponding patient sample (Figure 2A,C). Additional analysis of hot spot mutations in Phosphatidylinositol-4,5-Bisphosphate 3-Kinase Catalytic Subunit Alpha (*PI3KCA*) showed no alterations in any of the cell lines. Finally, copy number analysis showed a significant gain of *MDM2* in CDS17 and T-CDS17 cells which was not detected in the tumor sample and a homozygous deletion of *CDKN2A* (exon 3) in CDS11 cells and matched patient sample (Figure 2B,C).

3.3. WES of Chondrosarcoma Cell Lines and Clonal Evolution after In Vitro and In Vivo Growth

To better characterize the genomic alterations present in these cells lines, we performed WES in the CDS17 line (passage 14), its xenograft-derived line T-CDS17 (passage 5) and their matched normal (non-tumoral) and tumor patient samples. The average nucleotide coverage in WES studies was approximately 115X, being selected for further analyses only the variants presenting more than 15 reads. Data from WES analysis of tumor the sample were compared to that of normal tissue DNA to exclude germline alterations. Tumor and CDS17 samples showed similar number of somatic mutations (123 and 121 respectively) whereas the T-CDS17 cell line displayed a slightly higher number of mutations (169), corresponding most of them to SNV in the three samples (Figure 3A). All samples displayed a similar profile of SNV transitions and transvertions (Figure 3B and Figure S2A). Similar to other type of tumors, C > T and G > A transitions were the most common mutations found in all samples (Figure 3B). To analyze the genomic evolution of tumor cells after in vitro/in vivo growth adaptation, we used variant allele frequency data of tumors, CDS17 and T-CDS17 samples to delineate the different clonal populations in each sample using the PhyloWGS, and FishPlot software. This analysis retrieves 14 clusters which evolved among samples (Figure 3C,D). The tumor sample contains nine clusters presenting cellular prevalence values higher than 0.05. Among them, cluster 1 is the one including a higher number of SNVs and must be the founder clone since the set of mutations that contain is present in virtually all the tumors cells (cellular prevalence equal to 1) and the other clones seem to derive from it. Notably, the cellular prevalence of cluster 1 is maintained in CDS17 and T-CDS17 samples, thus suggesting that most variants, including driver mutations, are kept by in the cell lines. In addition, cluster 7 remained unchanged in a small proportion of cells in all samples. On the other hand, Clusters

2–4 were positively selected while Clusters 10–14 almost disappeared during the adaptation to in vitro culture, as seen by their variation in cellular prevalence in the CDS17 line. Moreover, Clusters 5 and 6 emerged in the cell line T-CDS17 with a cellular prevalence of 0.25 and 0.15 respectively and were likely acquired during the in vivo growth of tumor cells in immunodeficient mice (Figure 3C,D).

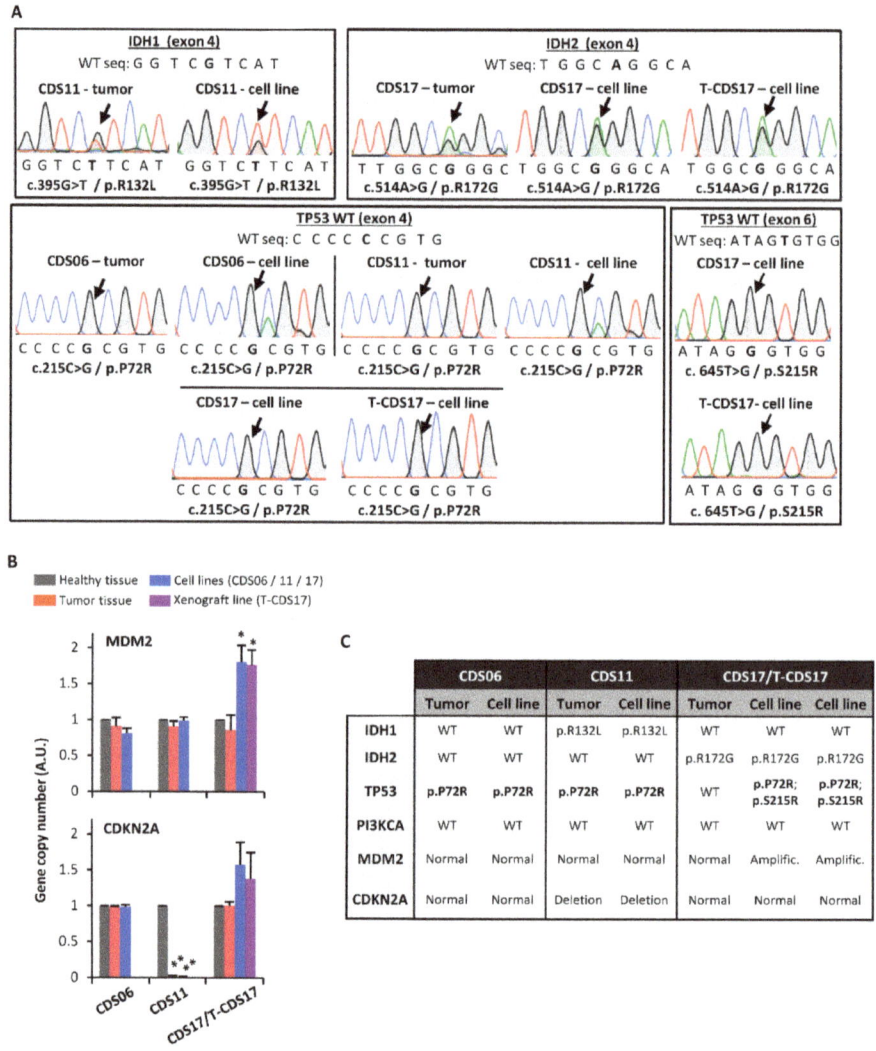

Figure 2. Genetic characterization of chondrosarcoma cell lines. (**A**) Sanger sequencing chromatograms showing mutations (black arrows) in *IDH1*, *IDH2*, and *TP53* genes present in the indicated tumors and cell lines. Reference wild type (WT) sequences are shown. (**B**) Gene copy numbers of the indicated genes were estimated by quantitative PCR on genomic DNA. Results are expressed relative to the corresponding healthy tissue sample and are the mean and standard deviation of three experiments (*: $p < 0.05$; **: $p < 0.005$; two-sided Student's *t*-test). (**C**) Summary of the genetic characterization of the indicated chondrosarcoma cell lines and tumor samples. Homozygous mutations are highlighted in bold.

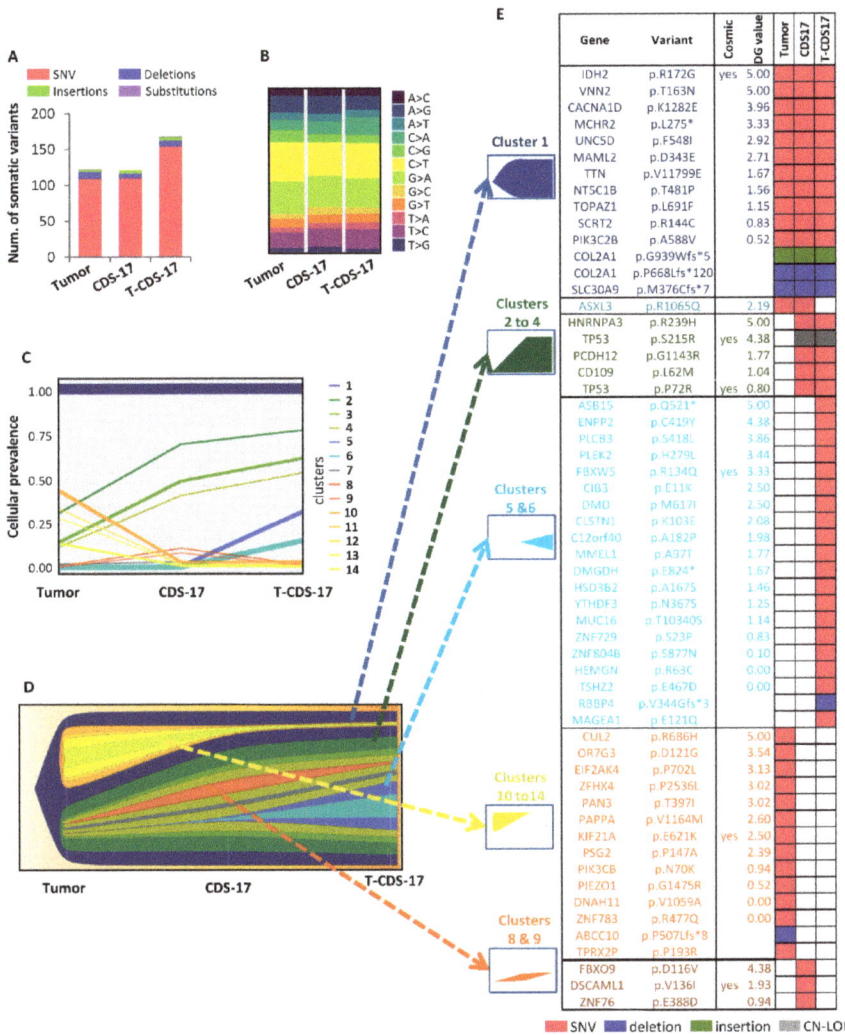

Figure 3. Clonal evolution of somatic mutations after in vitro and in vivo growth of chondrosarcoma cell lines. (**A**,**B**) Mutational burden data of a tumor patient sample and its derived cell lines CDS-17 and T-CDS17 obtained by whole exome sequencing (WES). The number and type of somatic mutations (**A**) and the profile of SNV transitions and transvertions (**B**) in each sample are shown. (**C**,**D**) Subclonal reconstruction was performed with PhyloWGS using WES data. The mean cellular prevalence estimates of mutation clusters in originating patient tumor sample and subsequent CDS17 and T-CDS17 cell lines are shown (**C**). Line widths represent the relative abundance of single nucleotide variants (SNVs) in each mutation cluster. Fish-plot representation of the different clusters in each sample is also shown (**D**). (**E**) List of non-synonymous somatic mutations detected in each cluster. Catalogue of Somatic Mutations in Cancer (COSMIC) status, DREAMgenics (DG) algorithm value, and mutation type are indicated.

To select the most relevant somatic mutations included in each group of clusters presenting similar trends we compared tumor versus normal, CDS17 versus tumor and T-CDS17 versus CDS17 samples and filter the results to select variants with non-synonymous effect on coded proteins which presented variant allele frequencies >0.035 in tumor, CDS17 or T-CDS17 samples and maximum allele frequencies <0.01 in population databases (dbSNP, ExAC, ESP, and 1000 Genomes) (Figure 3E). Using this approach, we found a group of 14 mutations included in cluster 1 which were mutated in all the samples. Among these mutations, only the c.514A > G transition (p.R172G) in *IDH2*, previously detected by Sanger sequencing (Figure 2A), was listed in the Catalogue of Somatic Mutations in Cancer (COSMIC). In addition, we also selected two different mutations in the *COL2A1* gene previously found in chondrosarcoma [5,6]. Mutations in the rest of genes were not previously described in cancer. Notably, some of these unreported variants, including SNVs in Vanin2 (*VNN2*), Calcium Voltage-Gated Channel Subunit Alpha1 D (*CACNA1D*), Melanin Concentrating Hormone Receptor 2 (*MCHR2*), Unc-5 Netrin Receptor D (*UNC5D*), or Mastermind Like Transcriptional Coactivator 2 (*MAML2*), showed high values in the 0 to 5 scale assigned by DREAMgenics (DG) value (integrated score of several predictive algorithms [34], see supplemental methods for details) used to predict deleterious mutations and, therefore, they might constitute new driver events in chondrosarcoma (Figures 3E and 4B). Another group of five mutated genes was filtered from variations included in Clusters 2–4, which become enriched in CDS17 and T-CDS17 cells. The most notably alterations in this group was the mutations p.S215R and p.P72R in *TP53*, previously detected by Sanger sequencing (Figure 2A), which was present in both alleles due to a copy-neutral (CN) loss of heterozygosity (LOH) event in chromosome 17 as detailed below. Most relevant variations emerging in T-CDS17 cells (Clusters 5 and 6) included mutations in 20 genes. Among them, a SNV in F-Box and WD Repeat Domain Containing 5 (*FBXW5*) is the only variation previously reported in COSMIC in tumor types different to chondrosarcoma (Figure 3E). Also, the set of variants of the tumor sample that were lost in CDS17 and T-CDS17 cells (Clusters 10–14) included a mutation in Kinesin Family Member 21A (*KIF21A*) previously reported in COSMIC for other types of tumor and other 13 unreported mutations. Finally, three mutations were filtered from variations contained in Clusters 8 and 9, which appear in a small fraction of CDS17 cells and disappeared again in T-CDS17 cells (Figure 3E). Besides the above described changes in somatic mutations, a major consequence of in vitro and in vivo growth of tumor cells was the emergence of structural alterations and copy number variants (CNV) leading to numerous LOH events in many mutations of CDS17 and T-CDS17 cells (Figure 4A,B). Most relevant structural alterations detected in CDS17 and T-CDS17 cells included a CN-LOH affecting chromosome 17, which would explain the homozygous mutations of the *TP53* gene (p.S215R and p.P72R) commented above. Analysis of variant frequencies in this chromosome showed that the CN-LOH affected the whole chromosome and is detected in virtually all cells, as indicated by the disappearance of almost all intermediate frequencies in CDS17 and T-CDS17 cells (Figure 4B,C). Similar CN-LOH events were detected in chromosome 16, although in this case the structural variation affects to only a subset of the cells, as seen by the shift in the intermediate frequencies of variants in CDS17 and T-CDS-17 cells as compared to normal and tumor samples. Noteworthy, the intermediate frequencies shift also indicated that the subpopulation presenting the CN-LOH in chromosome 16 increased in T-CDS17 as compared to CDS-17 cells (Figure 4B,C). Besides these CN variations, other LOH events were due to CNV in several chromosomes. Thus, a copy of chromosome 18 was lost in a subpopulation of CDS-17 cells and in the whole population of non-synonymous mutations undergoing LOH in each sample. COSMIC status, DG algorithm value, and mutation type are indicated.

After filtering LOH events using the criteria described above for somatic variants and including also other LOH variants with a recurrence in the COSMIC database higher than 10, we selected 24 mutations that underwent LOH in CDS17, 17 LOH events which emerged in T-CDS-17 and 5 mutations which were detected as LOH variations in CDS17 but not in T-CDS17 (Figure 4D). Altogether, these data indicate that these cell lines kept the most relevant driver mutations present in the founder clone of the tumor sample. In addition, the adaptation of tumor cells to in vitro cell culture and in vivo growth is accompanied by the gain/loss of additional point mutations and structural variants affecting different subclones of the cell lines.

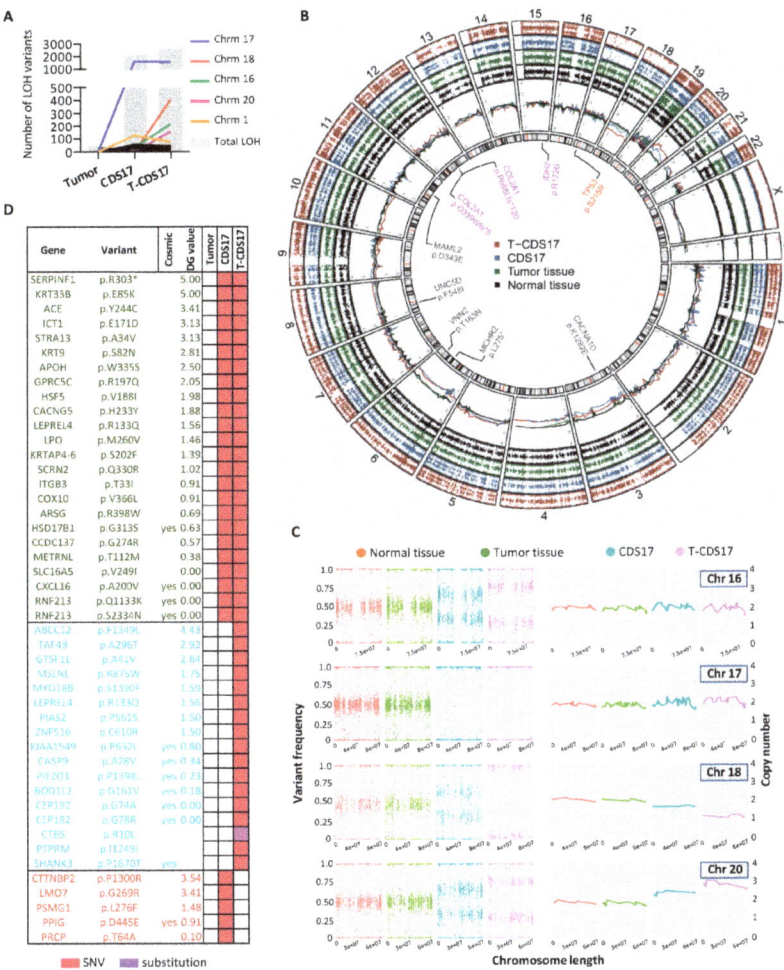

Figure 4. Genomic structural alterations after in vitro and in vivo growth of chondrosarcoma cell lines. (**A**) Number of LOH (total number and distribution between chromosomes) calculated from WES data of tumor, CDS17, and T-CDS17 samples. (**B**) Circular representation of the four samples sequenced through WES. Circles display from the inside outwards: (ring 1) chromosome ideogram, highlighting relevant previously reported (purple) or unreported (grey) somatic variants shared by tumor tissue, CDS17 and T-CDS17, as well as a TP53 homozygous mutation shared by CDS17 and T-CDS17 but not tumor tissue (orange); (ring 2) chromosome copy number (CN) of each sample based on normalized read counts; (rings 3–6) variant frequencies of common polymorphic positions (minimum allele frequency ≥0.01 in at least one major dbSNP population) in each sample. (**C**) Analysis of variant frequencies (left panels) and CN (right panels) extracted from (**B**) in the indicated chromosomes. Similar representations for other chromosomes are show in Figure S3B. (**D**) List of T-CDS17 cells. Conversely, a copy of chromosome 20 was gained in subset of CDS17 cells and in the entire population of T-CDS17 cells (Figure 4B,C). Finally, other copy number variations (CNVs) and/or shifts in variant frequencies affecting subpopulations of CDS-17 and/or T-CDS17 cells, was also detected in other chromosomes like 1, 2, 4, 5, 6, or 7 (Figure 4B and Figure S2B).

3.4. Analysis of CSC Subpopulations in New Chondrosarcoma Cell Lines

All the cell lines (CDS06, CDS11, CDS17, and T-CDS17) could be cultured as tumorspheres for at least two passages showing sphere forming frequencies between 0.20% and 0.28% in the first passage and between 0.1% and 0.16% in the second passage (Figure 5A and Table 1). Regarding the expression of CSC-related factors, CDS17 and T-CDS17 cells displayed high/medium levels of SOX2, while we could not detect SOX2 expression in CDS06 or CDS11 lines (Figure 5B). A similar pattern of expression was detected for ALDH1A1, while all the cell lines expressed ALDH1A3 (Figure 5B). According to the important contribution of these ALDH1A3 isoform to the Aldefluor activity [13], we detected Aldefluor positive cells in all lines in percentages ranging from 2.94% to 14.5% of the cells (Figure 5C). As previously shown in other sarcoma models [13], tumorsphere cultures of the CDS11 cell line are enriched in Aldefluor activity (Figure 5D). Furthermore, to confirm that Aldefluor could be used as a bone fide CSC marker in chondrosarcoma cell lines, we sorted T-CDS17 cells displaying high (ALDH^{high}) and low (ALDH^{low}) Aldefluor activity (Figure 5E) and inoculated several low cellular doses (LDA assays) subcutaneously into immunodeficient mice. We found low incidences of tumor growth after the inoculation of these cellular doses (we detected tumors in 4 out of 30 mice). In any case, ALDH^{low} cells developed only one tumor in the series where the higher number of cells was inoculated, whereas ALDH^{high} cells were able to develop three tumors, one per series. Using ELDA software to calculate the tumor initiation frequency of each population, we found that the ALDH^{high} subpopulation is three times more enriched in CSCs than the ALDH^{low} subpopulation (Figure 5F). Although, due to relatively low tumorigenicity of these cells when injected at low cellular doses, these results do not reach statistical significance, they clearly suggest that ALDH activity could be a suitable stem cell marker in these cells.

3.5. Invasion Ability of Chondrosarcoma Cell Lines

Using live cell time-lapse microscopy we found that spheroids of CDS11, CDS17, and T-CDS17—but not CDS06 cells—were able to invade 3D collagen matrices (Figure 6A,B). In accordance with its enhanced aggressiveness, T-CDS17 also displayed a significantly increased invasive potential when compared to the parental CDS17 cell line.

Deregulated SRC/FAK (Steroid receptor coactivator/Focal adhesion kinase) signaling is related to enhanced migration and invasion in many types of tumors and we previously found that several sarcoma models may invade through a mechanism depending on SRC/FAK signaling [30]. Here, we found that both the SRC inhibitor dasatinib or the FAK inhibitor PF-573228 were able to dose-dependently inhibit cell invasion, thus indicating that this mechanism is also mediating invasion in chondrosarcoma cell lines (Figure 6C–F).

4. Discussion

Chondrosarcomas are inherently resistant to conventional treatments and a range of new therapies aimed to target specific alterations are being currently tested [9,11,12]. Among them, the use of IDH inhibitors have not proved preclinical anti-tumor activity [49] and clinical trials including chondrosarcoma patients have not yet reported positive results [12].

Other therapeutic strategies that are being tested at clinical level include the targeting of signaling pathways controlled by hedgehog, SRC or PI3K/AKT/mTOR, as well as histone deacetylase inhibitors or anti-angiogenic agents, with only a few of them reporting partially encouraging results [12,50,51]. Altogether, there is an urgent need for more research aimed to find and test new therapies for advanced or unresectable chondrosarcomas.

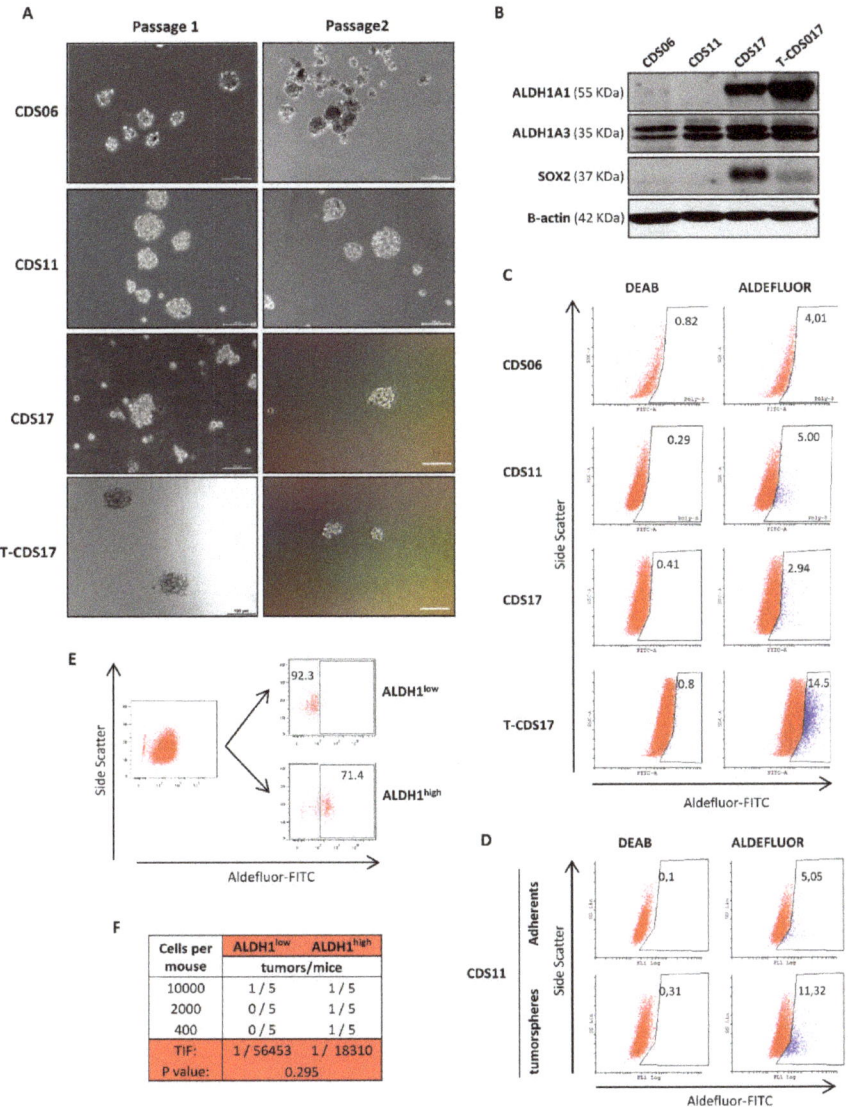

Figure 5. Characterization of cancer stem cell (CSC) subpopulations in chondrosarcoma cell lines. (**A**) Representative images of tumorspheres formed from the indicated cell lines in two successive passages. Scale bar = 100 μm. (**B**) Protein levels of Aldehyde Dehydrogenase 1 Family Member-A1 (ALDH1A1), -A3 (ALDH1A3), and Sex Determining Region Y-Box 2 (SOX2) in the indicated cell lines. β-actin levels were used as a loading control. (**C**) Aldefluor assay showing the activity of ALDH1 in the indicated cell lines. ALDH1 activity was blocked with the specific inhibitor N,N-diethylaminobenzaldehyde (DEAB) to establish the basal levels. (**D**) Comparison of Aldefluor activity in adherent and tumorsphere cultures of CDS11 cells. (**E**) Flow cytometry cell sorting of Aldefluor high (ALDH1^{high}) and low (ALDH1^{low}) populations in T-CDS17 cells. (**F**) Limiting dilution assay to evaluate tumor initiation frequency (TIF) of ALDH1^{high} and ALDH1^{low} T-CDS17 cells. The number of mice that grew tumors after 4 months and the total number of inoculated mice for each condition is indicated. TIF was calculated using ELDA software.

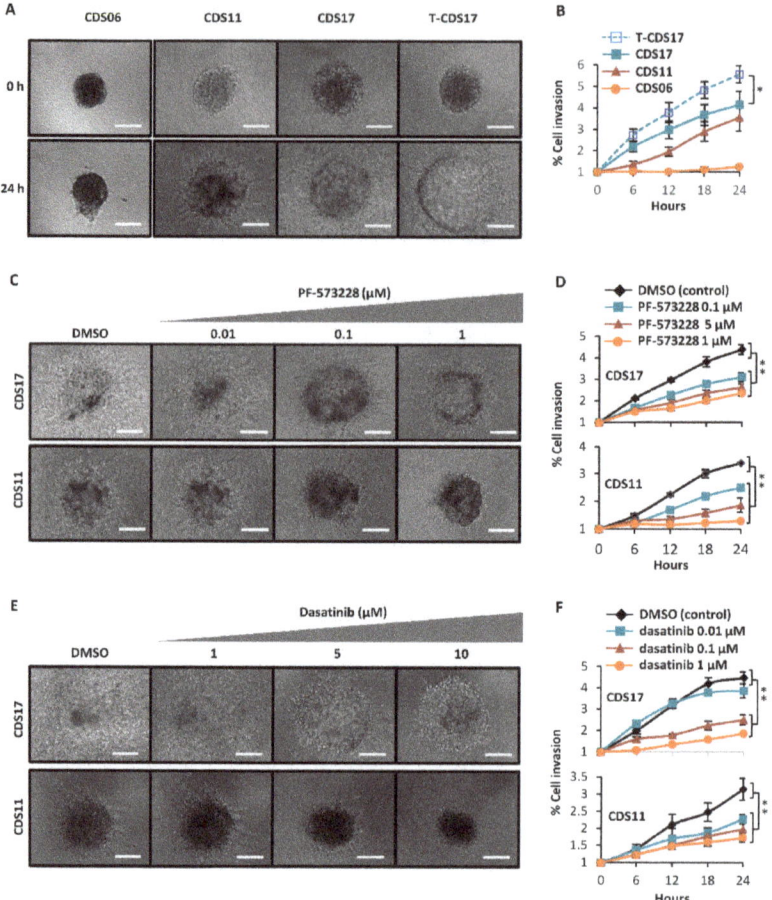

Figure 6. Invasive ability of chondrosarcoma cell lines. (**A,B**) Analysis of the invasive properties of the indicated cell lines using 3D spheroid invasion assays. Representative images of the 3D invading spheroids at the initial and final time points (**A**) and quantification of the invasive area (**B**) are presented. (**C,F**) Effect of increasing concentrations of PF-573228 (**C,D**) or dasatinib (**E,F**) on the invasive ability of CDS11 and CDS17 cells. Representative images of the 3D spheroids treated with the indicated concentrations of PF-573228 (**C**) or dasatinib (**E**) for 24 h and quantification of the invasive area after each treatment (**D,F**) are presented. Scale bars = 200 µm. Error bars represent the SD, and asterisks indicate statistically significant differences between the indicated series (* $p < 0.05$; ** $p < 0.01$; two-sided Student's t-test). (DMSO: Dimethyl sulfoxide).

Cell lines are easy to culture, relatively inexpensive and amenable to high-throughput screening models that have guided advances in cancer research for decades. Despite limitations, such as the accumulation of new mutations after endless in vitro culture [17], international studies reported that large panels of cell lines recapitulated the most relevant alterations of original tumors and, when using a relevant number of well characterized cell lines of a given cancer subtype, they were useful models to predict anti-cancer drug sensitivity and clinical outcomes [15,52–54]. These studies have contributed to retrieve the interest in substituting veteran endless passaged cell lines and replace them with new patient-derived cell lines which should be tagged with clinical information and include genomic characterization of both the cell line and the patient samples. These cell line models would complement more sophisticated models such as organoids or patient-derived xenografts [55].

Here we present four new chondrosarcoma cell lines with related clinical information and genetic characterization of the most common alterations (mutations in *IDH1*, *IDH2*, *TP53*, and *PI3KCA* and copy number variants in *MDM2* and *CDKN2*). All the alterations detected were also found in the original tumors with the exception of the *TP53* mutations and *MDM2* amplification found in CDS17 and T-CDS17 cell lines but not in tumor samples. This finding suggests that the loss of functional p53 could be a mechanism of adaptation to in vitro culture in chondrosarcoma cells. Our cell lines expand the panel of available chondrosarcoma cell lines (overviewed in Table S3). Of note, our study provides the first cell line (CDS06) derived from a secondary chondrosarcoma associated to a previous osteochondroma. In addition we add new dedifferentiated cchondrosarcoma cell lines with *IDH2* mutations to only one reported so far. Interestingly, none of previously published dedifferentiated lines described mutations in *IDH1* (Table S3).

Relevant for possible future applications in cancer research, three of the cell lines (CDS11, CDS17, and T-CDS17) were able to initiate tumors in vivo resembling the histology of the patient sample after inoculation in heterotopic and/or orthotopic sites. Some of these cell lines were also able to invade 3D matrices and all of them showed CSC-related features such as the ability to grow as tumorspheres or the presence of subpopulations with ALDH^{high} activity. Related to this, it has been previously shown that sarcoma cells increased their stemness and tumorigenic potential after being grown in mice [13,56]. Therefore cell line/xenograft line tandems, like the one formed by CDS17 and T-CDS17, constitute valuable models for studying/tracking cancer stem cells subpopulations during tumor progression [13]. These studies point ALDH1 as a relevant CSC-associated factor in different types of sarcoma [13,56]. Similarly, we found that the T-CDS17 cell line showed increased ALDH1 expression and activity, enhanced invasive ability and increased in vivo tumorigenic potential than its parental CDS17 cell line. Moreover, our results also suggest a role for ALDH1 as CSC marker in chondrosarcoma.

Our work also includes a WES analysis of CDS17 and T-CDS17 cells lines together with normal and tumor samples from the patient. This is the first time that a chondrosarcoma cell line and matched patient samples include such a level of genomic characterization. This analysis allowed us to know how the cell lines resemble the genomic diversity of the original tumor and also to track the genomic evolution of tumor cells during in vitro and in vivo growth. We found that the putative founder clone, that including a higher number of mutations and is present in all tumor cells, remains unaltered after in vitro cell culture (CDS17 cells) and in vivo growth (T-CDS17 cells). This clone includes previously known mutations, such as that previously found by Sanger sequencing in *IDH2* (R172G) [2,4] or mutations in *COL2A1* (G939Wfs*5 and P668Lfs*120) [5,6], as well as other unreported non-synonymous mutations presenting high scores in impact prediction algorithms, such as *VNN2*, *CACNA1D*, *MCHR2*, *UNC5D*, or *MAML2*, which possibly contribute to chondrosarcoma progression must be studied in detail.

Other mutations affecting different subclones appear or disappear during the adaptation of cells to in vitro/in vivo growth. Although not widely described for sarcomas, this genomic drift is in line with previous studies in other cancer types [57]. An important phenomenon related to the adaptation to growth conditions is the emergence of structural alterations in several chromosomes in CDS17 and T-CDS17 cells. The most relevant change was the CN-LOH affecting the chromosome 17 and responsible for appearance of homozygous mutations in *TP53*. Importantly, alterations in *TP53* were associated with aggressive behavior of chondrosarcomas [58] and similar LOH affecting chromosome 17 was detected in high grade chondrosarcomas [59]. Therefore, despite not being present in the original tumor, the CN-LOH in chromosome 17 detected in CDS17 and T-CDS17 resembles a naturally occurring mechanism for increasing aggressiveness in chondrosarcomas. Other structural variants, such as those detected chromosomes like 16, 18, or 20, affected a sequentially increased cell population in CDS17 and T-CDS17 cells. Given that T-CDS17 cells are more aggressive tan CDS17 cells, some of these structural alterations could be involved in the gain of malignancy in T-CDS17 cells. Whether these alterations occur also in patients during tumor progression or are only due to the adaptation of tumor cells to grow ex-vivo remains to be studied.

Although we could not be completely sure that all the genetic differences observed between CDS17 and T-CDS17 cell lines were due to the in vivo growth in mice and not to the ex-vivo expansion of T-CDS17, the fact that the genomic drift previously observed in patient-derived cell lines were mainly restricted to the first few passages [57] when the adaptation of cells to the in vitro growth conditions occurs, suggests that the new set of genetic alterations detected in T-CDS17 most likely emerged during the in vivo growth phase.

5. Conclusions

In summary, this study provides new patient-derived chondrosarcoma cell lines with clinical and genetic information from patients. These cell lines are suitable for studying CSC subpopulations and to generate in vivo models for this disease. Furthermore, a pioneering genomic analysis using a cell line (CDS17)/xenograft line (T-CDS-17) tandem model confirmed that these cell lines kept the most relevant mutations of the original tumor and described the genetic drift process that tumor cells underwent during the adaptation to in vitro and in vivo growth.

Supplementary Materials: The following are available online at http://www.mdpi.com/2077-0383/8/4/455/s1, Supplemental Materials and Methods, Figure S1: Computerized tomography scan (CT) at day 50 after intra-bone inoculation, Figure S2: WES analysis of chondrosarcoma cell lines, Table S1: Patient and tumor characteristics, Table S2: STR analysis for the indicated patient-derived primary cell lines and the corresponding tumor tissue of origin.

Author Contributions: Conceptualization, R.R.; Methodology, V.R., S.T.M., O.E., A.R., L.S., J.T., L.M.-C. and S.C.; Software, D.C. and G.R.O.; Validation, V.R. and S.T.M.; Formal analysis, V.R., S.T.M., D.C., G.R.O., S.C., and A.A.; Investigation, V.R., S.T.M., O.E., A.R., L.S., J.T., and L.M.-C.; Resources, R.R., A.A., and A.B.; Data curation, D.C. and C.A.-F.; Writing—original draft preparation, R.R.; Writing—review and editing, R.R., V.R., and S.T.M.; Supervision, R.R.; Funding acquisition, R.R.

Funding: This work was supported by the Agencia Estatal de Investigación (AEI) [MINECO/Fondo Europeo de Desarrollo Regional (FEDER) (SAF2016-75286-R to R.R.) and ISC III/FEDER: Miguel Servet Program (CPII16/00049 to R.R.), Sara Borrell Program (CD16/00103 to S.T.M.) and Consorcio CIBERONC (CB16/12/00390)] and the Spanish Group for Research on Sarcomas (GEIS) (project: GEIS-62). O.E. is recipient of a fellowship (Severo Ochoa Program) from PCTI-Asturias.

Acknowledgments: We thank Mario Garcia (Pharmacology laboratory, University of Oviedo) for his help with intra-tibia inoculations. We acknowledge the Spanish Group for Research on Sarcomas (GEIS), co-responsible institution for their support to the study. Finally, we acknowledge the Principado de Asturias BioBank (PT17/0015/0023), financed jointly by Servicio de Salud del Principado de Asturias, Instituto de Salud Carlos III and Fundación Bancaria Cajastur and integrated in the Spanish National Biobanks Network, for its collaboration.

Conflicts of Interest: The authors declare no competing financial interests.

References

1. Fletcher, C.; Bridge, J.; Hogendoorn, P.; Mertens, F. (Eds.) *WHO Classification of Tumours of Soft Tissue and Bone. Pathology and Genetics of Tumours of Soft Tissue and Bone*, 4th ed.; IARC Press: Lyon, France, 2013.
2. Amary, M.F.; Bacsi, K.; Maggiani, F.; Damato, S.; Halai, D.; Berisha, F.; Pollock, R.; O'Donnell, P.; Grigoriadis, A.; Diss, T.; et al. IDH1 and IDH2 mutations are frequent events in central chondrosarcoma and central and periosteal chondromas but not in other mesenchymal tumours. *J. Pathol.* **2011**, *224*, 334–343. [CrossRef]
3. Lu, C.; Venneti, S.; Akalin, A.; Fang, F.; Ward, P.S.; Dematteo, R.G.; Intlekofer, A.M.; Chen, C.; Ye, J.; Hameed, M.; et al. Induction of sarcomas by mutant IDH2. *Genes Dev.* **2013**, *27*, 1986–1998. [CrossRef]
4. Tinoco, G.; Wilky, B.A.; Paz-Mejia, A.; Rosenberg, A.; Trent, J.C. The biology and management of cartilaginous tumors: A role for targeting isocitrate dehydrogenase. *Am. Soc. Clin. Oncol. Educ. Book* **2015**, e648–e655. [CrossRef]
5. Tarpey, P.S.; Behjati, S.; Cooke, S.L.; Van Loo, P.; Wedge, D.C.; Pillay, N.; Marshall, J.; O'Meara, S.; Davies, H.; Nik-Zainal, S.; et al. Frequent mutation of the major cartilage collagen gene COL2A1 in chondrosarcoma. *Nat. Genet.* **2013**, *45*, 923–926. [CrossRef]

6. Totoki, Y.; Yoshida, A.; Hosoda, F.; Nakamura, H.; Hama, N.; Ogura, K.; Fujiwara, T.; Arai, Y.; Toguchida, J.; Tsuda, H.; et al. Unique mutation portraits and frequent COL2A1 gene alteration in chondrosarcoma. *Genome Res.* **2014**, *24*, 1411–1420. [CrossRef] [PubMed]
7. Schrage, Y.M.; Lam, S.; Jochemsen, A.G.; Cleton-Jansen, A.M.; Taminiau, A.H.; Hogendoorn, P.C.; Bovee, J.V. Central chondrosarcoma progression is associated with pRb pathway alterations: CDK4 down-regulation and p16 overexpression inhibit cell growth in vitro. *J. Cell. Mol. Med.* **2009**, *13*, 2843–2852. [CrossRef] [PubMed]
8. Boehme, K.A.; Schleicher, S.B.; Traub, F.; Rolauffs, B. Chondrosarcoma: A Rare Misfortune in Aging Human Cartilage? The Role of Stem and Progenitor Cells in Proliferation, Malignant Degeneration and Therapeutic Resistance. *Int. J. Mol. Sci.* **2018**, *19*. [CrossRef] [PubMed]
9. Bovee, J.V.; Cleton-Jansen, A.M.; Taminiau, A.H.; Hogendoorn, P.C. Emerging pathways in the development of chondrosarcoma of bone and implications for targeted treatment. *Lancet Oncol.* **2005**, *6*, 599–607. [CrossRef]
10. Brown, H.K.; Schiavone, K.; Gouin, F.; Heymann, M.F.; Heymann, D. Biology of Bone Sarcomas and New Therapeutic Developments. *Calcif. Tissue Int.* **2018**, *102*, 174–195. [CrossRef]
11. David, E.; Blanchard, F.; Heymann, M.F.; De Pinieux, G.; Gouin, F.; Redini, F.; Heymann, D. The Bone Niche of Chondrosarcoma: A Sanctuary for Drug Resistance, Tumour Growth and also a Source of New Therapeutic Targets. *Sarcoma* **2011**, *2011*, 932451. [CrossRef]
12. Polychronidou, G.; Karavasilis, V.; Pollack, S.M.; Huang, P.H.; Lee, A.; Jones, R.L. Novel therapeutic approaches in chondrosarcoma. *Future Oncol.* **2017**, *13*, 637–648. [CrossRef]
13. Martinez-Cruzado, L.; Tornin, J.; Santos, L.; Rodriguez, A.; Garcia-Castro, J.; Moris, F.; Rodriguez, R. Aldh1 Expression and Activity Increase During Tumor Evolution in Sarcoma Cancer Stem Cell Populations. *Sci. Rep.* **2016**, *6*, 27878. [CrossRef]
14. Tirino, V.; Desiderio, V.; Paino, F.; De Rosa, A.; Papaccio, F.; Fazioli, F.; Pirozzi, G.; Papaccio, G. Human primary bone sarcomas contain CD133+ cancer stem cells displaying high tumorigenicity in vivo. *FASEB J.* **2011**, *25*, 2022–2030. [CrossRef]
15. Goodspeed, A.; Heiser, L.M.; Gray, J.W.; Costello, J.C. Tumor-Derived Cell Lines as Molecular Models of Cancer Pharmacogenomics. *Mol. Cancer Res.* **2016**, *14*, 3–13. [CrossRef]
16. McDermott, U. Cancer cell lines as patient avatars for drug response prediction. *Nat. Genet.* **2018**, *50*, 1350–1351. [CrossRef]
17. Wilding, J.L.; Bodmer, W.F. Cancer cell lines for drug discovery and development. *Cancer Res.* **2014**, *74*, 2377–2384. [CrossRef]
18. Calabuig-Farinas, S.; Benso, R.G.; Szuhai, K.; Machado, I.; Lopez-Guerrero, J.A.; de Jong, D.; Peydro, A.; San Miguel, T.; Navarro, L.; Pellin, A.; et al. Characterization of a new human cell line (CH-3573) derived from a grade II chondrosarcoma with matrix production. *Pathol. Oncol. Res.* **2012**, *18*, 793–802. [CrossRef]
19. Farges, M.; Mazeau, C.; Gioanni, J.; Ettore, F.; Denovion, H.; Schneider, M. Establishment and characterization of a new cell line derived from a human chondrosarcoma. *Oncol. Rep.* **1997**, *4*, 697–700. [CrossRef]
20. Gil-Benso, R.; Lopez-Gines, C.; Lopez-Guerrero, J.A.; Carda, C.; Callaghan, R.C.; Navarro, S.; Ferrer, J.; Pellin, A.; Llombart-Bosch, A. Establishment and characterization of a continuous human chondrosarcoma cell line, ch-2879: Comparative histologic and genetic studies with its tumor of origin. *Lab. Investig.* **2003**, *83*, 877–887. [CrossRef]
21. Jagasia, A.A.; Block, J.A.; Qureshi, A.; Diaz, M.O.; Nobori, T.; Gitelis, S.; Iyer, A.P. Chromosome 9 related aberrations and deletions of the CDKN2 and MTS2 putative tumor suppressor genes in human chondrosarcomas. *Cancer Lett.* **1996**, *105*, 91–103. [CrossRef]
22. Kalinski, T.; Krueger, S.; Pelz, A.F.; Wieacker, P.; Hartig, R.; Ropke, M.; Schneider-Stock, R.; Dombrowski, F.; Roessner, A. Establishment and characterization of the permanent human cell line C3842 derived from a secondary chondrosarcoma in Ollier's disease. *Virchows Arch.* **2005**, *446*, 287–299. [CrossRef]
23. Kudawara, I.; Araki, N.; Myoui, A.; Kato, Y.; Uchida, A.; Yoshikawa, H. New cell lines with chondrocytic phenotypes from human chondrosarcoma. *Virchows Arch.* **2004**, *444*, 577–586. [CrossRef]
24. Kudo, N.; Ogose, A.; Hotta, T.; Kawashima, H.; Gu, W.; Umezu, H.; Toyama, T.; Endo, N. Establishment of novel human dedifferentiated chondrosarcoma cell line with osteoblastic differentiation. *Virchows Arch.* **2007**, *451*, 691–699. [CrossRef]

25. Kunisada, T.; Miyazaki, M.; Mihara, K.; Gao, C.; Kawai, A.; Inoue, H.; Namba, M. A new human chondrosarcoma cell line (OUMS-27) that maintains chondrocytic differentiation. *Int. J. Cancer* **1998**, *77*, 854–859. [CrossRef]
26. Monderer, D.; Luseau, A.; Bellec, A.; David, E.; Ponsolle, S.; Saiagh, S.; Bercegeay, S.; Piloquet, P.; Denis, M.G.; Lode, L.; et al. New chondrosarcoma cell lines and mouse models to study the link between chondrogenesis and chemoresistance. *Lab. Investig.* **2013**, *93*, 1100–1114. [CrossRef]
27. van Oosterwijk, J.G.; de Jong, D.; van Ruler, M.A.; Hogendoorn, P.C.; Dijkstra, P.D.; van Rijswijk, C.S.; Machado, I.; Llombart-Bosch, A.; Szuhai, K.; Bovee, J.V. Three new chondrosarcoma cell lines: One grade III conventional central chondrosarcoma and two dedifferentiated chondrosarcomas of bone. *BMC Cancer* **2012**, *12*, 375. [CrossRef]
28. Tornin, J.; Martinez-Cruzado, L.; Santos, L.; Rodriguez, A.; Nunez, L.E.; Oro, P.; Hermosilla, M.A.; Allonca, E.; Fernandez-Garcia, M.T.; Astudillo, A.; et al. Inhibition of SP1 by the mithramycin analog EC-8042 efficiently targets tumor initiating cells in sarcoma. *Oncotarget* **2016**, *7*, 30935–30950. [CrossRef]
29. Martinez-Cruzado, L.; Tornin, J.; Rodriguez, A.; Santos, L.; Allonca, E.; Fernandez-Garcia, M.T.; Astudillo, A.; Garcia-Pedrero, J.M.; Rodriguez, R. Trabectedin and Campthotecin Synergistically Eliminate Cancer Stem Cells in Cell-of-Origin Sarcoma Models. *Neoplasia* **2017**, *19*, 460–470. [CrossRef]
30. Tornin, J.; Hermida-Prado, F.; Padda, R.S.; Gonzalez, M.V.; Alvarez-Fernandez, C.; Rey, V.; Martinez-Cruzado, L.; Estupinan, O.; Menendez, S.T.; Fernandez-Nevado, L.; et al. FUS-CHOP Promotes Invasion in Myxoid Liposarcoma through a SRC/FAK/RHO/ROCK-Dependent Pathway. *Neoplasia* **2018**, *20*, 44–56. [CrossRef]
31. Estupinan, O.; Santos, L.; Rodriguez, A.; Fernandez-Nevado, L.; Costales, P.; Perez-Escuredo, J.; Hermosilla, M.A.; Oro, P.; Rey, V.; Tornin, J.; et al. The multikinase inhibitor EC-70124 synergistically increased the antitumor activity of doxorubicin in sarcomas. *Int. J. Cancer* **2018**. [CrossRef]
32. Rubio, R.; Abarrategi, A.; Garcia-Castro, J.; Martinez-Cruzado, L.; Suarez, C.; Tornin, J.; Santos, L.; Astudillo, A.; Colmenero, I.; Mulero, F.; et al. Bone environment is essential for osteosarcoma development from transformed mesenchymal stem cells. *Stem Cells* **2014**, *32*, 1136–1148. [CrossRef]
33. Bolger, A.M.; Lohse, M.; Usadel, B. Trimmomatic: A flexible trimmer for Illumina sequence data. *Bioinformatics* **2014**, *30*, 2114–2120. [CrossRef]
34. Cabanillas, R.; Dineiro, M.; Castillo, D.; Pruneda, P.C.; Penas, C.; Cifuentes, G.A.; de Vicente, A.; Duran, N.S.; Alvarez, R.; Ordonez, G.R.; et al. A novel molecular diagnostics platform for somatic and germline precision oncology. *Mol. Genet. Genomic Med.* **2017**, *5*, 336–359. [CrossRef]
35. Choi, Y.; Sims, G.E.; Murphy, S.; Miller, J.R.; Chan, A.P. Predicting the functional effect of amino acid substitutions and indels. *PLoS ONE* **2012**, *7*, e46688. [CrossRef]
36. Chun, S.; Fay, J.C. Identification of deleterious mutations within three human genomes. *Genome Res.* **2009**, *19*, 1553–1561. [CrossRef]
37. Davydov, E.V.; Goode, D.L.; Sirota, M.; Cooper, G.M.; Sidow, A.; Batzoglou, S. Identifying a high fraction of the human genome to be under selective constraint using GERP++. *PLoS Comput. Biol.* **2010**, *6*, e1001025. [CrossRef]
38. Deshwar, A.G.; Vembu, S.; Yung, C.K.; Jang, G.H.; Stein, L.; Morris, Q. PhyloWGS: Reconstructing subclonal composition and evolution from whole-genome sequencing of tumors. *Genome Biol.* **2015**, *16*, 35. [CrossRef]
39. Dong, C.; Wei, P.; Jian, X.; Gibbs, R.; Boerwinkle, E.; Wang, K.; Liu, X. Comparison and integration of deleteriousness prediction methods for nonsynonymous SNVs in whole exome sequencing studies. *Hum. Mol. Genet.* **2015**, *24*, 2125–2137. [CrossRef]
40. Jagadeesh, K.A.; Wenger, A.M.; Berger, M.J.; Guturu, H.; Stenson, P.D.; Cooper, D.N.; Bernstein, J.A.; Bejerano, G. M-CAP eliminates a majority of variants of uncertain significance in clinical exomes at high sensitivity. *Nat. Genet.* **2016**, *48*, 1581–1586. [CrossRef]
41. Kumar, P.; Henikoff, S.; Ng, P.C. Predicting the effects of coding non-synonymous variants on protein function using the SIFT algorithm. *Nat. Protoc.* **2009**, *4*, 1073–1081. [CrossRef]
42. Li, H.; Handsaker, B.; Wysoker, A.; Fennell, T.; Ruan, J.; Homer, N.; Marth, G.; Abecasis, G.; Durbin, R.; Genome Project Data Processing, S. The Sequence Alignment/Map format and SAMtools. *Bioinformatics* **2009**, *25*, 2078–2079. [CrossRef] [PubMed]
43. Miller, C.A.; McMichael, J.; Dang, H.X.; Maher, C.A.; Ding, L.; Ley, T.J.; Mardis, E.R.; Wilson, R.K. Visualizing tumor evolution with the fishplot package for R. *BMC Genom.* **2016**, *17*, 880. [CrossRef] [PubMed]

44. Puente, X.S.; Pinyol, M.; Quesada, V.; Conde, L.; Ordonez, G.R.; Villamor, N.; Escaramis, G.; Jares, P.; Bea, S.; Gonzalez-Diaz, M.; et al. Whole-genome sequencing identifies recurrent mutations in chronic lymphocytic leukaemia. *Nature* **2011**, *475*, 101–105. [CrossRef]
45. Reva, B.; Antipin, Y.; Sander, C. Predicting the functional impact of protein mutations: Application to cancer genomics. *Nucleic Acids Res.* **2011**, *39*, e118. [CrossRef] [PubMed]
46. Schwarz, J.M.; Cooper, D.N.; Schuelke, M.; Seelow, D. MutationTaster2: Mutation prediction for the deep-sequencing age. *Nat. Methods* **2014**, *11*, 361–362. [CrossRef] [PubMed]
47. Shihab, H.A.; Gough, J.; Mort, M.; Cooper, D.N.; Day, I.N.; Gaunt, T.R. Ranking non-synonymous single nucleotide polymorphisms based on disease concepts. *Hum. Genom.* **2014**, *8*, 11. [CrossRef]
48. European Nucleotide Archive repository. Available online: http://www.ebi.ac.uk/ena/data/view/PRJEB31233 (accessed on 28 February 2019).
49. Suijker, J.; Oosting, J.; Koornneef, A.; Struys, E.A.; Salomons, G.S.; Schaap, F.G.; Waaijer, C.J.; Wijers-Koster, P.M.; Briaire-de Bruijn, I.H.; Haazen, L.; et al. Inhibition of mutant IDH1 decreases D-2-HG levels without affecting tumorigenic properties of chondrosarcoma cell lines. *Oncotarget* **2015**, *6*, 12505–12519. [CrossRef]
50. Campbell, V.T.; Nadesan, P.; Ali, S.A.; Wang, C.Y.; Whetstone, H.; Poon, R.; Wei, Q.; Keilty, J.; Proctor, J.; Wang, L.W.; et al. Hedgehog pathway inhibition in chondrosarcoma using the smoothened inhibitor IPI-926 directly inhibits sarcoma cell growth. *Mol. Cancer Ther.* **2014**, *13*, 1259–1269. [CrossRef]
51. Heymann, D.; Redini, F. Targeted therapies for bone sarcomas. *Bonekey Rep.* **2013**, *2*, 378. [CrossRef]
52. Barretina, J.; Caponigro, G.; Stransky, N.; Venkatesan, K.; Margolin, A.A.; Kim, S.; Wilson, C.J.; Lehar, J.; Kryukov, G.V.; Sonkin, D.; et al. The Cancer Cell Line Encyclopedia enables predictive modelling of anticancer drug sensitivity. *Nature* **2012**, *483*, 603–607. [CrossRef]
53. Iorio, F.; Knijnenburg, T.A.; Vis, D.J.; Bignell, G.R.; Menden, M.P.; Schubert, M.; Aben, N.; Goncalves, E.; Barthorpe, S.; Lightfoot, H.; et al. A Landscape of Pharmacogenomic Interactions in Cancer. *Cell* **2016**, *166*, 740–754. [CrossRef]
54. Lee, J.K.; Liu, Z.; Sa, J.K.; Shin, S.; Wang, J.; Bordyuh, M.; Cho, H.J.; Elliott, O.; Chu, T.; Choi, S.W.; et al. Pharmacogenomic landscape of patient-derived tumor cells informs precision oncology therapy. *Nat. Genet.* **2018**, *50*, 1399–1411. [CrossRef]
55. Ledford, H. US cancer institute to overhaul tumour cell lines. *Nature* **2016**, *530*, 391. [CrossRef]
56. Golan, H.; Shukrun, R.; Caspi, R.; Vax, E.; Pode-Shakked, N.; Goldberg, S.; Pleniceanu, O.; Bar-Lev, D.D.; Mark-Danieli, M.; Pri-Chen, S.; et al. In Vivo Expansion of Cancer Stemness Affords Novel Cancer Stem Cell Targets: Malignant Rhabdoid Tumor as an Example. *Stem Cell Rep.* **2018**, *11*, 795–810. [CrossRef]
57. Ben-David, U.; Ha, G.; Tseng, Y.Y.; Greenwald, N.F.; Oh, C.; Shih, J.; McFarland, J.M.; Wong, B.; Boehm, J.S.; Beroukhim, R.; et al. Patient-derived xenografts undergo mouse-specific tumor evolution. *Nat. Genet.* **2017**, *49*, 1567–1575. [CrossRef]
58. Oshiro, Y.; Chaturvedi, V.; Hayden, D.; Nazeer, T.; Johnson, M.; Johnston, D.A.; Ordonez, N.G.; Ayala, A.G.; Czerniak, B. Altered p53 is associated with aggressive behavior of chondrosarcoma: A long term follow-up study. *Cancer* **1998**, *83*, 2324–2334. [CrossRef]
59. Yamaguchi, T.; Toguchida, J.; Wadayama, B.; Kanoe, H.; Nakayama, T.; Ishizaki, K.; Ikenaga, M.; Kotoura, Y.; Sasaki, M.S. Loss of heterozygosity and tumor suppressor gene mutations in chondrosarcomas. *Anticancer Res.* **1996**, *16*, 2009–2015.

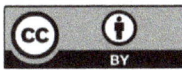

© 2019 by the authors. Licensee MDPI, Basel, Switzerland. This article is an open access article distributed under the terms and conditions of the Creative Commons Attribution (CC BY) license (http://creativecommons.org/licenses/by/4.0/).

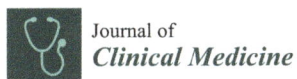
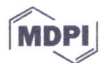

Article

Human Red Blood Cells as Oxygen Carriers to Improve Ex-Situ Liver Perfusion in a Rat Model

Daniele Dondossola [1,2,*], Alessandro Santini [3], Caterina Lonati [3,4], Alberto Zanella [2,3], Riccardo Merighi [4], Luigi Vivona [3], Michele Battistin [3], Alessandro Galli [3], Osvaldo Biancolilli [3], Marco Maggioni [5], Stefania Villa [6] and Stefano Gatti [4]

1. General and Liver Transplant Surgery Unit, Fondazione IRCCS Ca' Granda, Ospedale Maggiore Policlinico, 20019 Milan, Italy
2. Department of Pathophysiology and Transplantation, Università degli Studi of Milan, 20019 Milan, Italy; alberto.zanella1@unimi.it
3. Department of Anesthesia and Critical Care, Fondazione IRCCS Ca' Granda, Ospedale Maggiore Policlinico, 20019 Milan, Italy; alesantini85@gmail.com (A.S.); caterina.lonati@gmail.com (C.L.); preclinica@policlinico.mi.it (L.V.); battistin.michele@gmail.com (M.B.); alexgalli@hotmail.com (A.G.); osvaldo.biancolilli85@gmail.com (O.B.)
4. Center for Preclinical Research, Fondazione IRCCS Ca' Granda, Ospedale Maggiore Policlinico, 20019 Milan, Italy; riccardo.merighi92@gmail.com (R.M.); stefano.gatti@gmail.com (S.G.)
5. Pathology Department, Fondazione IRCCS Ca' Granda, Ospedale Maggiore Policlinico, 20019 Milan, Italy; marco.maggioni@policlinico.mi.it
6. Department of Transfusion Medicine and Hematology, Fondazione IRCCS Ca' Granda, Ospedale Maggiore Policlinico, 20019 Milan, Italy; stefania.villa@policlinico.mi.it
* Correspondence: dondossola.daniele@gmail.com; Tel.: +39-02-55033424

Received: 29 September 2019; Accepted: 5 November 2019; Published: 8 November 2019

Abstract: Ex-situ machine perfusion (MP) has been increasingly used to enhance liver quality in different settings. Small animal models can help to implement this procedure. As most normothermic MP (NMP) models employ sub-physiological levels of oxygen delivery (DO_2), the aim of this study was to investigate the effectiveness and safety of different DO_2, using human red blood cells (RBCs) as oxygen carriers on metabolic recovery in a rat model of NMP. Four experimental groups (n = 5 each) consisted of (1) native (untreated/control), (2) liver static cold storage (SCS) 30 min without NMP, (3) SCS followed by 120 min of NMP with Dulbecco-Modified-Eagle-Medium as perfusate (DMEM), and (4) similar to group 3, but perfusion fluid was added with human RBCs (hematocrit 15%) (BLOOD). Compared to DMEM, the BLOOD group showed increased liver DO_2 ($p = 0.008$) and oxygen consumption ($\dot{V}O_2$) ($p < 0.001$); lactate clearance ($p < 0.001$), potassium ($p < 0.001$), and glucose ($p = 0.029$) uptake were enhanced. ATP levels were likewise higher in BLOOD relative to DMEM ($p = 0.031$). $\dot{V}O_2$ and DO_2 were highly correlated ($p < 0.001$). Consistently, the main metabolic parameters were directly correlated with DO_2 and $\dot{V}O_2$. No human RBC related damage was detected. In conclusion, an optimized DO_2 significantly reduces hypoxic damage-related effects occurring during NMP. Human RBCs can be safely used as oxygen carriers.

Keywords: normothermic machine perfusion; rat; human red blood cells; oxygen consumption; oxygen delivery

1. Introduction

Liver machine perfusion (MP) was introduced in the clinical setting by Guarrera and colleagues [1] in 2009. Based on its ability to recondition, evaluate, and preserve liver grafts, MP showed a particular potential in reverting the detrimental impact of extended criteria donors (ECD) on post-liver transplant (LT) outcome and quality of life [2,3]. Among MPs, normothermic machine perfusion (NMP) represents the most promising technology due to its higher evaluation potential [4]. Further, NMP can be used in preclinical settings to evaluate other preservation or treatment techniques outside LT. In this last setting, NMP is defined as normothermic machine reperfusion (NMRP).

Since reactions elicited during ex-situ dynamic perfusion are largely unknown, technical and biological aspects of liver MP need to be extensively investigated through committed research. A number of animal models have been developed for this purpose. Because of their immediate translational value (e.g., appropriate human-like liver size), swine models have been broadly used in the start-up phase to rapidly translate preclinical results into the clinical setting. Conversely, small animal models can better be exploited to investigate subcellular mechanisms and changes associated with MP. To this purpose, based on low cost, reproducibility, and better understanding of subcellular events, rat models have been widely used [5].

Over the last ten years, 94 research papers were based on liver MP use in rodents. We reviewed all those reporting rat ex-situ perfusions with recirculating fluid and 39 of them described NMP/NMRP (Supplementary Materials: a brief review of the literature is provided in Tables S1 and S2). A large variability in NMP protocols among different research groups was evident. In particular, the potential usefulness of an oxygen carrier (OxC) during normothermic perfusion was not fully explored. While only few researchers used OxC perfusate for NMP or NMRP [6–16], most of them adopted a non-OxC model. The infrequent use of OxC could be related to the high number of rats needed to be used as blood donors (at least 3-4 animals/experiment) and unavailability of other oxygen carriers. However, while adequate oxygen delivery (DO_2) was observed in the absence of an oxygen carrier, the increased oxygen consumption ($\dot{V}O_2$) needed to control the reperfusion injury suggests the opportunity to increase DO_2 during reperfusion [8,17]. To this purpose, two main strategies may be adopted: use of non-cellular hemoglobin [18] or employment of other sources of blood [13]. While the first is limited by the restricted availability of these products, human blood cells can be easily procured for experimental use.

The aim of present research was optimization of procurement and perfusion procedures to obtain a safe and reproducible rat model of NMP. The study examined the potential protective role of improved DO_2 during NMP and evaluated the safety and efficacy of human red blood cell use. Indeed, the use of non-murine red blood cells can allow for the reduction of the number of animals/experiments in full respect of the 3Rs principles (Refinement, Reduction, and Replacement) [19].

2. Material and Methods

2.1. Animals and Study Design

Experiments were performed at the Center for Surgical Research, Fondazione IRCCS Ca' Granda Ospedale Maggiore Policlinico of Milan. Italian Institute of Health approved the experimental protocol (number 568EB.1). All animals received humane care in compliance with the Principles of Laboratory Animal Care formulated by the Federation of European Laboratory Animal Science Associations [20].

Adult Sprague-Dawley male rats weighing 240 to 330 g (Envigo RMS. S.R.L, Udine, Italy) were housed in a ventilated cage system (Tecniplast S.p.A., Varese, Italy) at 22 ± 1 °C, 55 ± 5% humidity, on a 12 h dark/light cycle, and were allowed free access to rat chow feed and water ad libitum. All efforts were made to minimize suffering.

A schematic workflow diagram of the investigation is shown in Figure 1. Twenty rats were randomly assigned to four experimental groups (n = 5/group): (1) *DMEM* whose livers were subjected to in-situ cold flushing, procured, cold stored for 30 min, and then ex-situ perfused for 120 min with a perfusion fluid without an oxygen carrier; (2) *BLOOD*, whose livers were subjected to all the procedures of the DMEM group, but NMP perfusion fluid included human red blood cells (RBC) as an oxygen carrier; (3) *Cold storage*, whose livers were subjected to in-situ cold flushing, procured, and then subjected to 30 min of cold storage; (4) *Native*, whose livers were procured immediately after anesthesia and suppressed.

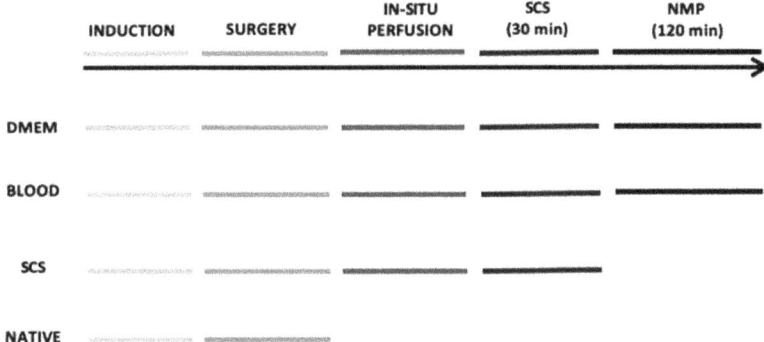

Figure 1. Schematic representation of the 4 experimental groups. DMEM and BLOOD groups performed all six steps of the timeline. Static cold storage (SCS) group underwent to all steps except for the normothermic machine perfusion, while Native group only to general anesthesia and surgery with liver tissue sampled at the end of the experiment.

2.2. Blood Group Typing and Compatibility Testing

Human blood used was collected in CPD (citrate-phosphate- dextrose), resuspended in SAGM (saline-adenine-glucose-mannitol), and leukoreduced at final hemtocrit of 60 ± 5%.

Blood samples of the Native group were tested for blood group typing. Blood was collected in K3-EDTA test tube and tested with 0 Rh (D) negative and AB Rh (D) negative human packed leukoreduced red blood cells and plasma. Direct blood group typing was performed with manual method using ABO Ortho BioVue Card (Ortho Clinical Diagnostics, Pencoed, UK) on 3% blood cells diluted in saline solution. Indirect blood group typing was manually performed on fresh plasma through Reverse Diluent Ortho BioVue Card with standard blood cells A1, B, and 0 (Affirmagen Ortho). We repeated the same analyses at 4 °C to enhance ABO antibody mediated activity.

Major compatibility (recipient serum versus donor red blood cells) and minor compatibility (donor plasma with the recipient red cells) were manually performed using Ortho BioVue with anti-IgG, C3d polyspecific Cards.

All rats resulted 0 Rh (D) negative at direct typing. Indirect blood group typing showed in one case anti-A and anti-B antibodies, while in two cases only anti-A antibodies were detected. Major compatibility was negative with 0 Rh (D) negative human red blood cells, while positive with AB Rh (D) negative donors. Minor compatibility was positive with both 0 Rh (D) negative and AB Rh (D) negative plasma of human donors. According to these results, in order to have the greatest incompatibility to highlight any damage from hemolysis, we decided to use AB Rh (D) positive packed leukoreduced red blood cells.

2.3. Reagents and Instruments

All experiments were carried out in sterile conditions and all instruments/drugs were kept sterile until use. The drugs, reagents, and instrumentation necessary to conduct this protocol are shown in Supplementary Materials (Tables S3 and S4).

2.4. Anesthesia, Surgery, and In-Situ Perfusion

A schematic overview of all experimental procedures is provided in Supplementary Materials (Figure S1). Rats were anesthetized by intraperitoneal injection of 80 mg/kg of sodic thiopentale and maintained in spontaneous breathing with an O_2 enriched air mixture by an open mask. The surgical procedure was carried on with a double-headed surgical microscope OPMI 1-F (Zeiss West Germany, Oberkochen, Germany). Procedure began with a xifo-pubic and bilateral subcostal incision. The hepatic pedicle was then exposed, and the bile duct was dissected. It was distally ligated with a 8-0 nylon tie and a customized cannula (tip: 24 G cannula Braun, Bethlehem, PA, USA; tube: PE-50, BD-Clay Adams, Becton, UK) was inserted through a choledotomy; the cannula was secured with a proximal 8-0 nylon tie. Subsequently, the portal vein was cannulated. Then, the pyloric vein was ligated (8-0 nylon) and transacted, and the main trunk of the portal vein was dissected until distally to the splenic vein. The portal vein was encircled with three 5-0 silk tie and unfractioned heparin (2 IU/g diluted in 1 mL of normal saline) was administered by tail IV injection. After three minutes, we ligated the portal vein distally to the splenic vein insertion and a 16 G cannula was inserted by venipuncture until the tip of the cannula reached the portal bifurcation. A blood retrograde flush was performed, and the in-situ perfusion system was connected. Then, the cannula was secured with a two silk tie and gently retracted to avoid obstruction of the right lobe portal vein branch. Rapid sternotomy was performed, the heart was removed, and the inferior vena cava (IVC) was transected. In-situ cold perfusion (4 °C) was started with 35 mL of Celsior solution (IGL, Lissieu, France) at a pressure of 30 cmH$_2$O. At the end of the perfusion, hepatectomy was completed and the liver graft was stored in 4 °C Celsior solution for 30 min. At the end of the cold storage and before NMP connection, the backtable was completed to free the superior vena cava (the liver was maintained on a refrigerated surface). All surgical times were recorded.

2.5. Surgical Procedure and In-Situ Perfusion

All procedures were carried out by an expert surgeon trained in microsurgery and ex-situ perfusion models. Time periods required for bile duct cannulation (from laparotomy to cannula placement in the bile duct), portal cannulation (from bile duct cannulation to portal cannula placement), in-situ cold-flush, liver procurement (from flushing to procurement), warm ischemia time (from the end of in-situ flush to the start of the cold storage), and liver connection to NMP (from end of SCS to connection to the circuit) were examined as indexes of technical success and reproducibility of the surgical procedure. The rats that were randomized to native group ($n = 5$) were not included in this analysis because they did not undergo any surgical procedure. There were no statistically significant differences among the "surgical" groups in terms of surgical preparation 37 ± 1 min for DMEM, 35 ± 2 min for BLOOD, and 35 ± 2 min for SCS. Cold flush lasted 60 ± 4 sec for DMEM, 71 ± 18 sec for BLOOD, and 61 ± 3 sec for SCS, while warm ischemia time 16 ± 1 min for DMEM, 16 ± 3 min for BLOOD, and 16 ± 2 min for SCS.

2.6. Ex-Situ Liver Perfusion

2.6.1. Perfusion Fluids Preparation

Perfusate composition is shown in Supplementary Materials (Table S5). DMEM perfusate was obtained by adding to DMEM, 4% human albumin, streptomycin and penicillin, glutamine, and insulin for a total volume of perfusate of 100 mL. Perfusion fluid was obtained according to Op den Dries and colleagues [13]. We added to DMEM 4% human albumin, streptomycin and penicillin, glutamine, insulin, heparin, and 15% hematocrit human RBC for a global volume of perfusate of 100 mL.

Human red cells were provided by the Blood Bank of our Institution (Department of Transfusion Medicine and Hematology). A packed red blood cell concentrate was prepared by centrifugation from one unit of a whole blood donation, which was unsuitable for human use because of an insufficient volume collected. The same unit (blood group: AB Rh+) was used throughout the experiment.

2.6.2. Normothermic Machine Perfusion Setup

The perfusion system (Figure 2) consisted of a customized circuit derived from the isolated lung perfusion system (Hugo Sachs Elektronik, Harvard Apparatus, March-Hugstetten, Germany) implemented and described by our laboratory [21–24]. It consisted of a reusable heated glass reservoir, a heated bubble trap, a circulating tube derived by an infusion system, an octagonal peristaltic pump, a polystyrene lid, and a single-use artificial lung (Supplementary Tables S3 and S4). The liver was placed onto the glass chamber modified to let the liver laid on the diaphragmatic surface on a modeled ad hoc, perforated parafilm. The liver was connected to the circuit through the portal vein cannula and the bile duct cannula to a 2 mL tube to collect bile. The chamber was closed to maintain humidity. Temperature inside the chamber was recorded with a 1.3 mm probe. The heat-exchanger was set at 40 °C to obtain a graft temperature of 37 °C. We carefully avoided air embolism during priming and liver connection. The artificial lung was ventilated with a 200 mL/min flow, with 95% FiO2 and 5% FiCO2.

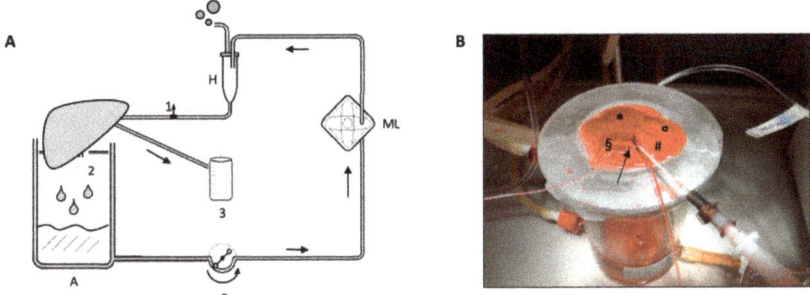

Figure 2. (**A**) Schematic representation of normothermic machine perfusion circuit. 1: pre-liver sampling stopcock; 2: post-liver sampling from IVC; 3: bile collection cuvette; A: heated glass reservoir; P: peristaltic pump; ML: membrane lung; H: heated exchanger and bubble trap. (**B**) Detail of the portal vein and bile duct cannula during ex-situ perfusion. Liver was laid on the diaphragmatic surface. Arrow: inferior vena cava; § right lateral lobe; * median lobe; ° left lateral lobe; # caudate lobe.

Circuit hemodynamic parameters were monitored using the Colligo system (Elekton, Milan, Italy). Portal vein and pre-lung pressures were recorded every 5 min during rewarming, and every 30 min during normothermic machine perfusion. Vascular resistances were calculated as mean portal vein pressure divided by blood flow in the portal vein (mL/min). Temperature was monitored by a thermo probe located between the lobes of the liver.

2.6.3. Ex-Vivo Liver Perfusion Protocol

The NMP-protocol lasted 150 min and divided into two phases. The first 30 min was called "rewarming", followed by 120 min of normothermic perfusion (Figure 3). In brief, after 30 min of static cold storage, the graft was connected to the NMP and the perfusion began. The portal flow was set at 5 mL/min and was increased by 5 mL/min every 5 min up to 30 mL/min or portal pressure of 8 cmH2O. At the beginning of the rewarming phase, the heat exchanger was set at 30 °C and the temperature was raised up to 40 °C to obtain a liver temperature of 37 °C after 30 min. During the normothermic phase temperature was maintained at 37 °C and portal flow remained unchanged.

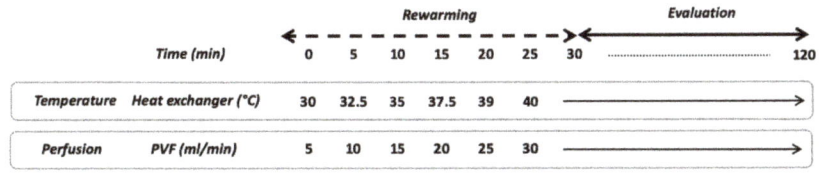

Figure 3. Schematic overview of NMP protocol. PVF, portal vein flow.

2.7. Perfusate Analysis

Perfusate samples were collected soon after grafting ex-situ reperfusion and then every 30 min during the normothermic phase. The concentration of gas, metabolites, hyaluronan (HA), electrolytes, hemoglobin, and cells were evaluated. Pre-liver stopcock was used for perfusate sampling, while post liver perfusate was collected directly from IVC. Bile was collected by gravity directly into a test tube and weighted.

2.8. Sample Processing and Analysis

Perfusate samples were centrifugated at 1500 rpm for 15 min at 4 °C (Haereus Multifuge 33R, Thermo Fisher Scientific, Whaltham). Supernatants were collected and stored at −20 °C for mediator concentration evaluation, whereas cell pellets were suspended in erythrocyte lysis buffer (0.155 M NH_4Cl, 10 mM $KHCO_3$, 0.1 mM Na_2EDTA, pH 7.4; all from MilliporeSigma, Frankfurter, Germany) and incubated for 10 min at 4 °C. A 10-min centrifugation at 2000 rpm was then performed. Recovered supernatants were used for free hemoglobin assessment, whereas pellets were suspended in 0.25 mL 13 PBS solution (MilliporeSigma, Frankfurter, Germany) for cell count and characterization.

Using a gas analyzer, acid-base balance (pH, pCO_2, pO_2), electrolytes (K^+, Na^+, Cl^-, Ca^{2+}), and metabolites (glucose and lactate) were evaluated (ABL 800 Flex; A. De Mori Strumenti, Milan, Italy).

At the beginning and end of the normothermic phase, perfusate samples were investigated for hepatocyte integrity (alanine-aminotransferase, ALT; aspartate-aminotransferase, AST; Lactate dehydrogenase, LDH), cholangiocellular damage (ALP, GGT), and blood count.

The concentration of total HA in outflow perfusate was determined by ELISA using a commercially available kit (sensitivity, 0.068 ng/mL; low standard, 0.625 ng/mL; R&D Systems, Minneapolis, MN, USA). The procedure was validated in preliminary experiments by using HA preparations with a known concentration and known average molecular mass (Select-HA HiLadder and LoLadder; Hyalose, Oklahoma City, OK, USA) [21–24].

Sodium Citrate concentration was measured by enzymatic assay using spectrophotometry (Citrate Assay Kit, Sigma-Aldrich, Saint Louis, USA). Millipore Amicon Ultra 0.5 mL 20 KDa were used to remove proteins. Thereafter, deproteinized samples were diluted 1:2 with citrate assay buffer and centrifugated at 14,000× g.

2.9. Tissue Analysis

Tissue samples were taken at the end of NMP in DMEM and BLOOD groups, at the end of cold storage in SCS group, and soon after laparotomy in group Native. Tissue samples ($n = 8$) were collected from the right median lobe: 1 sample was used for wet-to-dry ratio (W/D), 1 formalin fixed. Liver grafts were weighted at the end of static cold storage and the end of NMP.

2.10. Wet-to-Dry Ratio

A biopsy was weighed with an analytical balance, dried in an oven at 50 °C for 48 h, and then weighted [25]. Wet-to-dry ratio (W/D) was calculated and used as an index of edema. Livers procured from native and cold ischemia group were used as controls.

2.11. ATP Content Assessment

Liver samples were homogenized in trichloroacetic acid (MilliporeSigma, Frankfurter, Germany), then subjected to 10 min of centrifugation at maximum speed at 4 °C. Supernatants were diluted 1:30 using 0.1 M Tris-acetate, pH 7.75 (MilliporeSigma, Frankfurter, Germany). Next, 10 mL of each sample were dispensed in a blank 96-well plate and 90 mL of luciferin/luciferase reagent were added (Enliten ATP Assay System; Promega, Madison, WI, USA). Bioluminescent signals were immediately detected with a luminometer (Glomax Luminometer; Promega, Madison, WI, USA). ATP concentration was calculated by using a standard curve that ranged from 10,211 to 1025 M (rATP 10 mM; Promega, Madison, WI, USA). Results were expressed as concentration/wet tissue weight.

2.12. Histology

Liver samples were fixed in 4% formalin. Formalin-fixed-paraffin-embedded samples were stained with hematoxylin-eosin, Masson's trichrome, Periodic Acid Schiff (PAS) and reticulin histochemical staining, and CD31 immunohistochemical staining. Thirty random fields per slide were investigated to determine the necrosis area.

To evaluate liver tissue integrity, the histological samples were scored according to Brockman and colleagues [26] who demonstrated concordance among NMP results, histopathological analyses, and liver viability.

2.13. Evaluation of Liver Metabolism

The above-mentioned parameters and trends (glucose, lactates, potassium, and sodium citrate) were included in the liver metabolism evaluation. Citrate is metabolized by hepatocyte in the perivenular zone of hepatic lobule and its eventual decrease during the NMP procedure reflects active metabolism [27]. Equally, potassium uptake after the ischemic phase is indicative of an adequate reactivation of Na-K ATP dependent pumps in viable hepatocytes. The uptake ratio (($C_{start}-C_{end})/C_{start}$) was used to describe the variation of metabolic parameters during NMP.

Oxygen consumption ($\dot{V}O_2$) was measured using the modified Fick equation (Supplementary Figure S2). Pre-liver perfusate samples were intended as O_2 enriched perfusate (arterial blood of the Fick equation), whereas post-liver perfusate samples, collected directly from the IVC, were used for the calculation of venous oxygen content in the Fick equation.

2.14. Statistical Analysis

Statistical analysis was performed using SPSS statistics 25.0 software (IBM Corporation, Armonk, USA). Results are expressed as mean ± SEM. The sample size was determined considering a statistical test power of 0.80, with a alpha value of 0.05 and a minimum difference among groups of 0.40 with an expected SD of 0.20. Metabolic and viability parameters were analyzed by using 1-way repeated measures ANOVA. Conversely, 1-way ANOVA or Kruskal–Wallis test were used to evaluate ATP and uptake ratio results. Finally, linear regression analysis was used to correlate variables. Values of $p < 0.05$ were considered statistically significant.

3. Results

A total of 20 experiments were consecutively performed. Nineteen grafts are included in the analysis because one liver graft from the BLOOD group was discarded due to air embolism.

3.1. Perfusate Composition and Hemodynamic During NMP

Liver perfusion was started when the pH of the solution was at least 7.2. Table 1 shows the gas-analyses characteristics of the perfusate before graft connection to the NMP. Besides the differences due to the presence of red blood cells in the BLOOD group, pH, glucose, and bicarbonate concentration were statistically different at baseline gas-analyses between the groups. Baseline citrate concentration was 0.37 ± 0.05 mmol/L in the BLOOD group, while it was not detectable in the DMEM group.

During the rewarming phase, in which flow rate, temperature, and gas flow were gradually increased up to target value, there was a decrease in portal resistance in both groups (Figure 4). While in the rewarming phase portal resistance was not statistically different between the two groups ($p = 0.105$), during the normothermic phase, consistently with higher viscosity of the perfusing solution, it was higher in the BLOOD group ($p = 0.015$).

Table 1. Characteristics of the perfusion fluid in the two experimental groups: baseline blood-gas analyses before liver graft connection to NMP. Hb, hemoglobin; Htc, hematocrit; HbO$_2$, hemoglobin saturation; Gluc, glucose; Lac, lactate; na, not applicable. Results are expressed as mean ± SEM.

	DMEM (n = 5)	BLOOD (n = 4)	p
pH	7.38 ± 0.09	7.18 ± 0.09	0.042
pCO$_2$, mmHg	40.5 ± 8	49.5 ± 13	0.231
pO$_2$, mmHg	540.25 ± 26	446 ± 179	0.317
Hb, g/dL	-	4.4 ± 0.57	na
Htc, %	-	14 ± 2.00	na
HbO$_2$, %	0	96.25 ± 0.07	na
Gluc, g/dL	80 ± 0.50	136 ± 53	0.026
Lac, mmol/L	-	2.3 ± 1.7	na
K$^+$, mmol/L	4.15 ± 0.05	4.5 ± 1	0.427
Na$^+$, mmol/L	149 ± 1	147 ± 3	0.553
Ca^{2+}, mmol/L	0.72 ± 0.28	0.70 ± 0.05	0.342
Cl$^-$, mmol/L	121 ± 2.38	117 ± 5.00	0.522
HCO$_3^-$, mmol/L	23 ± 1.87	15 ± 1.00	0.011

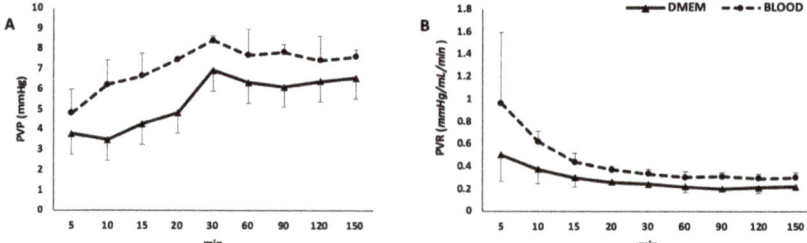

Figure 4. Portal vein pressure (**A**) and resistances (**B**). PVP, portal vein pressure; PVR, portal vein resistances.

3.2. Markers of Hepatocellular and Cholangiocellular Damage

Hepatocellular integrity was evaluated during the normothermic phase (Table 2). Even if transaminases (AST) and lactate-dehydrogenase (LDH) showed a trend toward increase, this was not significant ($p = 0.358$). Furthermore, there were no differences in AST and LDH levels between the groups (Figure S3). Potassium remained stable in DMEM, while it was reabsorbed in BLOOD ($p = 0.001$). Potassium uptake ratio was also higher in the BLOOD vs. DMEM group (Figure 5A). The total amount of bile collected was higher in BLOOD group (Figure 5B). Hyaluronan decreased during the perfusion ($p = 0.002$) without any differences between the groups ($p = 0.331$).

3.3. Evaluation of Liver Tissue Integrity

W/D ratio was not different between DMEM and BLOOD groups (DMEM 3.117 ± 0.136 vs. BLOOD 2.995 ±. 0.85, $p = 0.208$). Compared to SCS group (W/D 2.872 ± 0.128), parenchymal edema was increased in DMEM (vs SCS, $p = 0.029$), while W/D ratio was not statistically different in BLOOD (vs. SCS, $p = 0.275$). Liver histological architecture was preserved in all study groups (Figure 6). Both DMEM and BLOOD showed normal histology and the grade of post-reperfusion injury was not different between the study groups (Figure 5D). As expected, red blood cells were identified within sinusoids and vessels of BLOOD group specimens. Histopathological evaluation showed no sinusoidal obstructions, hemorrhages, or endothelial damage. PAS reaction on tissue samples identified a uniform distribution of glycogen in all hepatic zones of the lobule in BLOOD, while large areas of glycogen consumption were identified in the periportal spaces of DMEM.

Table 2. Main metabolic and biological characteristics of normothermic machine perfusion during normothermic phase in the two study groups. * compared to SCS group (2.872 ± 0.128) $p = 0.029$ in DMEM and $p = 0.275$ in BLOOD. ^ compared to SCS group (985.9 ± 102.6 pmol/mg) $p = 0.001$ in DMEM and $p = 0.012$ in BLOOD. Results are expressed as mean ± SEM.

	Normothermic Phase (30-150 min)				
	Min	DMEM (n = 5)	BLOOD (n = 4)	p (Graft)	p (Time)
AST, U/L/g	30	0.862 ± 0.769	0.739 ± 0.215	0.358	
	150	2.130 ± 1.591	2.273 ± 1.47		
Potassium mEq/L	30	5.45 ± 0.17	5.10 ± 0.62	0.657	0.01
	150	5.40 ± 0.43	4.40 ± 0.61		
Potassium uptake ratio		0.006 ± 0.051	0.138 ± 0.028	0.03	na
Bile, g	tot	1.165 ± 0.22	2.25 ± 0.48	0.237	
W/D ratio *		3.117 ± 0.136	2.995 ±. 0.85	0.208	
ATP, pmol/mg ^		327.3 ± 26.6	565.8 ± 56.6	0.031	
Glucose, mg/dL	30	313 ± 59	310 ± 12	0.008	<0.001
	150	364 ± 101	202 ± 26		
Glucose uptake ratio		−0.136 ± 0.154	0.346 ± 0.079	0.029	
Lactate, mmol/L	30	6.3 ± 0.5	4.5 ± 1.0	0.002	<0.001
	150	5.24 ± 1.2	1.6 ± 0.6		
Lactate uptake ratio		0.062 ± 0.359	0.643 ± 0.27	0.022	na
Citrate	30	na	0.37 ± 0.05		0.034
	150	na	0.29 ± 0.05		
Citrate uptake		na	0.228 ± 0.127		

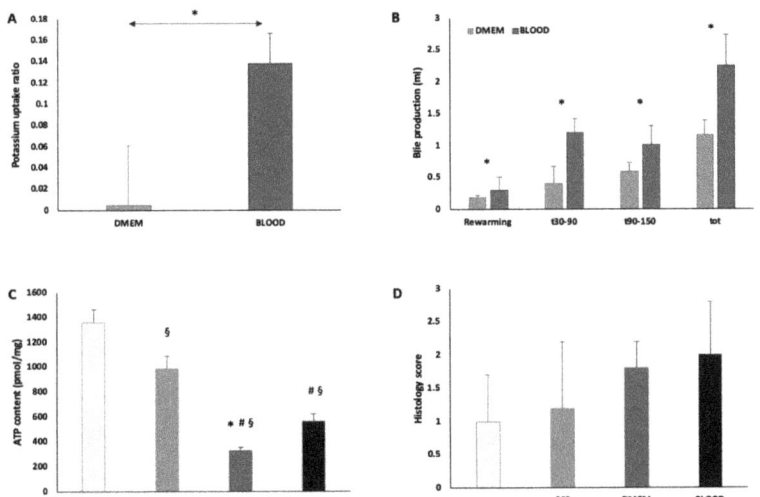

Figure 5. During ex-situ normothermic perfusion BLOOD group showed an increased potassium uptake ratio (* $p < 0.05$ DMEM vs. BLOOD) (**A**) and an increased bile production (* $p < 0.05$ DMEM vs. BLOOD) (**B**). These data suggest a more prompt and improved graft functional recovery, supported by the improved energetic pool at the end of NMP ($p < 0.05$, § vs. native, # vs. SCS, * vs. BLOOD) (**C**). NMP preserved parenchymal architecture in both experimental groups. In BLOOD group, the use of human red blood cells did not cause sinusoidal or parenchymal damage, consistently no trapped human red blood cells were found in sinusoids (**D**). Data are shown as mean ±SEM.

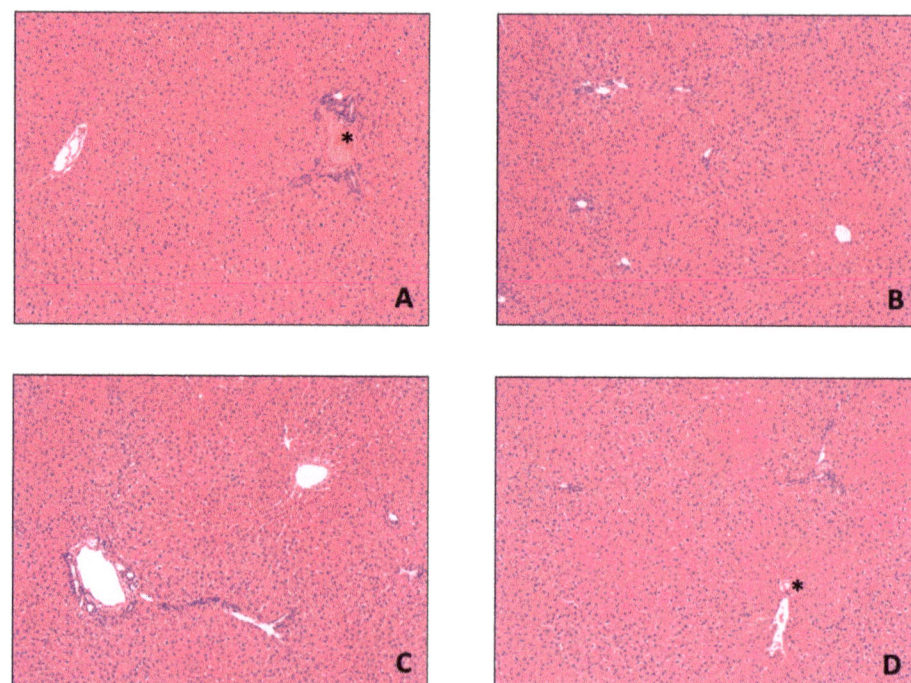

Figure 6. Histological examination of liver biopsies. Liver histological architecture was preserved in the four study groups ((**A**) Native (untreated/control) group; (**B**) SCS group; (**C**) DMEM group; (**D**) BLOOD group). As expected, red blood cells (*) can be found in Native and BLOOD group due to the presence of whole blood and blood based perfusate, respectively. Consistently, there were no hemorrhages or sinusoidal obstruction in BLOOD compared to the other groups. Sinusoidal architecture was preserved irrespective of the type of perfusion, as well as the rate of hepatocytes ploidy (6.2 ± 1.2/HPF). Hematoxylin and Eosin staining, 100× original magnification.

3.4. Liver Metabolism During NMP

During the normothermic phase, the metabolic function of the liver was evaluated to assess the performance of the two different types of perfusate (Table 2). The DO_2 of the BLOOD group was higher than in DMEM (DO_2: DMEM 0.405 ± 0.015 mL/min vs. BLOOD 1.685 ± 0.090 mL/min, $p < 0.001$) (Figure 7A). Equally, $\dot{V}O_2$ was higher in BLOOD group ($p = 0.001$). While DMEM $\dot{V}O_2$ did not change through the procedure, the BLOOD $\dot{V}O_2$ decreased over time (Figure 7B). The energetic load of liver tissue decreased during the 30 min of cold storage (native 1354.2 ± 109.1 pmol/mg vs. SCS 985.9 ± 102.6 pmol/mg, $p = 0.046$). At the end-NMP, ATP levels decreased independently of the presence of OxC (DMEM 327.3 ± 26.6 pmol/mg; BLOOD 565.8 ± 56.6 pmol/mg) compared to both SCS (DMEM vs. SCS, $p = 0.007$ and BLOOD vs. SCS, $p = 0.012$) and native (DMEM vs. native $p = 0.001$ and BLOOD vs. native $p = 0.003$) group, as indicated by a bioluminescent assay of liver homogenates. However, after 120 min of normothermia the grafts perfused with a blood based perfusate showed a statistically significant higher ATP ($p = 0.031$) (Figure 5C). Glucose during NMP was stable in DMEM group, while decreased in BLOOD group ($p < 0.001$), resulting in a greater concentration of glucose in perfusion fluid of DMEM group at the end of the experiment compared to the BLOOD group ($p = 0.008$) (Figure 7C). Glucose uptake ratio was higher in DMEM ($p = 0.029$). Lactates were higher at each time point ($p = 0.002$) and lactates uptake ratio was lower in DMEM (DMEM 0.062 ± 0.359 vs. BLOOD 0.643 ± 0.027, $p = 0.029$) (Figure 7D). Interestingly, during the ischemic phase ($DO_2 = 0$ mL/min), the estimated glucose uptake ratio was −0.280 ± 0.116, while the lactates uptake ratio was −0.180 ± 0.89. Citrate uptake ratio was 0.228 ± 0.127 in BLOOD group (it was not detectable in DMEM).

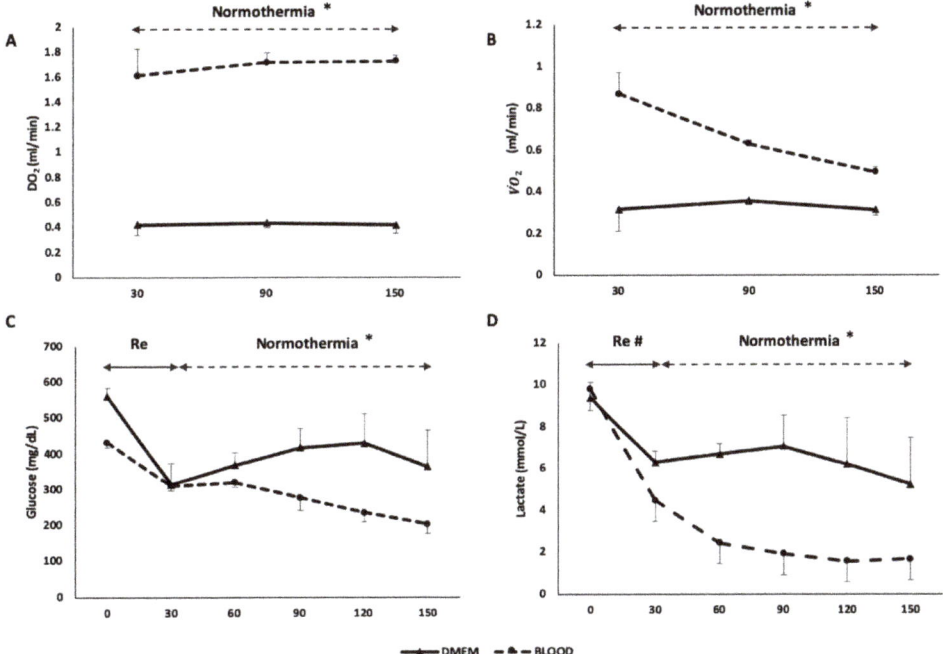

Figure 7. The use of human red blood cells as oxygen carrier resulted in an increased DO_2 in BLOOD group (* $p < 0.05$) (**A**) and a consequent improved $\dot{V}O_2$ (* $p < 0.001$) (**B**). Glucose was absorbed during normothermic phase in BLOOD group (* $p < 0.001$) (**C**) and lactates metabolism was increased during the whole procedure in BLOOD group (# $p < 0.05$) (**D**). These parameters suggest an improved metabolic function of the graft when a higher oxygen content was provided during perfusion. Re, rewarming; DO_2, delivery of oxygen; $\dot{V}O_2$, oxygen consumption. Data are shown as mean ± SEM.

The graft $\dot{V}O_2$ ($R^2 = 0.929$; $p < 0.001$) (Figure 8), the end-NMP tissue ATP content ($R^2 = 0.622$; $p = 0.020$) and the ability of the liver to clear lactates ($R^2 = 0.609$; $p = 0.022$) and glucose ($R^2 = 0.718$; $p = 0.008$) were directly related to the amount of oxygen delivered (DO_2). Equally, an increase in oxygen consumption ($\dot{V}O_2$) led to an increase in lactates clearance ($R^2 = 0.505$; $p = 0.048$) and glucose consumption ($R^2 = 0.597$; $p = 0.025$), while ATP levels showed only a trend toward a significant linear correlation with $\dot{V}O_2$ ($R^2 = 0.454$; $p = 0.067$). An increase of 1 pmol/mg of liver ATP produced an increase in lactates uptake ratio of 0.002 ± 0.001 ($R^2 = 0.641$; $p = 0.017$) and glucose uptake ratio of 0.003 ± 0.001 ($R^2 = 0.619$; $p = 0.021$).

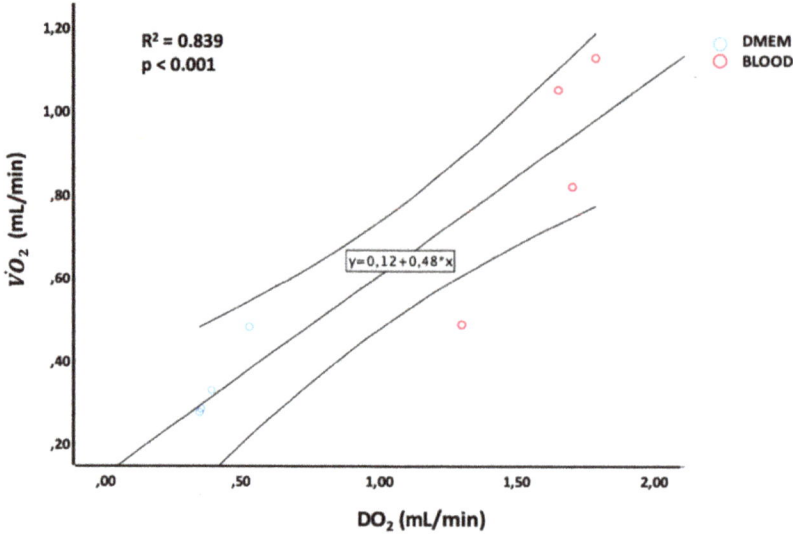

Figure 8. Linear regression between DO$_2$ and $\dot{V}O_2$ levels during ex-situ normothermic perfusion.

4. Discussion

The present research demonstrates that an optimized DO$_2$ reduces liver hypoxic damage during NMP. This significant result was achieved using human RBCs as oxygen carriers. Therefore, in addition to the beneficial effects on metabolic parameters, the study points at the use of human RBCs as a strategy to substantially reduce the number of animals employed in accordance with the 3Rs principles.

NMP is increasingly used in clinical settings [28–30] to evaluate, recondition, and preserve liver grafts, and this key strategy could be substantially improved by preclinical research, in particular by rodent models. Further, the use of NMRP, rather than LT to evaluate IRI without the use of a recipient, could reduce the number of animals employed. However, to expand their translational potential, these preclinical models need to be optimized and each experimental step should be carefully implemented [21].

We examined the influence of different perfusion solutions and the use of an oxygen carrier on graft reperfusion and viability. Results show that the addition of human RBCs [12,13] to NMP perfusate increases oxygen delivery and causes a faster and steeper restoration of liver metabolism. Indeed, the increased DO$_2$, achieved through the use of human RBCs, led to a more rapid clearance of lactate and partially counteracted the reduction in ATP content at the end of NMP.

Mischinger and colleagues [31] suggested in 1992 that ex-situ normothermic perfused livers do not need high DO$_2$. Based on this view, NMP set-up could be simplified by removing the OxC; namely, erythrocytes. Indeed, the general idea was that during NMP there was reduced ex-situ metabolic activity and a mitochondrial inhibition due to hypoxia-induced factors [32,33]. Conversely, other authors suggested that an optimized DO$_2$ during perfusion could result in a faster graft recovery after ischemia [34,35]. Autologous rat or human red blood cells can be used as oxygen carriers to increase DO$_2$. If rat blood is used, 3 to 4 donors are required to obtain a 15% hematocrit perfusate. Human blood enriched perfusate was used in ex-situ perfusions [12,13] of rat liver grafts, but the authors reported no clear advantage by using an OxC. Further, some papers showed a detrimental impact of human blood used during experiments on different animals [36].

In the present research, the use of human red blood cells and a dedicated membrane lung led to a higher DO$_2$ and a subsequent higher $\dot{V}O_2$ in the BLOOD group. Interestingly, our $\dot{V}O_2$ data are markedly higher relative to other reports (Table 3). The importance of $_2$ and DO$_2$ in our study is further supported by the positive linear regression between the main metabolic parameters and oxygen delivery and consumption. Indeed, early restoration of liver function and increased liver metabolism occurred in the BLOOD group with a better preservation of the energetic pool. The improved glucose and lactate uptake, and the increased glycogen and ATP tissue content, further indicate an upregulated metabolic status in the BLOOD group. The reduced potassium uptake and significant increase of W/D ratio at the end of perfusion (compared to SCS) in DMEM group likely depends on a more severe liver damage [37]. Furthermore, the direct relation between $DO_2/\dot{V}O_2$ and metabolic parameters suggests that the total amount of oxygen transported (DO_2) results in an increased ability to use oxygen ($\dot{V}O_2$) to generate energy (ATP) to sustain hepatocellular metabolism.

Table 3. Main metabolic parameters reported in literature during ex-situ normothermic perfusion on rats. Htc, hematocrit; pO_2, partial pressure of oxygen in perfusate; $\dot{V}O_2$, oxygen consumption; RBC, packed red blood cells or centrifugated red blood cells.

Author	Year	Blood Type	Htc	Blood Origin	pO_2	$\dot{V}O_2$ (max) (mL/min)
Dutkowski P	2006	full blood	6.4	rat	450	0.26
Izamis ML	2013	RBC	18	rat		0.5
Schlegel A	2014	full blood	15	rat	300–375	
Tolboom H	2012	RBC	18	rat		0.5
Tolboom H	2008	RBC	18	rat		0.4
Westerkamp AC	2015	RBC	25	human	450–600	

These data contradict the assumption of Mischinger and colleagues [31]. Furthermore, we deem that if DO_2 is not optimized with an OxC, NMP, or NMRP could result in a suboptimal ex-situ reperfusion procedure. The reason for the disparity between our data and previous observations [32,38] could depend on differences in ex-situ perfusion or other procedural steps.

The importance of adequate DO_2 is further highlighted in the rewarming phase. The BLOOD group showed an early $\dot{V}O_2$ peak with early lactate normalization. A higher DO_2 could help to overcome the oxygen debt accumulated during ischemia [17]. Although high O_2 levels during reperfusion could potentially lead to oxidative tissue injury causing a more pronounced tissue damage [39], we did not observe any change in this direction.

The safety of human RBCs used in this model is demonstrated by the absence of endothelial damage, sinusoid obstruction, extravascular hemorrhage, or parenchymal damage. An adequate wash-out of rat blood during perfusion and the virtual absence of human plasma can avoid incompatibility reactions and, therefore, reduce species-specific antibody reactions.

Furthermore, in our study, histological data confirm the preserved graft viability indicated by the metabolic evaluation. As recently suggested [40], we used a combination of different biomarkers to assess graft quality, and some of them (glucose and potassium uptake ratio, citrate clearance, hyaluronic acid clearance) are described in this research for the first time. Their interaction could be used in clinical or preclinical settings to evaluate graft viability.

Some limitations of the study deserve comment. First of all, the duration of the NMP was relatively short if compared to a clinical setting. While accelerated clearance and sinusoidal trapping of human RBCs were observed in rat transfusion models [41], we did not observe significant hemolysis due to human blood use, and no red blood cells were trapped within sinusoidal spaces. However, the exploitation of these types of perfusate should be tested in prolonged perfusion to confirm absence of blood related liver damage. Non-cellular hemoglobin was recently used in clinical NMP [18], and it should be tested in this setting.

In conclusion, this study provides a detailed description of a small animal model of NMP characterized by optimized liver function, liver metabolism, and absence of injury. Results suggest that OxC may be adopted with NMP or NMRP, in particular with expanded criteria grafts, to avoid the detrimental impact of low DO_2. In compliance with the 3R principle, human RBCs can be safely used to improve DO_2, but additional studies are needed to confirm the safety, effectiveness, and optimal administration protocol.

Supplementary Materials: The following are available online at http://www.mdpi.com/2077-0383/8/11/1918/s1, Table S1: brief review of ex-situ normothermic liver rat perfusion; Table S2: summary of the main characteristics of normothermic ex-situ perfusion protocols on rats published in literature; Table S3: reagents used during experiments; Table S4: instruments employed during experiments; Table S5: characteristics of the perfusion fluid in the two experimental groups; Figure S1: Schematic representation of experimental workflow; Figure S2: modified Fick equation used to calculate $\dot{V}O_2$ and DO_2 in our experiments; Figure S3: hepatocellular damage markers during normothermic machine perfusion.

Author Contributions: Conceptualization, D.D., C.L. and S.G.; Methodology, C.L., D.D., S.G., A.Z., R.M., A.S.; Formal Analysis, C.L., R.M., M.M., M.B., L.V., O.B., S.V.; Investigation, D.D., S.G., A.S., C.L., R.M., A.V.; Data Curation, A.S., D.D., C.L., R.M., V.L.; Writing—Original Draft Preparation, D.D., C.L.; Writing—Review & Editing, S.G., A.Z.; Supervision, S.G., A.Z.

Funding: The present study was supported by Fondazione Ca' Granda Ospedale Maggiore Policlinico, Milan, with the following grants: 5 × 1000–2014 "Ottimizzazione della procedura di perfusione di organi isolati a scopo di trapianto mediante modulazione del liquido di perfusione—Improvement of perfusion of isolated organs before transplantation through perfusion fluid optimization", 5 × 1000–2014 "Il benessere animale nella ricerca preclinica: strategie di implementazione—Implementation of strategies for laboratory animal care".

Acknowledgments: We thank "Associazione Italiana Copev per la prevenzione e cura dell'epatite virale Beatrice Vitiello—ONLUS" and "MILTA". Authors would like to thank Samata Oldoni for her valuable help.

Conflicts of Interest: The authors declare no conflict of interest.

References

1. Guarrera, J.V.; Henry, S.D.; Samstein, B.; Odeh-Ramadan, R.; Kinkhabwala, M.; Goldstein, M.J.; Ratner, L.E.; Renz, J.F.; Lee, H.T.; Brown, R.S.; et al. Hypothermic Machine Preservation in human liver transplantation: The first clinical series. *Am. J. Transplant.* **2010**, *10*, 372–381. [CrossRef] [PubMed]
2. Schlegel, A.; Kron, P.; Graf, R.; Clavien, P.A.; Dutkowski, P. Hypothermic Oxygenated Perfusion (HOPE) downregulates the immune response in a rat model of liver transplantation. *Ann. Surg.* **2014**, *260*, 931–937, discussion 937–938. [CrossRef] [PubMed]
3. Hessheimer, A.J.; Fondevila, C. Liver perfusion devices: How close are we to widespread application? *Curr. Opin. Organ Transplant.* **2017**, *22*, 105–111. [CrossRef] [PubMed]
4. Watson, C.J.E.; Jochmans, I. From "Gut Feeling" to Objectivity: Machine Preservation of the Liver as a Tool to Assess Organ Viability. *Curr. Transp. Rep.* **2018**, *5*, 72–81. [CrossRef]
5. Daniel, C.R.; Labens, R.; Argyle, D.; Licka, T.F. Extracorporeal perfusion of isolated organs of large animals—Bridging the gap between in vitro and in vivo studies. *ALTEX* **2018**, *35*, 77–98. [CrossRef]
6. Amersi, F.; Shen, X.; Anselmo, D.; Melinek, J.; Iyer, S.; Southard, D.J.; Katori, M.; Volk, H.; Busuttil, R.W.; Buelow, R.; et al. Ex Vivo Exposure to Carbon Monoxide Prevents Hepatic Ischemia/Reperfusion Injury Through p38 MAP Kinase Pathway. *Hepatology* **2002**, *35*, 815–823. [CrossRef]
7. Dutkowski, P.; Graf, R.; Clavien, P.A. Rescue of the Cold Preserved Rat Liver by Hypothermic Oxygenated Machine Perfusion. *Am. J. Transplant.* **2006**, *6*, 903–912. [CrossRef]
8. Perk, S.; Izamis, M.L.; Tolboom, H.; Uygun, B.; Berthiaume, F.; Yarmush, M.L.; Uygun, K. A metabolic index of ischemic injury for Perfusion-Recovery of cadaveric rat livers. *PLoS ONE* **2011**, *6*, e28518. [CrossRef]
9. Perk, S.; Izamis, M.L.; Tolboom, H.; Uygun, B.; Yarmush, M.L.; Uygun, K. A fitness index for transplantation of machine-perfused cadaveric rat livers. *BMC Res. Notes* **2012**, *5*, 325. [CrossRef]
10. Bruinsma, B.G.; Berendsen, T.A.; Izamis, M.L.; Yarmush, M.L.; Uygun, K. Determination and extension of the limits to static cold storage using subnormothermic machine perfusion. *Int. J. Artif. Organs* **2013**, *36*, 775–780. [CrossRef]
11. Schlegel, A.; Kron, P.; Graf, R.; Dutkowski, P.; Clavien, P.A. Warm vs. cold perfusion techniques to rescue rodent liver grafts. *J. Hepatol.* **2014**, *61*, 1267–1275. [CrossRef]

12. Westerkamp, A.C.; Mahboub, P.; Meyer, S.L.; Hottenrott, M.; Ottens, P.J.; Wiersema-buist, J.; Gouw, A.S.H.; Lisman, T.; Leuvenink, H.G.D.; Porte, R.J. End-Ischemic Machine Perfusion Reduces Bile Duct Injury In Donation After Circulatory Death Rat Donor Livers Independent of the Machine Perfusion Temperature. *Liver Transplant.* **2015**, *21*, 1300–1311. [CrossRef] [PubMed]
13. Op den Dries, S.; Karimian, N.; Westerkamp, A.C.; Sutton, M.E.; Kuipers, M.; Wiersema-Buist, J.; Ottens, P.J.; Kuipers, J.; Giepmans, B.N.; Leuvenink, H.G.D.; et al. Normothermic machine perfusion reduces bile duct injury and improves biliary epithelial function in rat donor livers. *Liver Transplant.* **2016**, *22*, 994–1005. [CrossRef] [PubMed]
14. Rigo, F.; De Stefano, N.; Navarro-tableros, V.; David, E.; Rizza, G.; Catalano, G.; Gilbo, N.; Maione, F.; Gonella, F.; Roggio, D.; et al. Extracellular Vesicles from Human Liver Stem Cells Reduce Injury in an Ex Vivo Normothermic Hypoxic Rat Liver Perfusion Model. *Trasplantation* **2018**, *102*, 205–210. [CrossRef] [PubMed]
15. Tolboom, H.; Milwid, J.M.; Izamis, M.L.; Uygun, K.; Berthiaume, F.; Yarmush, M.L. Sequential cold storage and normothermic perfusion of the ischemic rat liver. *Transplant. Proc.* **2008**, *40*, 1306–1309. [CrossRef] [PubMed]
16. Tolboom, H.; Izamis, M.-L.; Sharma, N.; Milwid, J.M.; Uygun, B.; Berthiaume, F.; Uygun, K.; Yarmush, M.L. Subnormothermic Machine Perfusion at Both 20°C and 30°C Recovers Ischemic Rat Livers for Successful. *Trasplantation* **2012**, *175*, 149–156. [CrossRef]
17. Bjerkvig, C.K.; Strandenes, G.; Eliassen, H.S.; Spinella, P.C.; Fosse, T.K.; Cap, A.P.; Ward, K.R. "Blood failure" time to view blood as an organ: How oxygen debt contributes to blood failure and its implications for remote damage control resuscitation. *Transfusion* **2016**, *56*, 182–189. [CrossRef]
18. Matton, A.P.M.; Burlage, L.C.; van Rijn, R.; de Vries, Y.; Karangwa, S.A.; Nijsten, M.W.; Gouw, A.S.H.; Wiersema-Buist, J.; Adelmeijer, J.; Westerkamp, A.C.; et al. Normothermic Machine Perfusion of Donor Livers Without the Need for Human Blood Products. *Liver Transplant.* **2018**, *24*, 528–538. [CrossRef]
19. Arck, P.C. When 3 Rs meet a forth R: Replacement, reduction and refinement of animals in research on reproduction. *J. Reprod. Immunol.* **2019**, *132*, 54–59. [CrossRef]
20. Guillen, J. FELASA Guidelines and Recommendations. *J. Am. Assoc. Lab. Anim. Sci.* **2012**, *51*, 311–321.
21. Bassani, G.A.; Lonati, C.; Brambilla, D.; Rapido, F.; Valenza, F.; Gatti, S. Ex vivo lung perfusion in the rat: Detailed procedure and videos. *PLoS ONE* **2016**, *11*, e0167898. [CrossRef] [PubMed]
22. Roffia, V.; De Palma, A.; Lonati, C.; Di Silvestre, D.; Rossi, R.; Mantero, M.; Gatti, S.; Dondossola, D.; Valenza, F.; Mauri, P.; et al. Proteome investigation of rat lungs subjected to Ex vivo perfusion (EVLP). *Molecules* **2018**, *23*, 3061. [CrossRef] [PubMed]
23. Lonati, C.; Bassani, G.A.; Brambilla, D.; Leonardi, P.; Carlin, A.; Favesani, A.; Gatti, S.; Valenza, F. Influence of ex vivo perfusion on the biomolecular profile of rat lungs. *FASEB J.* **2018**, *32*, 5532–5549. [CrossRef] [PubMed]
24. Lonati, C.; Bassani, A.; Brambilla, D.; Leonardi, P.; Carlin, A.; Maggioni, M.; Zanella, A.; Dondossola, D.; Fonsato, V.; Grange, C.; et al. Mesenchymal stem cell-derived extracellular vesicles improve the molecular phenotype of isolated rat lungs during ischemia/reperfusion injury. *J. Heart Lung Transplant.* **2019**, *24*, 1053–2498. [CrossRef]
25. Dondossola, D.; Lonati, C.; Rossi, G. Ex-vivo tissue determination of water fraction in associating liver partition with portal vein ligation for staged hepatectomy. *Surgery* **2018**, *163*, 971. [CrossRef]
26. Brockmann, J.; Reddy, S.; Coussios, C.; Pigott, D.; Guirriero, D.; Hughes, D.; Morovat, A.; Roy, D.; Winter, L.; Friend, P.J. Normothermic Perfusion: A New Paradigm for Organ Preservation. *Ann. Surg.* **2009**, *250*, 1–6. [CrossRef]
27. Kramer, L.; Bauer, E.; Joukhadar, C.; Strobl, W.; Gendo, A.; Madl, C.; Gangl, A. Citrate pharmacokinetics and metabolism in cirrhotic and noncirrhotic critically ill patients. *Crit. Care Med.* **2003**, *31*, 2450–2455. [CrossRef]
28. Ravikumar, R.; Jassem, W.; Mergental, H.; Heaton, N.; Mirza, D.; Perera, M.T.P.R.; Quaglia, A.; Holroyd, D.; Vogel, T.; Coussios, C.C.; et al. Liver Transplantation After Ex Vivo Normothermic Machine Preservation: A Phase 1 (First-in-Man) Clinical Trial. *Am. J. Transplant.* **2016**, *16*, 1779–1787. [CrossRef]
29. Banan, B.; Watson, R.; Xu, M.; Lin, Y.; Chapman, W. Development of a normothermic extracorporeal liver perfusion system toward improving viability and function of human extended criteria donor livers. *Liver Transpl.* **2016**, *22*, 979–993. [CrossRef]
30. Nasralla, D.; Coussios, C.C.; Mergental, H.; Akhtar, M.Z.; Butler, A.J.; Ceresa, C.D.L.; Chiocchia, V.; Dutton, S.J.; García-valdecasas, J.C.; Heaton, N.; et al. A randomized trial of normothermic preservation in liver transplantation. *Nature.* **2018**, *557*, 50–56. [CrossRef]

31. Mischinger, H.J.; Walsh, T.R.; Liu, T.; Rao, P.N.; Rubin, R.; Nakamura, K.; Todo, S.; Starzl, T.E.; Ph, D. An Improved Technique for Isolated Perfusion of Rat Livers and an Evaluation of Perfusates. *J. Surg. Res.* **1992**, *53*, 158–165. [CrossRef]
32. Riedel, G.L.; Scholle, J.L.; Shepherd, P.; Ward, W. Effects of hematocrit on oxygenation of the isolated perfused rat liver. *Am. J. Physiol.* **1983**, *245*, 769–774. [CrossRef] [PubMed]
33. Imber, C.J.; St Peter, S.D.; Lopez de Cenarruzabeitia, I.; Pigott, D.; James, T.; Taylor, R.; Mcguire, J.; Hughes, D.; Butler, A.; Rees, M.; et al. Advantages of normothermic perfusion over cold storage in liver preservation. *Transpation* **2002**, *73*, 701–709. [CrossRef] [PubMed]
34. Izamis, M.L.; Tolboom, H.; Uygun, B.; Berthiaume, F.; Yarmush, M.L.; Uygun, K. Resuscitation of Ischemic Donor Livers with Normothermic Machine Perfusion: A Metabolic Flux Analysis of Treatment in Rats. *PLoS ONE* **2013**, *8*, e69758. [CrossRef]
35. Dutkowski, P.; Furrer, K.; Tian, Y.; Graf, R.; Clavien, P.A. Novel Short-term Hypothermic Oxygenated Perfusion (HOPE) System Prevents Injury in Rat Liver Graft From Non-Heart Beating Donor. *Ann. Surg.* **2006**, *244*, 968–977. [CrossRef]
36. Osei-Hwedieh, D.O.; Kanias, T.; Croix, C.S.; Jessup, M.; Xiong, Z.; Sinchar, D.; Franks, J.; Xu, Q.; Novelli, E.M.; Sertorio, J.T.; et al. Sickle Cell Trait Increases Red Blood Cell Storage Hemolysis and Post-Transfusion Clearance in Mice. *EBioMedicine* **2016**, *11*, 239–248. [CrossRef]
37. Burlage, L.C.; Hessels, L.; Van Rijn, R.; Matton, A.P.M.; Fujiyoshi, M.; Van Den Berg, A.P.; Reyntjens, K.M.E.M.; Meyer, P.; De Boer, M.T.; De Kleine, R.H.J.; et al. Opposite acute potassium and sodium shifts during transplantation of hypothermic machine perfused donor livers. *Am. J. Transplant.* **2019**, *19*, 1061–1071. [CrossRef]
38. Orman, M.A.; Ierapetritou, M.G.; Androulakis, I.P.; Berthiaume, F. Metabolic Response of Perfused Livers to Various Oxygenation Conditions. *Biotechnol. Bioeng.* **2011**, *108*, 2947–2957. [CrossRef]
39. Granger, D.N.; Kvietys, P.R. Reperfusion injury and reactive oxygen species: The evolution of a concept. *Redox Biol.* **2015**, *6*, 524–551. [CrossRef]
40. Mergental, H.; Stephenson, B.T.F.; Laing, R.W.; Kirkham, A.J.; Neil, D.A.H.; Wallace, L.L.; Boteon, Y.L.; Widmer, J.; Bhogal, R.H.; Perera, M.T.P.R.; et al. Development of Clinical Criteria for Functional Assessment to Predict Primary Nonfunction of High-Risk Livers Using Normothermic Machine Perfusion. *Liver Transplant.* **2018**, *24*, 1453–1469. [CrossRef]
41. Straat, M.; Klei, T.; de Korte, D.; van Bruggen, R.; Juffermans, N. Accelerated clearance of human red blood cells in a rat transfusion model. *Intensive Care Med. Exp.* **2015**, *3*, 27. [CrossRef] [PubMed]

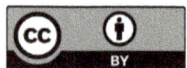

© 2019 by the authors. Licensee MDPI, Basel, Switzerland. This article is an open access article distributed under the terms and conditions of the Creative Commons Attribution (CC BY) license (http://creativecommons.org/licenses/by/4.0/).

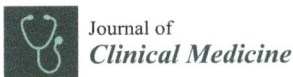
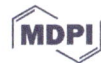

Review

Magnetic Resonance Imaging for Translational Research in Oncology

Maria Felicia Fiordelisi, Carlo Cavaliere, Luigi Auletta *, Luca Basso and Marco Salvatore

IRCCS SDN, Via Gianturco 113, 80143 Napoli, Italy; mfiordelisi@sdn-napoli.it (M.F.F.); carlocavaliere1983@yahoo.it (C.C.); lbasso@sdn-napoli.it (L.B.); direzionescientifica@sdn-napoli.it (M.S.)
* Correspondence: lauletta@sdn-napoli.it

Received: 1 October 2019; Accepted: 29 October 2019; Published: 6 November 2019

Abstract: The translation of results from the preclinical to the clinical setting is often anything other than straightforward. Indeed, ideas and even very intriguing results obtained at all levels of preclinical research, i.e., in vitro, on animal models, or even in clinical trials, often require much effort to validate, and sometimes, even useful data are lost or are demonstrated to be inapplicable in the clinic. In vivo, small-animal, preclinical imaging uses almost the same technologies in terms of hardware and software settings as for human patients, and hence, might result in a more rapid translation. In this perspective, magnetic resonance imaging might be the most translatable technique, since only in rare cases does it require the use of contrast agents, and when not, sequences developed in the lab can be readily applied to patients, thanks to their non-invasiveness. The wide range of sequences can give much useful information on the anatomy and pathophysiology of oncologic lesions in different body districts. This review aims to underline the versatility of this imaging technique and its various approaches, reporting the latest preclinical studies on thyroid, breast, and prostate cancers, both on small laboratory animals and on human patients, according to our previous and ongoing research lines.

Keywords: translational medicine; preclinical imaging; rodent models; oncology; magnetic resonance imaging

1. Introduction

Translational medicine is an interdisciplinary branch of biomedicine, which aims to translate results from preclinical (in vitro and in vivo) research to the clinical setting, the so-called "from bench to bedside" path [1]. Its main objective is to improve prevention, diagnosis, and treatment strategies for human diseases by filling the gap between the preclinical and the clinical setting. For fruitful translational research, it is fundamental that the discovery process, and the relative experimental design, is immediately aimed at its application in clinical practice [1,2].

In this context, the correct choice of the experimental model and the study design are a fundamental part of the translational plan, and they must be made carefully. In oncology, the use of animal models represents a still-irreplaceable step after in vitro studies. Indeed, they are an essential source of in vivo information, which validates in vitro results and improves their translational value [3–5]. Rodents, particularly mice, are the most used in vivo oncological models, thanks to their high genetic homology with humans, their easy genetic manipulability, and their fast reproductive cycle. Hence, their use allows for concluding studies in a relatively short time [3–7].

In vivo preclinical imaging makes possible noninvasive longitudinal studies; thus, achieving a reduction in the biological variability and a substantial decrease in the number of animals while maintaining the statistical power of the data [8–10]. Most imaging techniques for small animals are already the same used in clinical settings, i.e., computed tomography (CT), positron emission tomography (PET), high-frequency ultrasonography (HFUS) and magnetic resonance imaging (MRI), and hence, are readily translatable. In oncological research, these imaging modalities are useful in studying drug biodistribution, monitoring treatment response, and identifying new molecular targets and biomarkers for early tumor detection [3,11–15]. Preclinical scanners have to deal with smaller "subjects" with higher metabolic and physiological rates. Hence, dedicated scanners are designed to meet these needs in terms of higher spatial and temporal resolutions but still adopt the same physical and technological principles of their clinical counterparts, which lead to more direct and faster translatability of findings [15].

In this perspective, the MRI can be considered the least invasive and most comprehensive technique, from an anatomo-functional point of view, in the clinical setting. The preclinical MR scanners have to, as mentioned deal with a smaller field of view and higher spatial resolution, assured by the use of higher magnetic fields; e.g., up to 11.4 T. Nonetheless, novel sequences able to show specific pathophysiological features in oncologic disease might be directly translated to the clinic [9,16,17].

This work aimed to review the most recent scientific literature to highlight the translatability of MRI from preclinical animal studies to clinical oncology. In particular, we focused on thyroid, breast, and prostate cancer rodent models, according to our previous and ongoing research lines. Indeed, such histotypes display a significant impact both on clinical oncology and in preclinical research. Moreover, to underline the versatility of the MRI techniques, some preclinical studies on human patients have been reported, as well.

2. Animal Models in Oncology

Four broad categories of oncological small animal models are used: xenografts, orthotopic, patient-derived tumor xenografts (PDXs), and genetically engineered mouse models (GEMMs). As for spontaneous human cancer, chemical and radiation-induced murine models have also been developed, and they seem to behave more closely like human tumors [18,19]. Finally, specific considerations will be made about metastatic models. For most animal models, general anesthesia is usually needed, either to eliminate the stress and the pain linked to a surgical procedure, or to obtain immobility of the mouse. The other procedures are usually executable with physical restraint by personnel well-trained in handling animals [20].

2.1. Xenograft and Orthotopic Models

Subcutaneous and orthotopic xenograft models are based on cancer cell lines directly derived from human tumors. Such cell lines belong from primary, lymph nodes, or metastatic tumors; they are immortalized and usually well-defined from the genetic point of view [21,22]. Hence, they allow extremely reproducible experiments for growth rate, metastatic potential, histopathologic homogeneity, and biological behavior. For their growth in the host species, i.e., the mouse, the host itself has to be immunocompromised [3,22]. Depending on the cell line, various degrees of immune system "knock-out" might be necessary [23,24]. In general, these models summarize well, as mentioned, the histopathological features present in the original tumoral tissue, but the use of immunodeficient mice may hinder the study of the tumor–host immune interaction. Subcutaneous xenografts are more easily reproducible compared to orthotopic implantation, which usually requires invasive surgical procedures. However, xenografts are not representative of the original tumor in its native environment [21,25]. On the other hand, the use of orthotopic models reestablishes the interactions between the tumor and its origin organ and might recapitulate the metastatic behavior with sufficient penetrance and reproducibility. Nonetheless, a limit of orthotopic models, besides the lack of interaction with the host's immune system, is that they do not allow modeling the pre-neoplastic process since the cell line already has completely tumorous genetic and biological behavior [18,25,26]. Depending on the murine strain selected, these models might be less expensive than GEMMs [25,26]. These animal models, for their reproducibility, seem to be ideal for preclinical and translational studies concerning therapies for tumor growth and angiogenesis inhibition. Furthermore, they are useful for studying the pathogenetic aspects of cancer vascular invasion and metastasis [26–28].

Both xenograft and orthotopic models are used to replicate thyroid cancer. In the xenograft models, selected cell lines are injected into the subcutaneous tissue of immunodeficient mice. The selection of the appropriate cell line is important not only to fulfill the experimental aims but also because it has been demonstrated that among 40 thyroid cell lines, almost 40% are cross-contaminated or misidentified [29,30]. Hence, genetic evaluation of the chosen cell lines should always be performed [30,31]. The orthotopic model is more complex and requires microsurgery to inject tumor cells directly into the murine thyroid gland [25,26,32]. Recently, an HFUS-guided injection procedure has been presented and resulted in less invasiveness compared to the standard surgical procedure [33]. Such a procedure was easily reproducible for the orthotopic implantation of thyroid carcinoma cells and allowed for continuous monitoring of the disease, for a more extended period and with less contamination of other neck structures by the carcinomatous cells compared to the surgical approach [33]. In thyroid cancer research, the orthotopic model allows the understanding of the molecular and cellular mechanisms of thyroid cancer pathogenesis, improving the evaluation of new therapeutic compounds, and testing the effects of therapeutic interventions on both the primary tumor and metastases [34,35].

The xenograft and orthotopic mice models are widely used for investigating breast cancer. These are commonly produced by injecting subcutaneous tumor cells in the flank or orthotopically in the mammary fat pad of immunocompromised mice. The xenograft models allow one to study, in vivo, the tumor environment, and tumor growth, but the absence of an intact immune system profoundly affects tumor development, in particular, its early stages, and the progression of the metastatic process. Orthotopic models of breast cancer provide a more favorable microenvironment, but there are critical differences between human and mouse mammary stroma [36]. Commonly, these models involve athymic nude, severe combined immunodeficiency (SCID) and non-obese diabetic (NOD) SCID mice, which show genetic and immunological differences that mainly influence the induction and dissemination of metastases to organs. Indeed, natural killer (NK) cells and the remaining innate immune cells in nude and SCID mice probably contribute to the reduction of tumor engraftment, growth, and metastases in these models. On the other hand, NOD SCID and particularly NOD SCID gamma (NSG) represent a better background to study breast cancer metastases due to the lack of NK cells, and thus they could be considered ideal for the study of anti-metastatic treatments [37–39].

Prostatic cancer models are usually xenografts, in which tumor cells are inoculated subcutaneously, and the cellular lines mostly used are either androgen-independent (PC-3 and DU-145) or androgen-responsive (LNCaP) cells. Such a set of cell lines reproduces various features of the naturally occurring disease [40,41]. Orthotopic prostate tumor models are relevant to study the growth and metastasis of prostate cancer. Generally, tumor cells are injected into the prostates of immunodeficient mice; however, there is a low incidence of tumor formation due to technical difficulties that can be overcome by intratesticular inoculation [41–43].

The xenograft models of colon cancer are rarely used [44]. The orthotopic model represents an accurate reproduction of the human pathology and can be generated by the implantation of tumor cells, via a surgical celiotomy, under the cecal serosa. Alternatively, a model generated by trans-anal rectal injection has been developed, and it may allow a more accurate investigation of the inflammatory and immune responses, without the influence of previously-used abdominal surgery. The orthotopic colon cancer model is useful in inducing local tumor growth but is limited by a low rate of lymph node and hepatic metastases [45,46].

2.2. Patient-Derived Xenografts (PDX)

The PDX models are based on portions of primary tumors, are collected by biopsy or surgical excisions, and are transferred from the patient in immunodeficient mice by subcutaneous or orthotopic implantation. Since these models are derived directly from the patient's tumor, they have a great translational potential for the study and development of anticancer therapies in the perspective of personalized medicine. The main advantages of PDX are that they duplicate precisely, the original clinical tumor compared to long-established cell lines, and hence, they preserve the molecular, genetic, and histological heterogeneity of naturally occurring cancers [47–49]. These models have been shown to have a predictive value in the clinical outcome and are useful for studying novel or alternative drugs, in order to identify biomarkers for early predictive responses to the treatment, and thus, to guide therapeutic approaches in clinical patients. Furthermore, when this model is generated by an orthotopic implant, it often reproduces, as mentioned, the same metastatic process of the human disease. All these features give to PDX models, the ability to study metastases and the genetic evolution of a tumor [47–49]. There are some challenges concerning PDX models. Occasionally, to obtain a reasonable growth rate, they are propagated between different hosts; i.e., the graft is removed from one mouse and implanted in another one. During this passage, the stromal components of the mouse may become dominant over the human one; hence, limiting the translatability of results of the tested therapies. Moreover, the interaction of the tumor with the immunocompromised hosts does not allow studying the interaction with the immune system during the anticancer treatment, eventually hiding crucial therapeutic mechanisms [47,49,50]. Last but not least, the limitation of this model is linked to long bureaucratic waiting periods when obtaining the necessary authorization for animal experimentation. Only big governmental projects might be prepared from the perspective of a truly personalized medicine approach [48].

Concerning thyroid cancer, PDX mouse models accurately reproduce the tumor microenvironment and the biochemical interaction between tumor cells and stromal components, as previously mentioned [47]. However, particularly for medullary thyroid carcinomas, there are serious difficulties in generating a murine PDX model due to the slow tumor growth [51].

The PDX models of human breast cancer are gaining high relevance for preclinical evaluations of experimental therapeutics. In general, cells derived from patients are transplanted into a mammary fat pad of immunocompromised mice, particularly in NSG mice that are commonly used and better suited for PDX generation for their high engraftment rates [52,53].

The PDX models are used to highlight various aspects of prostate cancer in preclinical research. In particular, they are used to test individual responses to therapy, to clarify the angiogenetic pathways, and to identify new antimetastatic treatments. The tumor/human stroma interaction can support tumor growth and improve the onset of metastases resembling the naturally occurring disease. However, there are several issues during the orthotopic implantation, related to the size of the fragment and the choice of the implantation site, which have led to lower availability of PDX models of prostate cancer compared to other histotypes [41,54].

The PDX of colon cancer is generally generated using cultured primary cells derived from a patient's colon tumor, which are injected orthotopically into the cecal serosa. The direct transplantation of colon tumor tissue is being discarded, due to the bacterial contamination and the consequent septic shock in the immunocompromised host. Moreover, a significant amount of tissue is required, which can hardly be replaced in the event of engraftment failure. Nonetheless, PDX models of colon cancer allow the monitoring of tumor growth, metastatic evolution, and the pharmacological responses of individual patients [55,56].

2.3. Genetically Engineered Mouse Models (GEMMs)

The GEMMs play a significant role in cancer research, and they can be considered the most advanced animal models recapitulating human pathology [21,57]. The GEMMs develop tumors in situ, according to the gene(s) activated and/or deleted in immunocompetent, genetically manipulated, mice; the tumor growth in such models can be either spontaneous or molecularly-induced. These characteristics are extremely useful in studying the complex processes of carcinogenesis and also allow evaluating the interactions between tumor cells and the immune system in a more "natural" microenvironment [18,21]. These models better reflect human disease in terms of biological behavior, histology, and genetic accuracy, but they also show some disadvantages, such as variable penetrance, heterogeneous growth, and tumor latency, and they are expensive [4,13,15,21,57].

Transgenic thyroid cancer mouse models are widely used to study the numerous mutations already systematically identified in human specimens [25,32]. The GEMMs models represent a way to study carcinogenesis, tumor progression, and metastatization, and hence, responses to therapeutics. The use of these models of animals with intact immune systems, as well as the ability to histologically reproduce human tumors, allows the evaluation of different drugs at different stages of the disease during tumoral development. However, these models are not useful for evaluating antimetastatic therapies since they do not always reproduce the specific pathways of human disease [32,57]. They are also useful for the study of unconventional therapies, such as micro-RNA, small interfering-RNA, or immunotherapies, during the early events of tumor transformation and progression, and as a promising approach to customizing anticancer therapy [58].

The GEMMs models of breast cancer display many features of the human pathology, although they do not entirely recapitulate all its aspects, due to the complexity and heterogeneity of breast cancers. However, these models are invaluable for investigating the biology and pathogenesis of breast cancer, and they are especially helpful for elucidating the mechanisms that regulate the initiation and progression of this disease, as well as for understanding the genes involved in these phases [36,59]. Transgenic mouse models of breast cancer are developed in immunocompetent hosts, and therefore, they allow evaluating the cancer/host immune interaction. Some of these models spontaneously metastasize to the lungs, whereas the incidence of bone metastases is very low. Furthermore, there are some selective tissue promoters, such as the whey acidic protein and the mouse mammary tumor virus, which may be directed to the oncogenic expression of the mammary gland [36,60].

In the study of prostate cancer, GEMMs reproduce, in depth, its different stages, and their use has provided valuable information on tumor initiation and progression. These transgenic models have been divided into different categories. The first generation of GEMMs utilized probasin to produce the probasin-large T antigen transgenic mouse (LADY) and the transgenic adenocarcinoma of the mouse prostate (TRAMP) models, which both show an aggressive phenotype, often with metastatic bone involvement. On the other hand, the second generation GEMMs have integrated the single molecular changes observed in human diseases, such as the loss of phosphatase and TENsin homolog (PTEN) and Myc over-expression, but they seem to be unable to reproduce the different stages of prostate cancer [54,61].

A variety of GEMMs have been generated as models for colon cancer to understand how common, coexisting mutations cooperate in a natural environment. These transgenic models are useful for studying pathogenesis and testing potential therapeutic agents, although they do not show phenotypes similar to human diseases. Moreover, these models are not practical for studying colon cancer metastases [44,62].

2.4. Chemical and Radiation-Induced Models

These animal models are valuable tools to study mechanisms underlying human carcinogenesis. From that perspective, these murine models play an essential role in the interpretation of epidemiological observations: to assess the natural history, mechanism, and modifying factors of cancer development. Furthermore, these models allow evaluating the growth and histologic characteristics of the primary tumor and metastases. Nonetheless, they show high variability in terms of the time of onset and prevalence, as well as a long latency in metastatization; thus, influencing the number of animals required for a study [18,19].

Chemical agents or physical agonists and radiation, as well as the administration of known carcinogenic substances, have been used to induce thyroid cancer in mice. Mainly these are goitrogens that decrease thyroid hormone levels, resulting in alterations that then induce thyroid tumorigenesis. Furthermore, it is known that ionizing radiation is a determinant risk factor for thyroid cancer, but it is difficult to obtain a systematic and rapid model [63,64].

Radiation-induced mouse models and chemical carcinogenesis have been developed for the study of breast cancer. Through these models, the natural development of breast cancer linked to exposure to carcinogens has been evaluated. Radiation-induced models are relevant since radiation exposure is one of the epidemiologically-proven etiological factors of human breast cancer [65]. Moreover, chemical-induced breast cancer can be induced in some strains of rats by administering dimethylbenzanthracene and N-methyl-N-nitrosourea (MNU) [19,66].

Prostate cancer rodent models are rarely used. In particular, the most common is the chemically-induced, following the administration of methyl nitrosourea and testosterone in rats; these models infrequently recapitulate metastatization, and only will to the lymph nodes and lungs [66].

Chemically-induced colorectal cancer models were developed in mice following exposure to carcinogens, such as dimethylhydrazine, N-methyl-N-nitro-N-nitrosoguanidine, and MNU. The incidence depends on the dosage, duration, and frequency of administration; the route of administration; i.e., oral, subcutaneous, or intrarectal; and the timing of administration. These models are useful for studying the influence of diet on tumor development. However, the occurrence of cancer is low, making the use of a large number of animals necessary, and the metastatic phase is prolonged and infrequent [67].

2.5. Metastatic Models

The development of animal models of metastases is useful for the evaluation of new therapies that can prevent the metastatic phase or arrest the growth of metastasis already formed, and to identify new molecular targets. There are numerous approaches for the development of such models, including experimental metastases, spontaneous metastases, and the GEMMs' metastatic approach models [60,68]. Experimental metastasis models are established by direct injection of the selected cell line into the bloodstream through the tail vein or via intracardiac injection. Such an approach allows the diffusion of metastases to various organs, including the lungs, bones, brain, liver, and lymph nodes. The time-course is generally short, and the biology of metastases results is reproducible, but the injection site influences the target organ, and above all, this approach bypasses the early phases of the metastatic cascade [68]. The spontaneous metastasis model was derived from the orthotopic model, and more closely resembles the human pathology, providing the cascade of metastatic processes with adequate reproducibility [68,69]. The GEMMs' metastasis models show different degrees of penetrance and latency, and therefore, allow evaluating the metastatic process in a heterogeneous genetic background. Indeed, the activation or the loss of a gene may not replicate completely natural metastasis. Besides, the penetrance for the metastatic process is often low. Finally, long latency times and difficult recognition of metastases have been reported [68].

In thyroid cancer research, all the models above of metastatization are used. The orthotopic model is essential for evaluating the molecular mechanisms preceding metastatization. Often, the local invasion of neck's structures by the primary tumor, i.e., large vessels, the esophagus, and the trachea with consequent respiratory insufficiency or inability to feed, do not allow enough time to study metastases. On the other hand, most transgenic mouse models develop a limited number of spontaneous lung metastases, which are only detected post-mortem at the end of the experiment. Tail vein and intracardiac injections of thyroid cancer cell lines are used, as described in [32,70,71].

The orthotopic injection of cells into the mammary glands offers a comprehensive model of the metastatic process. A robust breast cancer metastasis model is obtained using immunocompromised NSG mice that facilitate understanding the mechanism underlying breast cancer metastatization [60,72,73]. Usually, this model causes a low incidence of bone metastasis, frequent in human beings. In any case, metastatization in mice models of breast cancer is strictly linked to the cell line used. Some transgenic models of breast cancer spontaneously metastasize to the lungs, but there is a very low incidence of bone metastases, probably due to the rapid progression of primary tumors [60].

Human prostate cancer cell lines have been orthotopically implanted into mice to study the different stages of cancer progression up to metastatization. This model also reproduces bone metastases, which, however, show a low incidence. Furthermore, the so-called mouse prostate reconstitution model is considered a valid approach for the development of bone micro-metastases. This model combines human neoplastic and non-neoplastic prostate cells with the murine urogenital sinus mesenchyme, and thus, the cells are implanted under the renal capsule of an immunodeficient mouse. This method allows for exploring the genetic pathogenesis of prostate cancer, but technical complexity often limits its use [60]. Most transgenic models of prostate cancer do not develop metastases or show a very low incidence, especially of bone metastases, often due to the rapid progressions of the primary tumors [60,66].

The metastatic colon cancer model is developed by orthotopic microinjection of human colon cancer cells directly in the subserosa of the cecum, via surgical celiotomy, or the injection into the portal vein. These traditional methods reproduce metastatic colonization of the liver and lungs and facilitate the study of the metastatic cascade that follows both qualitatively and quantitatively, the natural course. A noninvasive trans-anal model has been developed, with a trans-anal rectal injection of colon cancer cells after disruption of the mucosa with irritant agents administered via enema. This model allows assessing essential aspects of the development of metastases, without the negative influence of the surgical intervention. Transgenic metastasis models of colorectal cancer offer reproducible information on tumor onset and in the early phases of the metastatic process but have a low metastatic rate and limited dissemination to the target organs [74–78].

3. In Vivo Imaging

In clinical practice, CT, PET, ultrasonography, and MRI are essential for the diagnoses and monitoring of neoplastic diseases. In preclinical experimental models, these modalities provide functional and metabolic imaging and pathophysiological information beyond morphology, as well as the ability to study molecular events. In both clinical and preclinical areas, imaging modalities contribute to the oncology field by being reliable indicators for early tumoral responses to therapy, and they can guide effective therapies, or stratify patients [79,80]. General anesthesia is usually needed, in the case of imaging, to obtain immobility of the mouse, and to abolish the stress due to the loud noise, especially that produced by MRI [20].

3.1. Computed Tomography (CT)

In the clinical field, CT imaging has extensive applications in inflammation, angiography, cancer detection, and the evaluation of bone regeneration or toxicities. It provides useful anatomical details, but exposure to high radiation often limits the number of scans performed in the same patient. In preclinical research, this methodology, besides being particularly useful for the assessment of skeletal and lung abnormalities and cardiac function, is considered a robust technique for the quantitative evaluation of angiogenesis associated with solid tumors. The small animal CT has a high spatial resolution (up to 10 µm, in vivo) and relatively short imaging times. However, the employment of clinically-used contrast agents limits the repeated imaging in the same animal, in particular, due to the iodinated contrast, which is rapidly cleared from the blood, and therefore, should be administered repeatedly. Moreover, high dosages of this agent may result in nephrotoxicity, and its use may produce an ionization effect, resulting in radiation damage through reactive oxygen species [8,17,81–84].

3.2. Positron Emission Tomography (PET)

The PET has become a powerful tool for clinical diagnosis and preclinical research, and it plays an essential role in oncological research in monitoring metabolism, gene expression, cell proliferation, angiogenesis, hypoxia, and apoptosis, as well as for drug development [85]. Indeed, this modality, in the clinical setting, is used for tumor staging, to evaluate tumor response to therapies through the use of an radiolabeled imaging agent, such as [18F]-2-fluoro-2-deoxy-glucose [18F]-FDG for glucose metabolism or [18F]-fluoro-3'-deoxy-3'-L-fluorothymidine [18F]-FLT) for cell proliferation [86]. The PET also has a wide range of applications in preclinical research; for example, it allows investigating physiological and molecular mechanisms of human diseases, and evaluating novel radiolabeled imaging agents, and the biodistribution and the efficacy of new drugs in suitable animal models [87]. As for clinical scanning, preclinical PET devices provide excellent sensitivity (from 2% to 7%, depending on the energy window) and spatial resolution (1.2 mm, on average), but the main disadvantages are the lack of an anatomical parameter, usually overcome by associating a CT scan or MR scans. Moreover, the short half-life of most radioisotopes requires strict coordination between radiotracer production, delivery, and use in small animal models [83,84].

3.3. Single-Photon Emission Computed Tomography (SPECT)

Single-photon emission computed tomography (SPECT) is a functional, nuclear medicine technique based on the detection of gamma photons emitted by a radionuclide during its decay. SPECT employs a gamma camera, composed of detector crystals and a lead or tungsten collimator with multiple elongated holes—pinholes, which rotates around the subject and acquires multiple cross-sectional images. This technique is similar to PET, and it is widely employed in clinical routines, but it is less sensitive than PET. Indeed, the spatial resolution of clinical SPECT (8–10 mm) is lower than that of clinical PET (4–6 mm) [17,83]. The main advantage is the availability of several radiotracers (^{99m}Tc, ^{67}Ga, ^{111}In, and ^{123}I), which have relatively long half-lives compared to most PET radiotracers. In oncological research, SPECT tracers targeting angiogenesis, hypoxia, acidosis, and metabolic activity have been developed and applied [82]. In preclinical investigations, micro-SPECT has a higher spatial resolution (0.35–0.7 mm), compared to micro-PET, and as mentioned, the longer half-life of SPECT tracers is advantageous in terms of production and transport. On the other hand, in longitudinal studies, researchers have to wait for complete decay accordingly. The SPECT's main application is the study of the biodistribution and kinetics of novel radiopharmaceuticals. Indeed, preclinical PET scanners and radiopharmaceuticals showed a stronger ability to study tracers' kinetics compared to SPECT counterparts [82,83].

3.4. High-Frequency Ultrasonography (HFUS)

Compared to other molecular imaging modalities, HFUS represents a noninvasive, more cost-effective modality, with excellent temporal and spatial resolutions (up to 30 μm axial resolution and 70 μm lateral resolution). It shows the ability to obtain real-time anatomo-functional data rapidly. Moreover, this modality can be implemented by using microbubbles as a molecular-target contrast agent to enhance image quality and specificity. Ultrasound imaging is clinically used for routine screening examinations on breast, abdomen, neck, and other body districts, as well as for therapy monitoring. In this setting, over the last few years, the sensitivities and specificities of ultrasound devices to detect microbubbles have progressively improved. Indeed, beyond the frequent use of color or power dopplers, non-targeted microbubbles are used as intravascular contrast agents improving the detection and characterization of cancerous lesions, inflammatory processes, and cardiovascular pathologies [83,84,88]. In preclinical investigations, HFUS can be applied to monitor tumor growth and vasculature development, and in combination with contrast-enhanced microbubbles agents (CEMAs), is used to assess tumor angiogenesis, inflammation, and therapeutic effects. For example, the vascular endothelial growth factor receptor 2 (VEGFR2), which is a molecular marker of angiogenesis and is overexpressed on tumor vascular endothelial cells, is widely used in preclinical cancer research as a marker of therapy responsiveness [88–92]. Therefore, this modality could help enhance the translation of antiangiogenic agents and contribute positively to human patients' treatments [93].

3.5. Magnetic Resonance Imaging (MRI)

The MRI is a noninvasive imaging modality without ionizing radiation, which provides morphological images with excellent soft-tissue contrast and high spatial resolution. The MRI is one technique with multiple possible outcomes; indeed, depending on the sequences, it allows studying, other than the merely displaying the anatomy, of various aspects of the same lesion. In particular, diffusion of water molecules can be studied with diffusion-weighted sequences (DWI); spectroscopy allows detecting and quantifying small amounts of known molecules; angiographic sequences (like time-of-flight or phase contrast angiography) allow evaluating large blood vessels, even without the need of contrast agents, and so on [17,82–84]. The MRI has also proven to be useful in preclinical research, allowing the evaluation of biological processes at the molecular level in in vivo rodent models of diseases. The MRI needs complete immobility of the subject since even the respiratory and cardiac motions can induce substantial artifacts, reducing the quality and the information available from images; hence, requiring the use of respiratory gating to minimize the former effect [93].

The use of anesthesia may minimize animal motion, but some anesthetic agents may alter animal physiology, and thereby, potentially affect the biological processes under investigation [94]. Pre-anesthesia fasting times, the anesthetics, and their dose, may all impact biological processes. Pre-anesthetic fasting in mice is generally considered unnecessary, and prolonged fasting can cause hypoglycemia. However, in imaging studies, a full stomach may interfere with adjacent structures. From the metabolic point of view, fasting may display profound effects on glucose metabolism, and hence, for example, it may significantly influence the results of FDG-PET studies. Body temperature should be monitored and kept within thermoneutrality, since anesthesia induces more or less marked hypothermia, which can also negatively affect the quality of some molecular imaging procedures. The choice of the anesthetic protocol is paramount for particular MRI sequences as well. Indeed, anesthetics may display a significant impact on vascular tone and hemodynamics, masking or altering critical experimentally-related results. Nowadays, great drug selection is available, and the choice, as mentioned, should be in accordance to the specific experimental aims. Nonetheless, an ideal anesthetic agent should be easy to administer, produce a rapid and adequate immobilization, have limited side effects, and be reversible and safe for the animals [20,94].

On the other hand, significant technical challenges exist in the transfer of preclinical MRI sequences to the clinic, due to the higher strength of the magnetic fields used in preclinical settings. However, preclinical systems often lack the wide selection of coils available for medical use, and hence, they require the development of specific coils. Therefore, preclinical MRI is essential for the development and validation of novel techniques, but these technical and biological challenges can partly hinder translation [93,95].

3.6. Multimodality Imaging

The combination of different imaging methods, the so-called multimodal imaging approach, offers the opportunity to correlate the most advantageous capabilities of each method and provide complementary information while compensating for their limitations. In preclinical research, all possible combinations of molecular imaging techniques are usually employed. In human medicine, the first example is the PET/CT combination, which offers highly specific functional information, with an excellent anatomic co-registration. Such a system is used in preclinical imaging as well. Another fascinating combination is the PET/MRI, which has been used in the last few years, in both clinical and preclinical settings, even if with some critical technical drawbacks. In any case, the multimodal approach should offer an excellent anatomical resolution with functional information, allowing for a multiparametric evaluation within a single study [8,9,83,96–100].

4. Magnetic Resonance Imaging Sequences in the Translational Context

The MRI is one of the primary preclinical and clinical imaging modalities, ideal for non-invasive longitudinal studies and useful for monitoring multiple parameters. In the oncological field, MRI is suitable for the definition of lesions with a high spatial resolution and anatomical detail, allowing the identification of primary tumors and metastatic disease. Moreover, it is also useful for the evaluation of quantitative characteristics that provide physiological, biochemical, and molecular details able to predict the biological behavior of cancer [9,32,101]. Various MRI sequences have been successfully developed by preclinical research and translated into clinical applications, as described below. Indeed, the preclinical MRI scanners can be easily considered a translational platform, since both preclinical and clinical scanners work with the same hardware settings and with almost identical sequences [9,102]. However, it is always necessary to establish the reproducibility of the technique chosen before being introduced in the clinic.

As mentioned, the MRI offers the ability to evaluate numerous tumors' biological properties, such as angiogenesis, perfusion, pH, hypoxia, metabolism, and macromolecular content. Such biological features are used as indicators in preclinical research to monitor a cancer's response to therapy [93,95]. Moreover, the complementary nature of the information accessible, applying different MRI sequences in the same subject, can undoubtedly help cancer research; clinical management as well [101].

4.1. T1 and T2 Weighted Sequences

Image contrast in MRI acquisition is determined by tissue properties, sequence type, and sequence parameters. Several relaxation constants are used to describe the decay and recovery of the MR signal; in particular, the two most commonly used parameters are the T1 and T2, the so-called spin-lattice relaxation time (T1) and spin-spin relaxation time (T2), which are both weighted. Based on the T1 and T2 weighting, many sequences have been developed [103–105]. In clinical applications, the T1 and T2-weighted sequences are the standard for anatomical imaging, and they are useful in the oncology field, for the detection and evaluation of macroscopic changes in the lesion, and staging. In addition, exogenous contrast agents, such as gadolinium, manganese and iron-based contrast agents, can be applied to enhance the contrast between tissues or organs [104,106]. In preclinical studies, T1 and T2-weighted sequences are used for anatomical acquisition, with the employment of contrast agents as well [107].

4.1.1. Thyroid

In thyroid cancer, MRI texture analysis derived from conventional sequences reflects different histopathologic features and represents a possible association that can be used as a prognostic biomarker. Thirteen patients with histopathologically-confirmed thyroid carcinoma were enrolled and subjected to MRI acquisitions. The T1-precontrast and T2-weighted images were analyzed; overall, 279 texture features for each sequence were examined and correlated to the histopathological parameters Ki67 and p53, which are considered prognostic biomarkers. Several significant correlations were identified; indeed, sum square average features derived from T1-weighted images and entropy-based features derived from T2-weighted images are associated with p53 count in thyroid cancer. Similarly, different texture features derived from T1- and T2-weighted images showed associations with the Ki67 index. Hence, this relatively simple MRI technique, combined with texture analysis, does not replace histopathological examinations, but may be a novel, noninvasive modality for further characterizing thyroid cancer in clinical oncology [108].

The effects of the tyrosine kinase inhibitor gefitinib on MRI parameters, and the ability of such parameters to help schedule chemotherapy, were tested in a murine model of breast cancer. In this study, a xenograft model with BT474 cells (ductal carcinoma) was induced, and mice were treated with gefitinib either daily for ten days or "pulsed" for two consecutive days (higher dose for two administrations). The MRI acquisitions were performed at 2-day intervals over two weeks, and T1 and T2 weighted sequences were used to follow-up tumor volume. Moreover, diffusion and DCE MRI were performed, and relative results were reported in the respective paragraphs. Treatment with gefitinib resulted in significant tumor growth inhibition, both with pulsed and daily treatment. Hence, T1 and T2 proved to help evaluate growth inhibition but did not give any further information on which therapeutic protocol gave the best results [109].

4.1.2. Breast

In a preliminary study on breast cancer, the MRI texture analysis was used to analyze the correlation between textural features and tumor volume, and to distinguish the underlying molecular subtypes luminal A and B. Patients with histopathologically-proven, invasive, ductal breast cancer were selected. The first frame of T1 and T2-weighted sequences pre-contrast was acquired and followed by the administration of a gadolinium-based contrast agent. The data analyzed mainly in the pre-contrast images showed that luminal A and B types had different textural features. Luminal B types of cancer have, in fact, a more heterogeneous appearance in MR images compared to luminal A types. These subtypes also showed a difference in tumor volume, with luminal B types showing a larger volume than luminal A types. The MRI texture analysis, combining information from both T1 and T2-weighted images, may provide further information on the biological aggressiveness of breast tumors that may improve therapeutic efficacy and management [110].

4.1.3. Prostate

Anatomical MRI sequences may improve the accuracy of evaluating prostate volume, especially in subjects under hormonal treatment. The T2-weighted MRI was performed to evaluate the normal prostate volume in male C57/BL6 mice. The mice underwent castration, and they were repeatedly imaged to follow the castration-induced regression of the prostate. In addition to the T2-weighted sequence, a chemical shift-selective sequence (CHESS) was performed to suppress abdominal fat signal, and hence, to improve prostate distinction. Forty days after castration, each mouse was treated daily with the androgen dihydrotestosterone (DHT) subcutaneously (s.c.) to induced prostate re-growth. These sequences, in particular, the CHESS, allowed good discrimination of both the prostate margins and the ventral lobe from the dorsal and lateral lobes. Hence, this approach may improve the ability to differentiate the prostate from surrounding tissues and to better visualize the boundaries of the organ, even in human patients [111].

4.2. Dynamic Contrast-Enhanced

The most common MRI methods available to quantify perfusion, hemodynamic, and vascular properties of a tissue, are the dynamic contrast-enhanced (DCE) MRI and the arterial spin labeling (ASL) methods [93]. The DCE MRI represents an indirect measure of angiogenesis that evaluates the dynamic passage of a contrast agent through the tumor vessels to derive pharmacokinetic properties, measuring the contrast agent extravasation rate (Ktrans) and volume fraction (ve) of the extracellular extravascular space (EES), as thoroughly described elsewhere [93,112–114]. Such methods have been used to monitor perfusion, as a marker of responsiveness to antiangiogenic treatments, both in preclinical and clinical trials, in terms of either efficacy or early identification of treatment failure [14,99,115–120]. Therefore, the clinical ability of this method is remarkable not only for the functional information on the tumor vascularization pattern but also for the chemotherapy planning, monitoring response, and implementing a new line of therapies [121].

4.2.1. Breast

In the preclinical model of ductal breast cancer with BT474 cells previously described (see 4.1 T1 and T2 Weighted Sequences, [109]), the DCE was also performed at 2-day intervals over two weeks. Transendothelial permeability (Kps), and fractional plasma volume (fPV) were measured. Tumor Kps decreased with pulsed treatment but then rebounded and increased with daily treatment. Tumor fPV increased in both treated groups, subsequently decreasing with pulsed treatment. Therefore, such quantitative MRI parameters may provide a sensitive measure to distinguish treatment regimens, and they might be useful for determining correct treatment scheduling, and hence, enhance chemotherapeutic efficacy [109].

In a preliminary study of breast cancer in human patients, the predictive ability of MRI was demonstrated using the DCE or DWI methods to predict tumor response following neoadjuvant therapy (NAT). This model integrated the heterogeneity of MRI-derived parameters (i.e., efflux rate constant—*Kep*, and ADC, as further described in the respective paragraph) with the hormone receptor status (i.e., estrogen receptor—ER, progesterone receptor—PR, and human epidermal growth factor receptor 2—HER2) and clinical data which were obtained before and after the first cycle of NAT. Thirty-three breast cancer patients underwent neoadjuvant chemotherapy, and therefore, were scanned for DW and DCE-MRI in the following three time-points: before NAT, after the first cycle of NAT, and after all NAT cycles. The median number of treatment cycles was 14 cycles. After completion of NAT, the pathological complete response (pCR) and nonresponse (non-pCR) were determined at the time of surgery. Twelve patients exhibited a pCR, and twenty-one patients were non-pCR. For patients with pCRs, the mean Kep had decreased between the pre and post-first NAT cycles, while for a non-pCR patient, Kep increased. Measurements after all NAT cycles were not obtainable in pCR patients since there was no residual tumor identifiable in the MRI scan. The immunohistochemical evaluation of hormone receptor status has defined the molecular subtypes of breast cancer for all patients; indeed, among the thirty-three patients, nine, six, eight, and ten patients are classified into luminal A, B, HER2, and basal subtypes, respectively. The MRI approach in question seems to accurately predict a treatment response right after a single cycle of therapy. Moreover, this method may improve the accuracy of evaluating a tumor's response to NAT, showing a higher predictive power than models based on tumor size changes, and it may be used as a short-term surrogate marker of outcome in breast cancer patients [122].

4.2.2. Prostate

Male BALB/c nude mice were implanted subcutaneously with the human-derived, androgen-sensitive CWR22 cell line, to evaluate the predictive capacity of DCE in a prostate cancer xenograft mouse model. These mice received combinations of androgen-deprivation therapy, obtained by surgical castration and/or radiotherapy. The MRI sequences applied were DCE and DWI, which will be discussed in the dedicated paragraph, and they were performed pre-radiation, and on day one and nine; the ADC value, the K^{trans}, tumor volume, and PSA were used to measure the therapeutic response. The K^{trans} and PSA showed a high level of correlation with treatment response, and thus, this parameter might be included in the evaluation of treatment responses in prostate cancer patients [123].

4.3. Arterial Spin Labeling

As mentioned, the ASL is a noninvasive and quantitative technique that allows perfusion measurement without requiring the administration of a contrast agent. This technique uses arterial blood water as an endogenous diffusible tracer by "labeling" it; i.e., by inverting the magnetization of the blood with radiofrequency pulses. As a result, studies can be repeated in the same subject over time [93,101,124–127]. Measurement of tumor blood flow with this technique is strongly helpful for tumor grading and evaluation of anticancer treatment [124,126]. The ASL is widely used in the preclinical and clinical fields, but in the latter case, it is still an emerging technique and has not yet replaced more invasive procedures, such as contrast-enhanced MRI, probably due to the complexity of the method and the relatively high sensitivity to motion artifacts [124].

Breast

ASL might gain a significant impact on the diagnosis and therapy management of breast cancer, thanks to its ability to quantify perfusion without the use of contrast agents, as examined in a pilot study. Quantification of perfusion of normal fibroglandular tissue and breast cancer using a flow-sensitive, alternating-inversion, recovery-balanced, steady-state free precession (FAIR TrueFISP) ASL sequence was performed in twenty-two individuals, including eighteen patients with suspected breast tumors and four healthy controls, in addition to the routine clinical imaging protocol. The definitive diagnosis was obtained by histology after biopsy or surgery. The results showed that ASL perfusion was successfully acquired in thirteen of eighteen tumor patients and all healthy controls. The mean ASL perfusion of invasive ductal carcinoma tissue was significantly higher than the perfusion of the normal breast parenchyma and invasive lobular carcinoma. No significant difference was found between the mean ASL perfusion of the normal breast parenchyma and invasive lobular carcinoma tissue.

Hence, these results indicate that ASL perfusion can differentiate malignant lesions from normal breast parenchyma as well as breast tumor types. This MRI modality may be useful to detect early changes in response to neoadjuvant chemotherapy, and the signal changes proportional to the blood flow may represent a property that allows identifying potential biological markers, and consequently, developing targeted therapies. Furthermore, image acquisition can be repeated without the concern of cumulative doses of paramagnetic contrast agent, and in patients with renal insufficiency, who may not be safely injected with contrast agents [128].

4.4. Blood Oxygen Level-Dependent Functional Magnetic Resonance Imaging

The blood oxygen level-dependent (BOLD) functional MRI (fMRI) provides information on changes in oxygenation in tissue to measure the hemodynamic response. The BOLD "contrast" reflects a variation in the transverse relaxation rate of tissue, and the paramagnetic effects influence it by the concentration of deoxyhemoglobin [93,129]. Generally speaking, this technique is heavily used to study cerebral activity, but it has the potential to evaluate metabolism, angiogenesis, and variations of oxygenation in tumors, as well. Indeed, in preclinical models and human tumors, it has been applied as a noninvasive method to monitor antiangiogenic therapies [129,130]. However, BOLD provides an indirect estimate of oxygen delivery and has a variable and scarce relationship with tumor tissue hypoxia, which is a significant negative prognostic factor. The ability to "map" hypoxia might help therapy planning and predicts treatment failure; thus, driving early changes of therapeutic strategy [131–133]. Furthermore, BOLD measurements are influenced by variations in vessel caliber, by the presence of hemorrhage and movement artifacts, which hinders its implementation as a clinical biomarker of hypoxia and its readiness to translate into clinical use [131,132].

Breast

The BOLD MRI method has been employed as a simple, noninvasive method to assess tumor oxygenation during a preliminary observational study. Eleven patients with locally advanced breast cancer were enrolled for preoperative neoadjuvant chemotherapy with doxorubicin and cyclophosphamide for four cycles. Of these, seven patients completed all chemotherapy treatments and underwent MRI before, during, and after chemotherapy. Breast tumor response was divided into complete response, partial, and stable response based on clinical palpation. The BOLD study applied a 6-min oxygen-breathing challenge; BOLD contrast enhancement was observed in all tumors, but patients with complete responses showed a significantly higher BOLD before the start of chemotherapy compared with both partial or stable response; furthermore, there was no significant difference between latter groups. The correlation between high BOLD response and better treatment outcome suggests that this may be an excellent, noninvasive prognostic tool for cancer management, providing early predictive information on the response to chemotherapy [134].

4.5. Oxygen-enhanced Magnetic Resonance Imaging

Oxygen-enhanced (OE) MRI is an alternative in vivo technique to quantify and map changes, distributions, and the extent of oxygen concentrations in tumors. In OE-MRI, the longitudinal relaxation rate is used to evaluate changes in the level of molecular oxygen dissolved in blood plasma or interstitial tissue. Therefore, the measured variations are proportional to the variation of oxygen concentration in the tissue. This method allows the noninvasive identification, quantification, and mapping of tumor hypoxia with MRI in vivo, making the technique suitable for rapid clinical translation [131,133]. Indeed, tumor hypoxia and oxygen dynamics have been correlated to aggressiveness and therapeutic resistance in many tumors [135].

Prostate

In a preclinical study for prostate cancer, this technique was used as a potential predictive biomarker of radiation-therapy response. Dunning R3327-AT1 prostate tumors were surgically implanted subcutaneously in the flank of adult male syngeneic Copenhagen rats; nineteen days after implantation, OE-MRI was performed before each irradiation (2Fx15 Gy). The tumors were irradiated approximately 24 h after OE-MRI experiments. Before and during radiotherapy, the anesthetized animals inhaled either air or oxygen for at least 15 min. The OE-MRI and irradiation were repeated a week later, and the tumor growth delay was determined by the time required to achieve double-time volume (VDT) and quadruple time volume (VQT). Moreover, during hypofractionated radiotherapy, the BOLD and tissue oxygen-level dependent (TOLD) contrast, and the quantitative responses of relaxation rates (R1 and R2) were applied. The semi-quantitative parameters showed a significant correlation between the average TOLD and BOLD responses for single tumors before and after the irradiation. For the R1 and R2 rates, there were no significant differences before irradiation, but there was a significant difference between air and oxygen breathing. Tumors in oxygen-breathing animals expressed a more significant growth delay than tumors in the air group during irradiation. Therefore, the inhalation of oxygen during hypofractionated radiotherapy significantly improved radiation-therapy response, and OE-MRI may be added to routine clinical MRI for patient stratification and the personalization of radiotherapy treatment planning [135].

4.6. Diffusion-Weighted Imaging

Diffusion-weighted imaging (DWI) is an MRI approach used to evaluate the diffusion rate of water molecules within tissues without the use of exogenous contrast agents [14]. The diffusion of water molecules and the degree of mobility are expressed quantitatively by the apparent diffusion coefficient (ADC), which can estimate the changes in cellularity and the integrity of cell membranes [99,136,137]. In particular, DWI is suited for the characterization of the tumor and for monitoring treatment response. Indeed, the variations in the ADC can demonstrate changes in the physiology of the tumors following therapeutic interventions, and therefore, ADC may be a potential biomarker of treatment efficacy [99,118,137–139]. The DWI has shown its value in tumor monitoring in both preclinical cancer models and clinical patients [101,138,140,141].

Preclinical assessments of early responses to therapy have been evaluated in breast and prostate cancer models, and in lymph node sites as a potential alternative method for detecting metastatic lesions. Primary applications of DWI are tumor detection and differentiation from non-tumor tissues, differentiation of malignant from benign lesions, and monitoring and prediction of treatment responses [137]. Hence, this technique may also be a noninvasive imaging biomarker of tumor aggressiveness for better stratification of patients with poor prognosis [138,139]. Indeed, this technique is being considered the standard of care for prostate and liver cancer, in which the different ADC measurements can predict tumor aggressiveness [14,93,139,142]. Additionally, in breast and thyroid cancers, ADC is considered an imaging biomarker able to differentiate malignant and benign lesions, and it has also been shown to predict the response to neoadjuvant chemotherapy in the former histotype [101,143]. Furthermore, DWI has been evaluated as a possible alternative to PET/CT for the detection of metastatic lesions [14,93,139,142].

4.6.1. Thyroid

It has been shown that DWI and ADC maps, have the potential to distinguish malignant and benign nodules in the thyroid, since this technique can assess the different cellular architectures of tumors [144]. Differences in ADC were evaluated between benign and malignant nodules, correlating ADC to cytological results by fine-needle aspiration. The study included 36 patients with thyroid gland nodules and 24 healthy patients, all of whom were examined with DWI sequences. In the nodular patient group, there were 27 cases of benign nodules and nine cases diagnosed as thyroid gland malignancy; in total, 52 benign nodules and 16 malignant nodules were examined. The ADC values were significantly different between benign and malignant nodules, and from healthy thyroid tissues in the controls. In the benign group, the ADC value of thyroid nodules was increased while in the malignant group, it was reduced; in the healthy thyroid tissue, the ADC value was within the normal range. The reduction in the ADC observed in most malignant lesions was linked to the decrease in extracellular/extravascular space due to cellular proliferation, as confirmed by cytology. These results showed that DWI provides useful and promising results on the nature of a thyroid nodule, and it may have a role in the selection of nodules that should undergo needle aspiration cytology [143].

Similarly, DWI ADC mapping was performed on 14 patients with malignant thyroid nodules diagnosed by ultrasound and verified by biopsy. In these patients, 13 nodules were malignant, as shown with biopsy evidence, and five nodules were benign. Malignant nodules had significantly lower ADC values than the benign ones, confirming previous results [145].

In a preliminary study, the employment of DWI was investigated using a readout-segmented multishot EPI (RESOLVE) sequence to differentiate between well-differentiated and undifferentiated subgroups of thyroid carcinomas. Moreover, the correlations between this technique and histopathologic data, such as the Ki-67 index and p53 expression, were evaluated. Indeed, Ki-67 represents a histopathologic parameter associated with cell proliferation, whereas p53 is considered a marker of tumor aggressiveness. Fourteen patients received preoperative MRI scans, including DWI-RESOLVE, and T1 and T2 conventional sequences before and after contrast-medium administration (gadopentetate dimeglumine). Four patients showed follicular thyroid carcinoma; four patients, papillary thyroid carcinoma; and six patients, undifferentiated thyroid carcinomas. The results showed that the mean ADC values were significantly lower in undifferentiated carcinomas compared with follicular and papillary carcinomas. A decrease in ADC mean values inversely correlated with an increase in Ki-67, while the increase in p53 expression was correlated to an increased in ADC mean values. Therefore, DWI seems able to distinguish between differentiated and undifferentiated thyroid carcinomas. This approach, once further validated, might help to preselect optimal therapeutic strategies in the presurgical phase [144].

4.6.2. Breast

The DWI and magnetic resonance spectroscopy (MRS) were able to detect early tumor responses in triple-negative breast cancer (TNBC) mouse xenografts after combination therapy with TRA-8, a monoclonal antibody targeted to the apoptosis receptor, and carboplatin, a standard chemotherapeutic agent. The therapeutic efficacy was assessed by monitoring tumor volume, first ADC changes, and lipid concentration through the fat–water ratio (FWR) MRS. Two different TNBC xenograft models, implanted either with 2LMP or SUM159 cell lines, were treated intraperitoneally with either carboplatin, TRA-8, or their combination. The MRI acquisitions with DWI and MRS were performed before, during, and at the end of the therapeutic protocol. Combination therapy with TRA-8 and carboplatin showed significantly reduced tumor growth in both 2LMP and SUM159 TNBC models compared to both single-drug treatments, and the therapeutic efficacy was verified histologically, as witnessed by a significant increase of apoptotic cell density. Substantial changes in ADC were detected only three days after the initiation of TRA-8 or combination therapy, while significant changes in FWR required seven days for detection. Both ADC and FWR changes were confirmed as useful imaging biomarkers to evaluate the therapeutic efficacy, but ADC changes may be used as an earlier predictor. This imaging protocol might be translated into clinical trials testing these or similar drugs, since early assessment is useful for preventing unnecessary/ineffective treatments and, hence, to improve outcomes [146].

In the preclinical model of ductal breast cancer with BT474 cells previously described (see 4.1 T1 and T2 Weighted Sequences, [109]), ADC was also tested as a predictor of gefitinib efficacy. Tumor ADC increased in all treated groups. Therefore, as mentioned, the parameters included in the study, specifically Kps and fPV from DCE and ADC from DWI, may all provide, in combination, a more sensitive approach to determining the right treatment plan [109].

A mouse model of a breast cancer brain metastasis was developed to optimize a longitudinal MRI and MRS method for analyzing the pathogenic aspects of brain metastasis, since cerebral metastasis showed a high incidence in breast carcinoma patients. Brain metastases were generated by the intra-carotid injection of human mammary carcinoma cells 435-Br1, a brain metastasis variant of the parental cell line MDA-MB-435. Different MRI approaches were used to characterize the morphological and metabolic development patterns of brain metastases, including T2 and contrast enhanced-T1 weighted images, DWI, and MRS imaging. The acquired data were then combined with the histological analyses of the dissected brains. As a result, nine out of thirteen mice developed MR-detectable abnormal masses (single or multiple) in the brain parenchyma within 20 to 62 days after injection. Two additional animals had brain metastases detected only by histological analysis. The ADC maps correctly differentiated the edema and disorders of cerebrospinal fluid circulation areas from metastases, in addition to the MRS results that have been discussed in the dedicated paragraph. This imaging approach might be considered helpful in early detection and differentiation of brain metastases from other cerebral abnormalities [147].

In the preliminary study of breast cancer in human patients already described (see 4.2 Dynamic Contrast-Enhanced [122]), the DWI method was used to predict tumors' responses following neoadjuvant therapy (NAT), in conjunction with DCE. After completion of NAT, the pathologic complete response (pCR) and nonresponse (non-pCR) were determined at the time of surgery. The mean ADC was increased between the first two time points for the same pCR, while no noticeable change in mean ADC was observed for the non-pCR patient. The MRI approach described may improve the accuracy of evaluating the tumor response to NAT, showing a higher predictive power than models based on tumor size changes, and it may be used as an early marker of outcome in breast cancer patients [122].

4.6.3. Prostate

In a prostate cancer xenograft mice model, DWI was tested as a predictor of the efficacy of docetaxel, a cytostatic and cytotoxic antineoplastic drug. The LnCaP cell line, derived from the lymph node metastasis of a human prostatic adenocarcinoma was used, since it secretes the prostate-specific antigen (PSA). Serum PSA levels and tumor volumes were used to measure tumor response noninvasively. Results showed a good response of the xenograft to docetaxel, and serum PSA was confirmed as a useful biomarker of therapy response, but changes in ADC represented an earlier indicator of therapeutic response. This approach should be validated in the clinic to correctly manage the therapeutic regimen, especially for second-line therapies that show reduced response rates and higher toxicity [148].

In the study described before (see 4.2 Dynamic Contrast-Enhanced [123]), mice bearing prostate cancer xenografts underwent, as mentioned, DWI acquisitions pre-radiation, and on day one and nine after. The ADC values, volumes, and PSA levels revealed significant correlations with treatment response. The combination of all parameters, including the K^{trans} obtained with the DCE, successfully predicted treatment response with a high correlation coefficient. Therefore, the combination of such parameters with standard clinical parameters may improve the predictive power for the therapeutic outcome in prostate cancer patients, and it might be applied for the personalization of therapeutic approaches [123].

A multiparametric analysis to evaluate in vivo vascularization, metabolism, and physiological characteristics that are permissive for the occurrence of metastases has been tested in a prostate cancer xenograft models using noninvasive MRI and MRS. A human prostate cancer xenograft model implanted s.c. or orthotopically in the prostate was used. The tumors were derived from PC-3 human prostate cells inoculated s.c. in the right flank of SCID mice; the intact tumor tissue obtained from subcutaneous tumors was harvested and re-implanted s.c. in the flank or orthotopically with a microsurgical method of SCID mice. These mouse models underwent MRI acquisitions, including T1-weighted with the administration of albumin-Gd-DTPA, multislice DWI for evaluation of vasculature, and MRS for metabolic maps of total choline and lactate/lipid and extracellular pH (pHe). As the results showed, the tumors in the orthotopic site were identifiable by the hyperintense signal detected in DWI compared to the s.c., and they showed higher vascular volume and higher permeability, as well. In the metastases' characterizations, several lung nodules were observed in mice with orthotopically-implanted tumors, and only a few small clusters of cells were observed in the lungs of mice with xenografts. Therefore, the higher metastatization rate of orthotopic tumors might be linked to the higher vascular volume and permeability. These data confirm the profound influence of the tumor microenvironment on the metastatization process and the feasibility of identifying noninvasive clinically translatable parameters that may contribute to determining risk factors for metastases formation in patients. Future translational studies are necessary to validate these observations further [149].

4.7. Diffusion Kurtosis Imaging

Diffusion kurtosis imaging (DKI) has been applied to many body-districts, showing a higher capability in differentiating between benign and malignant tumors, and in predicting treatment responses compared to conventional DWI. From the DKI model, the diffusion coefficient (D) and the diffusional kurtosis (K) are derived, which provide more information on the tissue structure than DWI. Indeed, the parameter D evaluates the tissue diffusion and seems to be more accurate than ADC; the K parameter seems to be more sensitive to irregular and heterogeneous cellular environments, but less sensitive to cell density.

Thyroid

In a preliminary study, the usefulness of DKI compared to DWI was investigated in thyroid lesions, also assessing the correlation of such MRI parameters with histopathologic features. Fifty-eight patients with thyroid nodules detected by ultrasound underwent MRI examination, including T1 and T2-weighted imaging, conventional DWI, and DKI. Histopathological analysis was performed with the evaluation of Ki-67 and vascular endothelial growth factor (VEGF), since Ki-67 is a cell proliferation protein and is considered a neoplastic marker, as mentioned above, and the VEGF is a cytokine that induces angiogenesis and is related to angiogenesis in tumors. Fifty-eight thyroid lesions were found, including twenty-four papillary thyroid cancers, twenty-one adenomas, seven nodular goiters, and six cases of Hashimoto's thyroiditis. Malignant lesions showed significantly higher mean ADC and D values and lower K values compare to benign lesions. The number of positively-stained VEGF and Ki-67 cells was significantly higher in the malignant group. The DKI-derived D parameter showed the strongest correlation with both Ki-67 and VEGF. Therefore, DKI should be considered advantageous over the conventional DWI for the diagnosis of thyroid lesions with better diagnostic accuracy [150].

4.8. Magnetic Resonance Spectroscopy

Magnetic resonance spectroscopy (MRS) allows the identification of different atomic nuclei, such as hydrogen, carbon, phosphorus, and fluorine, in specific regions of interest; thus, providing functional and biochemical information on a wide range of biological processes. For example, among the cellular metabolites measured with MRS, there is choline contained in cell membranes, creatine and glucose involved in energy production, and alanine and lactate that are typically increased in some tumors [83]. In clinical applications, it is a noninvasive method for the assessment of tumor biochemistry and physiology to identify the early changes in response to therapy, as well as for grading and staging of cancer [93,151,152]. In many preclinical studies, e.g., in breast or colon cancer, this method is used to track intra-tumor changes during therapy, and the levels of the metabolites measured may represent a potential noninvasive marker to check tumor response [153–155].

4.8.1. Thyroid

Proton (H) MRS and DWI-ADC mapping (see 4.6 Diffusion-Weighted Imaging, [145]) were performed on 14 patients with malignant thyroid nodules diagnosed by ultrasonography and verified by biopsy. In these patients, 13 nodules were malignant with biopsy evidence, and five nodules were benign. Intra-nodular choline (Cho) peak, Cho/creatine (Cr) ratio, and ADC values of malignant nodules were evaluated and compared to those of benign nodules. Malignant nodules had significantly higher Cho peak amplitudes and a higher Cho/Cr ratio than benign ones. Hence, the use of H-MRS may be added to other imaging approaches in the evaluation of thyroid nodules and the determination of their nature. It might help to establish adequate treatments at an early stage, reducing the morbidity and mortality of the disease, and, at the same time, avoiding unnecessary surgical interventions in patients with benign lesions. Nonetheless, there are technical difficulties in performing MRS on thyroid glands, or other neck structures, concerning tumor movement due to swallowing and breathing, substantial differences in magnetic susceptibility between the neck and the air in the trachea, and the contamination of spectra by adjacent fat [145].

4.8.2. Breast

In the TNBC xenograft mouse models previously described (see 4.6 Diffusion-Weighted Imaging, [146]), MRS was associated with DWI to detect early tumor response after combination therapy with TRA-8 and carboplatin. The therapeutic efficacy was assessed by monitoring tumor volume, ADC changes, and lipid concentration through the fat–water ratio (FWR) MRS. The MRI acquisitions with DWI and MRS were performed before, during, and at the end of the therapeutic protocol. Significant changes in FWR required seven days for detection. Both ADC and FWR changes were confirmed as useful imaging biomarkers to evaluate the therapeutic efficacy, but ADC changes were detected earlier than FWR. This imaging protocol should be translated into clinical trials to improve outcomes by stopping ineffective therapies [146].

In the brain metastasis model previously described (see 4.6 Diffusion-Weighted Imaging, [147]), MRS was again added to DWI. A single-voxel MRS was used to analyze the metabolic patterns of the lesions in ten subjects. Only eight out of ten mice had brain metastases, and just two of them showed a field homogeneity good enough and a correct voxel position inside the lesion. However, when the lesions increased in size and infiltrated the brain parenchyma, the spectral changes indicated the replacement of the healthy tissue pattern with the tumor tissue pattern. The data proved a decrease in N-acetyl aspartate (NAA) as the earliest sign of metastasis growth, followed by a decrease in Cho and Cr levels. Those results suggest that this approach, in addition to DWI, may help in discriminating brain metastasis growth and the classification of distinct progression stages, and it might open the way to its use in the diagnosis and therapy monitoring [147].

Phosphorus (^{31}P) MRS was used to quantify the levels of phosphorylated metabolites in breast cancer tissue. In particular, phosphocholine (PCho), glycerophosphocholine (GPC), phosphoethanolamine (PEtn), and glycerophosphoethanolamine (GPE) may be considered valuable biomarkers for the diagnosis and noninvasive monitoring of therapies both in preclinical studies and in the clinical phase. To this end, the metabolic response to the oral treatment with phosphatidylinositol-3-kinase/mammalian target of the rapamycin (PI3K/mTOR) inhibitor BEZ235 was evaluated in basal-like (MAS98.12) and luminal-like (MAS98.06) breast xenograft models. These models were established by direct implantation of primary human breast cancer tissues in the mammary fat pad of immunodeficient mice, and then serially transplanted in BalbC nu/nu mice. As a result, a significant increase in GPC and PCho was found in basal-like xenografts, whereas PEtn decreased. No significant changes were observed in phosphorylated metabolites in luminal-like xenografts, which did not respond to treatment with BEZ235. These data demonstrate the usefulness of 31P MRS in the metabolic profiling of breast cancer subtypes and the evaluation of the metabolic response to targeted anticancer drugs [156].

In a pilot study, the use of MRS was tested for monitoring breast cancer therapy. Indeed, such neoplastic tissue contains high levels of choline-containing compounds (tCho). The changes in tCho concentration were determined to predict the early clinical response to neoadjuvant chemotherapy in the first 24 h after initial treatment in patients with locally advanced breast cancer. Sixteen women, aged 18 to 80 years, with biopsy-confirmed, locally advanced breast cancer, were enrolled. Thirteen patients received combined doxorubicin hydrochloride and cyclophosphamide treatment that was administered on day one, with additional doses at 21-day intervals for a total of 64 days. Patients underwent MRS before treatment, within 24 h after the first dose, and then after the fourth dose. As a result, eight out of thirteen patients showed a significant correlation between changes in tCho concentration and lesion-size reduction. These patients had a lower tCho level within 24 h after the first dose compared to baseline and a further decrease in the tCho concentration after the fourth dose of the combined therapy. The other five patients out of the thirteen showed no changes and had a baseline tCho concentration less than or equal to that measured within 24 h after the first dose. Therefore, MRS may be used to assess early response to neoadjuvant chemotherapy and to customize an effective regimen for individual patients [157].

4.8.3. Prostate

In the prostate cancer model described (see 4.6 Diffusion-Weighted Imaging, [148]), MRS was applied to obtain metabolic maps of total choline and lactate/lipid ratio, and extracellular pH (pHe). Total choline and lactate/lipid levels were significantly higher in orthotopic compared with xenograft tumors, whereas the pHe maps showed a significantly lower pH in orthotopic tumors compared with subcutaneous tumors. As already stated, such an imaging approach may prove to be extremely helpful in studying the tumor microenvironment, demonstrating changes that might be linked the metastatization process, like in this case, total choline and a more acidic extracellular pH. Once validated, these techniques may also support the development of novel strategies to reduce metastatization [148].

4.9. Chemical Exchange Saturation Transfer

Chemical exchange saturation transfer (CEST) is an MRI method to detect low concentrations of metabolites for probing specific molecular and physiological events. The sensitivity of this approach is enhanced by the use of a set of new specific contrast agents, and endogenous as well as exogenous molecules can be used. Indeed, a variety of molecules have been demonstrated as potential contrast agents in this technique, including small diamagnetic molecules, paramagnetic ions complexes, liposomes, nanoparticles, and hyperpolarized gases [158–160]. The CEST applications in the clinic aim to monitor different metabolites, such as glycogen concentration (glycoCEST), glycosaminoglycans levels (gagCEST), or glutamate (gluCEST). Moreover, this is a valid imaging modality for detecting and monitoring the progression of tumors and assessing their responses to therapy by avoiding exposing the patient to radiation [159,161,162]. In preclinical studies, CEST has been used to measure the rate of metabolites' uptakes, such as glycogen and glucose, which are hallmarks of the tumor microenvironment. The evaluation of extracellular pH (acidoCEST), which is linked to the increase in lactic acid production after an increase in glycolysis, may be used for assessing tumor aggressiveness and early responses to treatments that inhibit glycolytic metabolism [161,163,164]. The CEST measurement of glucose metabolism (glucoCEST) in tumor mouse models allows studying the tumor microenvironment, and it may represent a potential replacement of the PET approach [159,164].

4.9.1. Breast

The CEST has been proposed as a new molecular imaging approach to detect glucose or its analogs in the diagnosis of tumors. D-glucose and deoxy-D-glucose (2DG) were commonly employed to that end, but their toxicity at high concentrations precludes their clinical use and limits preclinical applications. A preliminary experiment was conducted to examine the validity of 3-O-methyl-D-glucose (3OMG) as a nontoxic alternative, which has been demonstrated to be able to detect tumors in several models of murine and human breast cancer. Moreover, this method was compared with glucoCEST and [18F]-FDG PET on the same animals. Orthotropic tumors were induced in mice by injecting human MDA-MB-231 or MCF7 cells. The CEST MRI sequences were performed on mice before and after the administration (intravenous, intraperitoneal, or oral) of 3OM. The same animals were then injected with [18F]-FDG for PET imaging, and D-glucose for glucoCEST after a specific time. The results showed that the CEST MRI following the administration of 3OMG produced patterns that reflected the metabolic activity of tumors and clearly distinguished them from other body districts. A marked 3OMG-CEST MRI contrast was obtained, and the most aggressive breast cancer models produced the highest CEST contrast. The contrast reached its maximum at 20 min post administration and lasted for more than one hour, without any difference in effect levels or timing between the three routes of administration. The 3OMG CEST method compared to the glucoCEST showed a higher CEST contrast than D-glucose. Moreover, a good correlation was found between 3OMG CEST contrast and FDG uptake, providing clear validation of this technique. Therefore, the validation of the 3OMG-CEST MRI method in the clinic would offer significant advantages for evaluation, detection, and monitoring of tumors' progressions, and assessing their responses to therapy, avoiding radiation exposure [161].

4.9.2. Prostate

The CEST approach, using amide proton transfer (APT) MR imaging, was used in a preliminary study to localize prostate cancer better and to detect the difference in cancer aggressiveness, discriminating between cancerous and non-cancerous tissues. The APT MRI does not require the injection of a contrast agent since it uses endogenous amide protons in tissue, which allows detecting micromolar concentrations of mobile proteins with high sensitivity. Therefore, the applicability of this imaging modality to the detection of prostate cancer was based on the high rate of tumor cell proliferation and on the cellular density of this tumor, which leads to high levels of mobile proteins. In this study, twelve patients with biopsy-proven prostate cancer scheduled for prostatectomy were enrolled and underwent T2 and APT MRI acquisitions. The APT ratio in the tumor zone was significantly higher than that in the benign regions of the peripheral zone; hence, distinguishing them. Such results were confirmed by both the T2-weighted imaging and histopathological findings. The CEST APT imaging technique may, thus, represent a potential approach to detecting and discriminating between low and high-grade prostate cancer, and it might be more specific compared with DCE or DWI sequences [164].

4.10. Short Tau Inversion Recovery

The short tau inversion recovery (STIR), is an inversion recovery sequence, which is a spin-echo sequence with a 180° preparation pulse to flip the longitudinal magnetization into the opposite direction. In this case, to generate an MR signal, the longitudinal magnetization is then converted to transverse magnetization through the application of a 90° pulse. The time between the change from 180° to 90°, or inversion time in such sequences, is kept short, between 130 and 150 ms.

Breast

In a preliminary clinical experience, the usefulness of whole-body turbo STIR sequence was assessed to detect liver, brain, and bone metastases as a single examination in breast cancer patients, in alternative to conventional techniques. Seventeen patients with biopsy-proven breast cancer and suspected metastatic disease were included in this study and underwent both whole-body STIR-MRI and conventional imaging, such as MR brain imaging with spin-echo; T1 and T2-weighted CT and ultrasound scanning; and bone scintigraphy. Three patients were found to be free of metastases in both conventional and STIR imaging. In eleven out of seventeen patients, appendicular or axial skeletal metastases were identified, with a good correlation between findings in whole-body STIR and scintigraphy. Hepatic metastases were found in five patients using whole-body STIR, of which only three patients' finding correlated with CT and ultrasound findings. Metastases and brain abnormalities were found in four patients via both whole-body STIR and dedicated brain MRI. Therefore, this pilot evaluation, even if performed on a small cohort of patients, showed that STIR acquisition might represent an accurate, convenient, and cost-effective staging method during the long-term follow-up of breast cancer patients [165].

5. Conclusions

Translational research must be supported by a real interdisciplinary, synergistic collaboration to avoid the inconveniences and ineffectiveness of the methods, in order to emphasize the benefits of patients in a robust translational application. In order for an experimental imaging methodology to be successfully translated into clinical practice, it must have a substantial and immediate impact on application to the patient, and therefore, be easily accessible. The development and use of animal models of cancer and its integration with molecular imaging tools may enhance the clinical translatability of preclinical studies focused on the clinical implementation of MRI methodologies in the management of tumor diseases from the diagnoses to therapeutics' evaluations and follow-up monitoring. From that perspective, it should be borne in mind that there is not a single ideal mouse model that recapitulates all features of the human pathology. Hence, the development and choice of the appropriate model must comply with the experimental, or from a translational perspective, with the direct clinical needs. Thus, it is fundamental to evaluating which the characteristics that may influence clinical efficacy are; i.e., histopathologic features, immune system interaction, carcinogenesis, angiogenesis, tumor progression, and metastatic potential. Indeed, as described, each model has its peculiarities, and all might be considered complementary to each other. Finally, the best combination of the appropriate experimental model and the careful choice of imaging modalities with clinical homologs might accelerate the reduction in the gap between preclinical and clinical studies. The high translational ability of MRI, among the other imaging techniques, due to the high similarity in terms of hardware and software between experimental and clinical scanners, should strengthen the efforts in evaluating how far this technique can go for the diagnosis and management of cancer patients.

Author Contributions: M.F.F. searched for literature and drafted the manuscript; C.C. coordinated the research group and selected the papers to be included; L.A. revised the manuscript and formatted it for submission; L.B. wrote the technical parts in the manuscript; M.S. coordinated the research group and revised the manuscript.

Funding: This research was funded by "Ricerca Corrente", Italian Ministry of Health.

Conflicts of Interest: The authors declare no conflict of interest.

References

1. Cohrs, R.J.; Martin, T.; Ghahramani, P.; Bidaut, L.; Higgins, P.J.; Shahzad, A. Translational medicine definition by the european society for translational medicine. *New Horiz. Transl. Med.* **2015**, *2*, 86–88. [CrossRef]
2. Rubio, D.M.; Schoenbaum, E.E.; Lee, L.S.; Schteingart, D.E.; Marantz, P.R.; Anderson, K.E.; Platt, L.D.; Baez, A.; Esposito, K. Defining translational research: Implications for training. *Acad. Med.* **2010**, *85*, 470–475. [CrossRef] [PubMed]
3. De Jong, M.; Maina, T. Of mice and humans: Are they the same?—Implications in cancer translational research. *J. Nucl. Med.* **2010**, *51*, 501–504. [CrossRef] [PubMed]
4. De Jong, M.; Essers, J.; Van Weerden, W.M. Imaging preclinical tumour models: Improving translational power. *Nat. Rev. Cancer* **2014**, *14*, 481–493. [CrossRef]
5. Denayer, T.; Stöhr, T.; Van Roy, M. Animal models in translational medicine: Validation and prediction. *New Horiz. Transl. Med.* **2014**, *2*, 5–11. [CrossRef]
6. Emes, R.D.; Goodstadt, L.; Winter, E.E.; Ponting, C.P. Comparison of the genomes of human and mouse lays the foundation of genome zoology. *Hum. Mol. Genet.* **2003**, *12*, 701–709. [CrossRef]
7. Suzuki, Y.; Yamashita, R.; Shirota, M.; Sakakibara, Y.; Chiba, J.; Mizushima-Sugano, J.; Nakai, K.; Sugano, S. Sequence comparison of human and mouse genes reveals a homologous block structure in the promoter regions. *Genome Res.* **2004**, *14*, 1711–1718. [CrossRef]
8. Koo, V.; Hamilton, P.W.; Williamson, K. Non-invasive in vivo imaging in small animal research. *Cell Oncol.* **2006**, *28*, 127–139.
9. Cunha, L.; Horvath, I.; Ferreira, S.; Lemos, J.; Costa, P.; Vieira, D.; Veres, D.S.; Szigeti, K.; Summavielle, T.; Màthè, D.; et al. Preclinical imaging: An essential ally in modern biosciences. *Mol. Diagn. Ther.* **2014**, *18*, 153–173. [CrossRef]
10. Mejia, J.; Camargo Miranda, A.C.; Ranucci Durante, A.C.; de Oliveira, L.R.; de Barboza, M.R.F.F.; Taboada Rosell, K.; Pereira Jardim, D.; Holthausen Campos, A.; dos Reis, M.A.; Forli Catanoso, M.; et al. Preclinical molecular imaging: Development of instrumentation for translational research with small laboratory animals. *Einstein* **2016**, *14*, 408–414. [CrossRef]
11. Lewis, J.S.; Achilefu, S.; Garbow, J.R.; Laforest, R.; Welch, M.J. Small animal imaging: Current technology and perspectives for oncological imaging. *Eur. J. Cancer* **2002**, *38*, 2173–2188. [CrossRef]
12. Pomper, M.G. Translational molecular imaging for cancer. *Cancer Imaging* **2005**, *5*, S16–S26. [CrossRef]

13. Workman, P.; Aboagye, E.O.; Balkwill, F.; Balmain, A.; Bruder, G.; Chaplin, D.J.; Double, J.A.; Everitt, J.; Farningham, D.A.H.; Glennie, M.J.; et al. Guidelines for the welfare and use of animals in cancer research. *Br. J. Cancer* **2010**, *102*, 1555–1577. [CrossRef]
14. Kircher, M.F.; Hricak, H.; Larson, S.M. Molecular imaging for personalized cancer care. *Mol. Oncol.* **2012**, *6*, 182–195. [CrossRef]
15. Wolf, G.; Abolmaali, N. Preclinical molecular imaging using PET and MRI. *Mol. Imaging Oncol.* **2013**, *187*, 257–310.
16. Grassi, R.; Cavaliere, C.; Cozzolino, S.; Mansi, L.; Cirillo, S.; Tedeschi, G.; Franchi, R.; Russo, P.; Cornacchia, S.; Rotondo, A. Small animal imaging facility: New perspectives for the radiologist. *Radiol. Med.* **2009**, *114*, 152–167. [CrossRef] [PubMed]
17. James, M.L.; Gambhir, S.S. A molecular imaging primer: Modalities, imaging agents, and applications. *Physiol. Rev.* **2012**, *92*, 897–965. [CrossRef]
18. Talmadge, J.E.; Singh, R.K.; Fidler, I.J.; Raz, A. Murine models to evaluate novel and conventional therapeutic strategies for cancer. *Am. J. Pathol.* **2007**, *170*, 793–804. [CrossRef] [PubMed]
19. Imaoka, T.; Nishimura, M.; Iizuka, D.; Daino, K.; Takabatake, T.; Okamoto, M.; Kakinuma, S.; Shimada, Y. Radiation-induced mammary carcinogenesis in rodent models: what's different from chemical carcinogenesis? *J. Radiat. Res.* **2009**, *50*, 281–293. [CrossRef]
20. Gargiulo, S.; Greco, A.; Gramanzini, M.; Esposito, S.; Affuso, A.; Brunetti, A.; Vesce, G. Mice anesthesia, analgesia, and care, part I: Anesthetic considerations in preclinical research. *ILAR J.* **2012**, *53*, E55–E69. [CrossRef] [PubMed]
21. Becher, O.J.; Holland, E.C. Genetically engineered models have advantages over xenografts for preclinical studies. *Cancer Res.* **2006**, *66*, 3355–3359. [CrossRef] [PubMed]
22. Lunardi, A.; Nardella, C.; Clohessy, J.C.; Pandolfi, P.P. Of model pets and cancer models: An introduction to mouse models of cancer. *Cold Spring Harb. Protoc.* **2014**, *1*, 17–31. [CrossRef] [PubMed]
23. Teicher, B.A. Tumor models for efficacy determination. *Mol. Cancer Ther.* **2006**, *5*, 2435–2443. [CrossRef] [PubMed]
24. Schreiber, R.D.; Old, L.J.; Smyth, M.J. Cancer Immunoediting: Integrating Immunity's Roles in Cancer Suppression and Promotion. *Science* **2011**, *331*, 1565–1570. [CrossRef]
25. Kim, S. Animal models of cancer in the head and neck region. *Clin. Exp. Otorhinolaryngol.* **2009**, *2*, 55–60. [CrossRef]
26. Antonello, Z.A.; Nucera, C. Orthotopic mouse models for the preclinical and translational study of targeted therapies against metastatic human thyroid carcinoma with BRAFV600E or wild-type BRAF. *Oncogene* **2014**, *33*, 5397–5404. [CrossRef]
27. Rubio-Viqueira, B.; Hidalgo, M. Direct in vivo xenograft tumor model for predicting chemotherapeutic drug response in cancer patients. *Clin. Pharm. Ther.* **2009**, *85*, 217–221. [CrossRef]
28. Jung, J. Human Tumor Xenograft Models for Preclinical Assessment of Anticancer Drug Development. *Toxicol. Res.* **2014**, *30*, 1–5. [CrossRef]
29. Schweppe, R.E.; Klopper, J.P.; Korch, C.; Pugazhenthi, U.; Benezra, M.; Knauf, J.A.; Fagin, J.A.; Marlow, L.A.; Copland, J.A.; Smallridge, R.C.; et al. Deoxyribonucleic acid profiling analysis of 40 human thyroid cancer cell lines reveals cross-contamination resulting in cell line redundancy and misidentification. *J. Clin. Endocrinol. Metab.* **2008**, *93*, 4331–4341. [CrossRef]
30. Schweppe, R.E. Thyroid cancer cell lines: Critical models to study thyroid cancer biology and new therapeutic targets. *Front. Endocrinol.* **2012**, *3*, 81. [CrossRef]
31. Saiselet, M.; Floor, S.; Tarabichi, M.; Dom, G.; Hébrant, A.; van Staveren, W.G.C.; Maenhaut, C. Thyroid cancer cell lines: An overview. *Front. Endocrinol.* **2012**, *3*, 133. [CrossRef] [PubMed]
32. Greco, A.; Auletta, L.; Orlandella, F.M.; Iervolino, P.L.C.; Klain, M.; Salvatore, G.; Mancini, M. Preclinical imaging for the study of mouse models of thyroid cancer. *Int. J. Mol. Sci.* **2017**, *18*, 2731. [CrossRef] [PubMed]
33. Greco, A.; Albanese, S.; Auletta, L.; Mirabelli, P.; Zannetti, A.; D'Alterio, C.; Di Maro, G.; Orlandella, F.M.; Salvatore, G.; Soricelli, A.; et al. High-Frequency Ultrasound-Guided injection for the generation of a novel orthotopic mouse model of human thyroid carcinoma. *Thyroid* **2016**, *26*, 552–558. [CrossRef] [PubMed]
34. Kim, S.; Park, Y.W.; Schiff, B.A.; Doan, D.D.; Yazici, Y.; Jasser, S.A.; Younes, M.; Mandal, M.; Bekele, B.N.; Myers, J.N. An Orthotopic Model of Anaplastic Thyroid Carcinoma in Athymic Nude Mice. *Clin. Cancer Res.* **2005**, *11*, 1713–1721. [CrossRef] [PubMed]

35. Nucera, C.; Nehs, M.A.; Mekel, M.; Zhang, X.; Hodin, R.; Lawler, J.; Nose, V.; Parangi, S. A novel orthotopic mouse model of human anaplastic thyroid carcinoma. *Thyroid* **2009**, *19*, 1077–1084. [CrossRef] [PubMed]
36. Vargo-Gogola, T.; Rosen, J.M. Modelling breast cancer: One size does not fit all. *Nat. Rev. Cancer* **2007**, *7*, 659–672. [CrossRef]
37. Dewan, M.Z.; Terunuma, H.; Ahmed, S.; Ohba, K.; Takada, M.; Tanaka, Y.; Toi, M.; Yamamoto, N. Natural killer cells in breast cancer cell growth and metastasis in SCID mice. *Biomed. Pharm.* **2005**, *59*, s375–s379. [CrossRef]
38. Beckhove, P.; Schutz, F.; Diel, I.J.; Solomayer, E.F.; Bastert, G.; Foerster, J.; Feuerer, M.; Bai, L.; Sinn, H.P.; Umansky, V.; et al. Efficient engraftment of human primary breast cancer transplants in nonconditioned NOD/SCID mice. *Int. J. Cancer* **2003**, *105*, 444–453. [CrossRef]
39. Puchalapalli, M.; Zeng, X.; Mu, L.; Anderson, A.; Glickman, L.X.; Zhang, M.; Sayyad, M.R.; Mosticone Wangensteen, S.; Clevenger, C.V.; Koblinski, J.E. NSG mice provide a better spontaneous model of breast cancer metastasis than athymic (nude) mice. *PLoS ONE* **2016**, *11*, e0163521. [CrossRef]
40. Van Weerden, W.M.; Bangma, C.; de Wit, R. Human xenograft models as useful tools to assess the potential of novel therapeutics in prostate cancer. *Br. J. Cancer* **2009**, *100*, 13–18. [CrossRef]
41. Tuomela, J.; Härkönen, P. Tumor models for prostate cancer exemplified by fibroblast growth factor 8-induced tumorigenesis and tumor progression. *Reprod. Biol.* **2014**, *14*, 16–24. [CrossRef] [PubMed]
42. Bastide, C.; Bagnis, C.; Mannoni, P.; Hassoun, J.; Bladou, F. A Nod Scid mouse model to study human prostate cancer. *Prostate Cancer Prostatic Dis.* **2002**, *5*, 311–315. [CrossRef] [PubMed]
43. Koshida, K.; Konaka, H.; Imao, T.; Egawa, M.; Mizokami, A.; Namiki, M. Comparison of two in vivo models for prostate cancer: Orthotopic and intratesticular inoculation of LNCaP or PC-3 cells. *Int. J. Urol.* **2004**, *11*, 1114–1121. [CrossRef] [PubMed]
44. Jackstadt, R.; Sansom, O.J. Mouse models of intestinal cancer. *J. Pathol.* **2016**, *238*, 141–151. [CrossRef] [PubMed]
45. Thalheimer, A.; Illert, B.; Bueter, M.; Gattenlohner, S.; Stehle, D.; Gasser, M.; Thiede, A.; Waaga-Gasser, A.M.; Meyer, D. Feasibility and Limits of an Orthotopic Human Colon Cancer Model in Nude Mice. *Comp. Med.* **2006**, *56*, 105–109. [PubMed]
46. Donigan, M.; Norcross, L.S.; Aversa, J.; Colon, J.; Smith, J.; Madero-Visbal, R.; Li, S.; McCollum, N.; Ferrara, A.; Gallagher, J.T.; et al. Novel Murine Model for Colon Cancer: Non-Operative Trans-Anal Rectal Injection. *J. Surg. Res.* **2009**, *154*, 299–303. [CrossRef]
47. Tentler, J.J.; Tan, A.C.; Weekes, C.D.; Jimeno, A.; Leong, S.; Pitts, T.M.; Arcaroli, J.J.; Messersmith, W.A.; Eckhardt, S.G. Patient-derived tumour xenografts as models for oncology drug development. *Nat. Rev. Clin. Oncol.* **2012**, *9*, 338–350. [CrossRef]
48. Siolas, D.; Hannon, G.J. Patient-Derived Tumor Xenografts: Transforming clinical samples into mouse models. *Cancer Res.* **2013**, *73*, 5315–5319. [CrossRef]
49. Hidalgo, M.; Amant, F.; Biankin, A.V.; Budinská, E.; Byrne, A.T.; Caldas, C.; Clarke, R.B.; De Jong, S.; Jonkers, J.; Mælandsmo, G.M.; et al. Patient derived xenograft models: An emerging platform for translational cancer research. *Cancer Discov.* **2014**, *4*, 998–1013. [CrossRef]
50. Greco, A.; Albanese, S.; Auletta, L.; De Carlo, F.; Salvatore, M.; Howard, C.M.; Claudio, P.P. Advances in molecular preclinical therapy mediated by imaging. *Q. J. Nucl. Med. Mol. Imaging* **2017**, *61*, 76–94.
51. Vitale, G.; Gaudenzi, G.; Circelli, L.; Manzoni, M.F.; Bassi, A.; Fioritti, N.; Faggiano, A.; Colao, A. Animal models of medullary thyroid cancer: State of the art and view to the future. *Endocr. Relat. Cancer* **2017**, *24*, R1–R12. [CrossRef] [PubMed]
52. Zhang, X.; Claerhout, S.; Prat, A.; Dobrolecki, L.E.; Petrovic, I.; Lai, Q.; Landis, M.D.; Wiechmann, L.; Schiff, R.; Giuliano, M.; et al. A renewable tissue resource of phenotypically stable, biologically and ethnically diverse, patient-derived human breast cancer xenograft models. *Cancer Res.* **2013**, *73*, 4885–4897. [CrossRef] [PubMed]
53. Zhang, X.; Lewis, M.T. Establishment of Patient-Derived Xenograft (PDX) Models of human breast cancer. *Curr. Protoc. Mouse Biol.* **2013**, *3*, 21–29. [CrossRef] [PubMed]
54. Rea, D.; del Vecchio, V.; Palma, G.; Barbieri, A.; Falco, M.; Luciano, A.; De Biase, D.; Perdonà, S.; Facchini, G.; Arra, C. Mouse models in prostate cancer translational research: From xenograft to PDX. *BioMed Res. Int.* **2016**, *2016*, 9750795. [CrossRef]

55. Puig, I.; Chicote, I.; Tenbaum, S.P.; Arqués, O.; Herance, J.R.; Gispert, J.D.; Jimenez, J.; Landolfi, S.; Caci, K.; Allende, H.; et al. A personalized preclinical model to evaluate the metastatic potential of patient-derived colon cancer initiating cells. *Clin. Cancer Res.* **2013**, *19*, 6787–6801. [CrossRef]
56. Sook Seol, H.; Kang, H.; Lee, S.I.; Kim, N.E.; Kim, T.I.; Chun, S.M.; Kim, T.W.; Yu, C.S.; Suh, Y.A.; Singh, S.R.; et al. Development and characterization of a colon PDX model that reproduces drug responsiveness and the mutation profiles of its original tumor. *Cancer Lett.* **2014**, *345*, 56–64. [CrossRef]
57. Cook, N.; Jodrell, D.I.; Tuveson, D.A. Predictive in vivo animal models and translation to clinical trials. *Drug Discov. Today* **2012**, *17*, 253–260. [CrossRef]
58. Valeri, N.; Braconi, C.; Gasparini, P.; Murgia, C.; Lampis, A.; Paulus-Hock, V.; Hart, J.R.; Ueno, L.; Grivennikov, S.I.; Lovat, F.; et al. MicroRNA-135b Promotes cancer progression by acting as a downstream effector of oncogenic pathways in colon cancer. *Cancer Cell* **2014**, *24*, 469–483. [CrossRef]
59. Kim, J.B.; O'Hare, M.J.; Stein, R. Models of breast cancer: Is merging human and animal models the future? *Breast Cancer Res.* **2004**, *6*, 22–30. [CrossRef]
60. Simmons, J.K.; Hildreth, B.E.; Supsavhad, W.; Elshafae, S.M.; Hassan, B.B.; Dirksen, W.P.; Toribio, R.E.; Rosol, T.J. Animal Models of Bone Metastasis. *Vet. Pathol.* **2015**, *52*, 827–841. [CrossRef]
61. Grabowska, M.M.; DeGraff, D.J.; Yu, X.; Jin, R.J.; Chen, Z.; Borowsky, A.D.; Matusik, R.J. Mouse Models of Prostate Cancer: Picking the Best Model for the Question. *Cancer Metastasis Rev.* **2014**, *33*, 377–397. [CrossRef]
62. Taketo, M.M.; Edelmann, W. Mouse models of colon cancer. *Gastroenterology* **2009**, *136*, 780–798. [CrossRef] [PubMed]
63. Boltze, C.; Brabant, G.; Dralle, H.; Gerlach, R.; Roessner, A.; Hoang-Vu, C. radiation-induced thyroid carcinogenesis as a function of time and dietary iodine supply: An in vivo model of tumorigenesis in the rat. *Endocrinology* **2002**, *143*, 2584–2592. [CrossRef]
64. Rusinek, D.; Krajewska, J.; Jarząb, M. Mouse models of papillary thyroid carcinoma—Short review. *Endokrynol. Pol.* **2016**, *67*, 212–223. [CrossRef] [PubMed]
65. Rivina, L.; Davoren, M.J.; Schiestl, R.H. Mouse models for radiation-induced cancers. *Mutagenesis* **2016**, *31*, 491–509. [CrossRef] [PubMed]
66. Rosol, T.J.; Tannehill-Gregg, S.H.; LeRoy, B.E.; Mandl, S.; Contag, C.H. Animal models of bone metastasis. *Cancer Treat. Res.* **2004**, *118*, 47–81.
67. Heijstek, M.W.; Kranenburg, O.; Borel Rinkes, I.H.M. Mouse models of colorectal cancer and liver metastases. *Dig. Surg.* **2005**, *22*, 16–25. [CrossRef]
68. Khanna, C.; Hunter, K. Modeling metastasis in vivo. *Carcinogenesis* **2005**, *26*, 513–523. [CrossRef]
69. Hoffman, R.M. Orthotopic metastatic mouse models for anticancer drug discovery and evaluation: A bridge to the clinic. *Investig. New Drug* **1999**, *17*, 343–359. [CrossRef]
70. Zhang, L.; Gaskins, K.; Yu, Z.; Xiong, Y.; Merino, M.J.; Kebebew, E. An in vivo mouse model of metastatic human thyroid cancer. *Thyroid* **2014**, *24*, 695–704. [CrossRef]
71. Morrison, J.A.; Pike, L.A.; Lund, G.; Zhou, Q.; Kessler, B.E.; Bauerle, K.T.; Sams, S.B.; Haugen, B.R.; Schweppe, R.E. Characterization of thyroid cancer cell lines in murine orthotopic and intracardiac metastasis models. *Horm. Cancer* **2015**, *6*, 87–99. [CrossRef] [PubMed]
72. Iorns, E.; Drews-Elger, K.; Ward, T.M.; Dean, S.; Clarke, J.; Berry, D.; El Ashry, D.; Lippman, M. A new mouse model for the study of human breast cancer metastasis. *PLoS ONE* **2012**, *7*, e47995. [CrossRef] [PubMed]
73. Camorani, S.; Hill, B.S.; Fontanella, R.; Greco, A.; Gramanzini, M.; Auletta, L.; Gargiulo, S.; Albanese, S.; Lucarelli, E.; Cerchia, L.; et al. Inhibition of bone marrow-derived mesenchymal stem cells homing towards triple-negative breast cancer microenvironment using an anti-PDGFRβ aptamer. *Theranostics* **2017**, *7*, 3595–3607. [CrossRef] [PubMed]
74. Cui, J.H.; Krueger, U.; Henne-Bruns, D.; Kremer, B.; Kalthoff, H. Orthotopic transplantation model of human gastrointestinal cancer and detection of micrometastases. *World J. Gastroenterol.* **2001**, *7*, 381–386. [CrossRef]
75. Cespedes, M.V.; Espina, C.; Garcia-Cabezas, M.A.; Trias, M.; Boluda, A.; Gomez del Pulgar, M.T.; Sancho, F.J.; Nistal, M.; Lacal, J.C.; Mangues, R. Orthotopic microinjection of human colon cancer cells in nude mice induces tumor foci in all clinically relevant metastatic sites. *Am. J. Pathol.* **2007**, *3*, 1077–1085. [CrossRef]
76. Donigan, M.; Loh, B.D.; Norcross, L.S.; Li, S.; Williamson, P.R.; DeJesus, S. A metastatic colon cancer model using nonoperative transanal rectal injection. *Surg. Endosc.* **2010**, *24*, 642–647. [CrossRef]
77. Rajput, A.; Agarwal, E.; Leiphrakpam, P.; Brattain, M.G.; Chowdhury, S. Establishment and validation of an orthotopic metastatic mouse model of colorectal cancer. *ISRN Hepatol.* **2013**, *2013*, 206875. [CrossRef]

78. Young Oh, B.; Kyung Hong, H.; Lee, W.Y.; Cho, Y.B. Animal models of colorectal cancer with liver metastasis. *Cancer Lett.* **2017**, *387*, 114–120.
79. Wong, F.C.; Kim, E.E. A review of molecular imaging studies reaching the clinical stage. *Eur. J. Radiol.* **2009**, *70*, 205–211. [CrossRef]
80. Fruhwirth, G.O.; Kneilling, M.; de Vries, I.J.M.; Weigelin, B.; Srinivas, M.; Aarntzen, E.H.J.G. The potential of in vivo imaging for optimization of molecular and cellular anti-cancer immunotherapies. *Mol. Imaging Biol.* **2018**, *20*, 696–704. [CrossRef]
81. Badea, C.T.; Drangova, M.; Holdsworth, D.W.; Johnson, G.A. In vivo small animal imaging using micro-CT and digital subtraction angiography. *Phys. Med. Biol.* **2008**, *53*, R319–R350. [CrossRef] [PubMed]
82. Kagadis, G.C.; Loudos, G.; Katsanos, K.; Langer, S.G.; Nikiforidis, G.C. In vivo small animal imaging: Current status and future prospects. *Med. Phys.* **2010**, *37*, 6421–6442. [CrossRef] [PubMed]
83. Chen, Z.Y.; Wang, Y.X.; Lin, Y.; Zhang, J.S.; Yang, F.; Zhou, Q.L.; Liao, Y.Y. Advance of molecular imaging technology and targeted imaging agent in imaging and therapy. *BioMed Res. Int.* **2014**, *2014*, 819324. [CrossRef]
84. Gabrielson, K.; Maronpot, R.; Monette, S.; Mlynarczyk, C.; Ramot, Y.; Nyska, A.; Sysa-Shah, P. In vivo imaging with confirmation by histopathology for increased rigor and reproducibility in translational research: A review of examples, options, and resources. *ILAR J.* **2018**, *59*, 80–98. [CrossRef] [PubMed]
85. Lauber, D.T.; Fulop, A.; Kovacs, T.; Szigeti, K.; Mathe, D.; Szijarto', A. State of the art in vivo imaging techniques for laboratory animals. *Lab. Anim.* **2017**, *51*, 465–478. [CrossRef] [PubMed]
86. Van Es, S.C.; Venema, C.M.; Glaudemans, A.W.J.M.; Lub-de Hooge, M.N.; Elias, S.G.; Boellaard, R.; Hospers, G.A.P.; Schröder, C.P.; de Vries, E.G.E. Translation of new molecular imaging approaches to the clinical setting: Bridging the gap to implementation. *J. Nucl. Med.* **2016**, *57*, 96S–104S. [CrossRef] [PubMed]
87. Rowland, D.J.; Lewis, J.S.; Welch, M.J. Molecular Imaging: The application of small animal positron emission tomography. *J. Cell. Biochem.* **2002**, *39* (Suppl. 39), 110–115. [CrossRef]
88. Kiessling, F.; Fokong, S.; Koczera, P.; Lederle, W.; Lammers, T. Ultrasound microbubbles for molecular diagnosis, therapy, and theranostics. *J. Nucl. Med.* **2012**, *53*, 345–348. [CrossRef]
89. Loveless, M.E.; Li, X.; Huamani, J.; Lyshchik, A.; Dawant, B.; Hallahan, D.; Gore, J.C.; Yankeelov, T.E. A Method for Assessing the Microvasculature in a Murine Tumor Model Using Contrast-Enhanced Ultrasonography. *J. Ultrasound Med.* **2008**, *27*, 1699–1709. [CrossRef]
90. Palmowski, M.; Huppert, J.; Hauff, P.; Reinhardt, M.; Schreiner, K.; Socher, M.A.; Hallscheidt, P.; Kauffmann, G.W.; Semmler, W.; Kiessling, F. Vessel fractions in tumor xenografts depicted by flow- or contrast-sensitive three-dimensional high-frequency doppler ultrasound respond differently to antiangiogenic treatment. *Cancer Res.* **2008**, *68*, 7042–7049. [CrossRef]
91. Willmann, J.K.; Paulmurugan, R.; Chen, K.; Gheysens, O.; Rodriguez-Porcel, M.; Lutz, A.M.; Chen, I.Y.; Chen, X.; Gambhir, S.S. US imaging of tumor angiogenesis with microbubbles targeted to vascular endothelial growth factor receptor type 2 in mice. *Radiology* **2008**, *246*, 508–518. [CrossRef] [PubMed]
92. Zhao, L.; Zhan, Y.; Rutkowski, J.L.; Feuerstein, G.Z.; Wang, X. Correlation between 2- and 3-dimensional assessment of tumor volume and vascular density by ultrasonography in a transgenic mouse model of mammary carcinoma. *J. Ultrasound Med.* **2010**, *29*, 587–595. [CrossRef] [PubMed]
93. Hormuth, D.A.; Sorace, A.G.; Virostko, J.; Abramson, R.G.; Bhujwalla, Z.M.; Enriquez-Navas, P.; Gillies, R.; Hazle, J.D.; Mason, R.P.; Quarles, C.C.; et al. Translating preclinical MRI methods to clinical oncology. *J. Magn. Reson. Imaging* **2019**. [CrossRef] [PubMed]
94. Hildebrandt, I.J.; Su, H.; Weber, W.A. Anesthesia and other considerations for in vivo imaging of small animals. *ILAR J.* **2008**, *49*, 17–26. [CrossRef]
95. Brockmann, M.A.; Kemmling, A.; Groden, C. Current issues and perspectives in small rodent magnetic resonance imaging using clinical MRI scanners. *Methods* **2007**, *43*, 79–87. [CrossRef]
96. Pichler, B.J.; Wehrl, H.F.; Kolb, A.; Judenhofer, M.S. PET/MRI: The next generation of multi-modality imaging? *Semin. Nucl. Med.* **2008**, *38*, 199–208. [CrossRef]
97. Pichler, B.J.; Kolb, A.; Nagele, T.; Schlemmer, H.P. PET/MRI: Paving the way for the next generation of clinical multimodality imaging applications. *J. Nucl. Med.* **2010**, *51*, 333–336. [CrossRef]
98. Judenhofer, M.S.; Cherry, S.R. Applications for Preclinical PET/MRI. *Semin. Nucl. Med.* **2013**, *43*, 19–29. [CrossRef]

99. De Souza, R.; Spence, T.; Huang, H.; Allen, C. Preclinical imaging and translational animal models of cancer for accelerated clinical implementation of nanotechnologies and macromolecular agents. *J. Control. Release* **2015**, *219*, 313–330. [CrossRef]
100. Auletta, L.; Gramanzini, M.; Gargiulo, S.; Albanese, S.; Salvatore, M.; Greco, A. Advances in multimodal molecular imaging. *Q. J. Nucl. Med. Mol. Imaging* **2017**, *61*, 19–32.
101. Kauppinen, R.A.; Peet, A.C. Using magnetic resonance imaging and spectroscopy in cancer diagnostics and monitoring. Preclinical and clinical approaches. *Cancer Biol. Ther.* **2011**, *12*, 665–679. [CrossRef] [PubMed]
102. Felder, J.; Celik, A.A.; Choi, C.H.; Schwan, S.; Shah, N.J. 9.4 T small animal MRI using clinical components for direct translational studies. *Transl. Med.* **2017**, *15*, 264. [CrossRef] [PubMed]
103. Scherzinger, A.L.; Hendee, W.R. Basic principles of magnetic resonance imaging an update. *West J. Med.* **1985**, *143*, 782–792. [PubMed]
104. Moser, E.; Stadlbauer, A.; Windischberger, C.; Quick, H.H.; Ladd, M.E. Magnetic resonance imaging methodology. *Eur. J. Nucl. Med. Mol. Imaging* **2009**, *36*, S30–S41. [CrossRef]
105. Mills, A.F.; Sakai, O.; Anderson, S.W.; Jara, H. Principles of quantitative MR imaging with illustrated review of applicable modular pulse diagrams. *RadioGraphics* **2017**, *37*, 2083–2105. [CrossRef]
106. Chavhan, G.B.; Babyn, P.S.; Thomas, B.; Shroff, M.M.; Haacke, E.M. Principles, techniques, and applications of T2*- based MR imaging and its special applications. *RadioGraphics* **2009**, *29*, 1433–1449. [CrossRef]
107. Pautler, R.G. Mouse MRI: Concepts and applications in physiology. *Physiology* **2004**, *19*, 168–175. [CrossRef]
108. Meyer, H.J.; Schob, S.; Hohn, A.K.; Surov, A. MRI texture analysis reflects histopathology parameters in thyroid cancer—A first preliminary study. *Transl. Oncol.* **2017**, *10*, 911–916. [CrossRef]
109. Aliu, S.O.; Wilmes, L.J.; Moasser, M.M.; Hann, B.C.; Li, K.L.; Wang, D.; Hylton, N.M. MRI methods for evaluating the effects of tyrosine kinase inhibitor administration used to enhance chemotherapy efficiency in a breast tumor xenograft model. *J. Magn. Res. Imaging* **2009**, *29*, 1071–1079. [CrossRef]
110. Holli-Helenius, K.; Salminen, A.; Rinta-Kiikka, I.; Koskivuo, I.; Brück, N.; Boström, P.; Parkkola, R. MRI texture analysis in differentiating luminal A and luminal B breast cancer molecular subtypes—A feasibility study. *BMC Med. Imaging* **2017**, *17*, 69. [CrossRef]
111. Nastiuk, K.L.; Liu, H.; Hamamura, M.; Muftuler, L.T.; Nalcioglu, O.; Krolewski, J.J. In vivo MRI volumetric measurement of prostate regression and growth in mice. *BMC Urol.* **2007**, *7*, 12. [CrossRef]
112. Ullrich, R.T.; Jikeli, J.F.; Diedenhofen, M.; Böhm-Sturm, P.; Unruh, M.; Vollmar, S.; Hoehn, M. In-vivo visualization of tumor microvessel density and response to anti-angiogenic treatment by high resolution MRI in mice. *PLoS ONE* **2011**, *6*, e19592. [CrossRef]
113. Khalifa, F.; Soliman, A.; El-Baz, A.; El-Ghar, M.A.; El-Diasty, T.; Gimel'farb, G.; Ouseph, R.; Dwyer, A.C. Models and methods for analyzing DCE-MRI: A review. *Med. Phys.* **2014**, *41*, 124301. [CrossRef]
114. Fiordelisi, M.F.; Auletta, L.; Meomartino, L.; Basso, L.; Fatone, G.; Salvatore, M.; Mancini, M.; Greco, A. preclinical molecular imaging for precision medicine in breast cancer mouse models. *Contrast Media Mol. Imaging* **2019**, *2019*, 8946729. [CrossRef]
115. Pickles, M.D.; Lowry, M.; Manton, D.J.; Gibbs, P.; Turnbull, L.W. Role of dynamic contrast enhanced MRI in monitoring early response of locally advanced breast cancer to neoadjuvant chemotherapy. *Breast Cancer Res. Treat.* **2005**, *91*, 1–10. [CrossRef]
116. Ah-See, M.L.W.; Makris, A.; Taylor, N.J.; Harrison, M.; Richman, P.I.; Burcombe, R.J.; Stirling, J.J.; d'Arcy, J.A.; Collins, D.J.; Pittam, M.R.; et al. Early changes in functional dynamic magnetic resonance imaging predict for pathologic response to neoadjuvant chemotherapy in primary breast cancer. *Clin. Cancer Res.* **2008**, *14*, 6580–6589. [CrossRef]
117. Howe, F.A.; Mcphail, L.D.; Griffiths, J.R.; Mcintyre, D.J.O.; Robinson, S.P. Vessel size index magnetic resonance imaging to monitor the effect of antivascular treatment in a rodent tumor model. *Int. J. Radiat. Oncol. Biol. Phys.* **2008**, *71*, 1470–1476. [CrossRef]
118. Xu, J.; Li, K.; Smith, R.A.; Waterton, J.C.; Zhao, P.; Ding, Z.; Does, M.D.; Manning, H.C.; Gore, J.C. A comparative assessment of preclinical chemotherapeutic response of tumors using quantitative non-Gaussian diffusion MRI. *Magn. Reson. Imaging* **2017**, *37*, 195–202. [CrossRef]
119. Dassler, K.; Scholle, F.D.; Schütz, G. Dynamic Gadobutrol-Enhanced MRI predicts early response to antivascular but not to antiproliferation therapy in a mouse xenograft model. *Magn. Reson. Med.* **2014**, *71*, 826–1833. [CrossRef]

120. Rajendran, R.; Huang, W.; Tang, A.M.Y.; Liang, J.M.; Choo, S.; Reese, T.; Hentze, H.; van Boxtel, S.; Cliffe, A.; Rogers, K.; et al. Early detection of antiangiogenic treatment responses in a mouse xenograft tumor model using quantitative perfusion MRI. *Cancer Med.* **2014**, *3*, 47–60. [CrossRef]
121. Cho, H.J.; Ackerstaff, E.; Carlin, S.; Lupu, M.E.; Wang, Y.; Rizwan, A.; O'Donoghue, J.; Ling, C.C.; Humm, J.L.; Zanzonico, P.B.; et al. Noninvasive multimodality imaging of the tumor microenvironment: Registered dynamic magnetic resonance imaging and positron emission tomography studies of a preclinical tumor model of tumor hypoxia. *Neoplasia* **2009**, *11*, 247–259. [CrossRef]
122. Kang, H.; Hainline, A.; Arlinghaus, L.R.; Elderidge, S.; Li, X.; Abramson, V.G.; Chakravarthy, A.B.; Abramson, R.G.; Bingham, B.; Fakhoury, K.; et al. Combining multiparametric MRI with receptor information to optimize prediction of pathologic response to neoadjuvant therapy in breast cancer: Preliminary results. *J. Med. Imaging* **2018**, *5*, 011015. [CrossRef]
123. Røe, K.; Kakar, M.; Seierstad, T.; Ree, A.H.; Olsen, D.R. Early prediction of response to radiotherapy and androgen-deprivation therapy in prostate cancer by repeated functional MRI: A preclinical study. *Radiat. Oncol.* **2011**, *6*, 65. [CrossRef]
124. Golay, X.; Hendrikse, J.; Lim, T.C.C. Perfusion imaging using arterial spin labeling. *Top. Magn. Reson. Imaging* **2004**, *15*, 10–27. [CrossRef]
125. Rajendran, R.; Lewa, S.K.; Yonga, C.X.; Tana, J.; Wangb, D.J.J.; Chuanga, K.H. Quantitative mouse renal perfusion using arterial spin labeling. *NMR Biomed* **2013**, *26*, 1225–1232. [CrossRef]
126. Alsop, D.V.; Detre, J.A.; Golay, X.; Günther, M.; Hendrikse, J.; Hernandez-Garcia, L.; Lu, H.; MacIntosh, B.J.; Parkes, L.M.; Smits, M.; et al. Recommended implementation of arterial spin-labeled perfusion mri for clinical applications: A consensus of the ISMRM perfusion study group and the european consortium for ASL in dementia. *Magn. Reson. Med.* **2015**, *73*, 102–116. [CrossRef]
127. Johnson, S.P.; Ramasawmy, R.; Campbell-Washburn, A.E.; Wells, J.A.; Robson, M.; Rajkumar, V.; Lythgoe, M.F.; Pedley, R.B.; Walker-Samuel, S. Acute changes in liver tumour perfusion measured non-invasively with arterial spin labelling. *Br. J. Cancer* **2016**, *114*, 897–904. [CrossRef]
128. Buchbender, S.; Obenauer, S.; Mohrmann, S.; Martirosian, P.; Buchbender, C.; Miese, F.R.; Wittsack, H.J.; Miekley, M.; Antoch, G.; Lanzman, R.S. Arterial spin labelling perfusion MRI of breast cancer using FAIR TrueFISP: Initial results. *Clin. Radiol.* **2013**, *68*, e123–e127. [CrossRef]
129. Rakow-Penner, R.; Daniel, B.; Glover, G.H. Detecting blood oxygen level-dependent (bold) contrast in the breast. *J. Magn. Res. Imaging* **2010**, *32*, 120–129. [CrossRef]
130. Al-Hallaq, H.A.; Fan, X.; Zamora, M.; River, J.N.; Moulder, J.E.; Karczmar, G.S. Spectrally inhomogeneous BOLD contrast changes detected in rodent tumors with high spectral and spatial resolution MRI. *NMR Biomed.* **2002**, *15*, 28–36. [CrossRef]
131. O'Connor, J.P.B.; Naish, J.H.; Parker, G.J.M.; Waterton, J.C.; Watson, Y.; Jayson, G.C.; Buonaccorsi, G.A.; Cheung, S.; Buckley, D.L.; Mcgrath, D.M.; et al. Preliminary study of oxygen-enhanced longitudinal relaxation in MRI: A potential novel biomarker of oxygenation changes in solid tumors. *Int. J. Radiat. Oncol. Biol. Phys.* **2009**, *75*, 1209–1215. [CrossRef]
132. Linnik, I.V.; Scott, M.L.J.; Holliday, K.F.; Woodhouse, N.; Waterton, J.C.; O'Connor, J.P.B.; Barjat, H.; Liess, C.; Ulloa, J.; Young, H.; et al. Noninvasive tumor hypoxia measurement using magnetic resonance imaging in murine U87 glioma xenografts and in patients with glioblastoma. *Magn. Res. Med.* **2014**, *71*, 1854–1862. [CrossRef]
133. O'Connor, J.P.B.; Boult, J.K.R.; Jamin, Y.; Babur, M.; Finegan, K.G.; Williams, K.J.; Little, R.A.; Jackson, A.; Parker, G.J.M.; Reynolds, A.R.; et al. Oxygen-enhanced mri accurately identifies, quantifies, and maps tumor hypoxia in preclinical cancer models. *Cancer Res.* **2016**, *76*, 787–795. [CrossRef]
134. Jiang, L.; Weatherall, P.T.; McColl, R.W.; Tripathy, D.; Mason, R.P. Blood Oxygenation Level-Dependent (BOLD) contrast magnetic resonance imaging (MRI) for prediction of breast cancer chemotherapy response: A pilot study. *J. Magn. Res. Imaging* **2013**, *37*, 1083–1092. [CrossRef]
135. White, D.A.; Zhang, Z.; Li, L.; Gerberich, J.; Stojadinovic, S.; Peschke, P.; Mason, R.P. Developing Oxygen-Enhanced Magnetic Resonance Imaging as a Prognostic Biomarker of Radiation Response. *Cancer Lett.* **2016**, *380*, 69–77. [CrossRef]
136. Zhao, M.; Pipe, J.G.; Bonnett, J.; Evelhoch, J.L. Early detection of treatment response by diffusion weighted H-NMR spectroscopy in a murine tumour *in vivo*. *Br. J. Cancer* **1996**, *73*, 61–64. [CrossRef]

137. Koh, D.M.; Collins, D.J. Diffusion-Weighted MRI in the Body: Applications and Challenges in Oncology. *Am. J. Roentgenol.* **2007**, *188*, 1622–1635. [CrossRef]
138. Ross, B.D.; Moffat, B.A.; Lawrence, T.S.; Mukherji, S.K.; Gebarski, S.S.; Quint, D.J.; Johnson, T.D.; Junck, L.; Robertson, P.L.; Muraszko, K.M.; et al. Evaluation of cancer therapy using diffusion magnetic resonance imaging. *Mol. Cancer Ther.* **2003**, *2*, 581–587.
139. Curvo-Semedo, L.; Lambregts, D.M.J.; Maas, M.; Beets, G.L.; Caseiro-Alves, F.; Beets-Tan, R.G.H. Diffusion-Weighted MRI in rectal cancer: Apparent diffusion coefficient as a potential noninvasive marker of tumor aggressiveness. *J. Magn. Res. Imaging* **2012**, *35*, 1365–1371. [CrossRef]
140. Moffat, B.A.; Hall, D.E.; Stojanovska, J.; McConville, P.J.; Moody, J.B.; Chenevert, T.L.; Rehemtulla, A.; Ross, B.D. Diffusion imaging for evaluation of tumor therapies in preclinical animal models. *Magn. Reson. Mater. Phys. Biol. Med.* **2004**, *17*, 249–259. [CrossRef]
141. Padhani, A.R.; Liu, G.; Mu-Koh, D.; Chenevert, T.L.; Thoeny, H.C.; Takahara, T.; Dzik-Jurasz, A.; Ross, B.D.; Van Cauteren, M.; Collins, D.; et al. Diffusion-weighted magnetic resonance imaging as a cancer biomarker: Consensus and recommendations. *Neoplasia* **2009**, *11*, 102–125. [CrossRef]
142. Li, X.; Abramson, R.G.; Arlinghaus, L.R.; Kang, H.; Chakravarthy, A.B.; Abramson, V.G.; Farley, J.; Mayer, I.A.; Kelley, M.C.; Meszoely, I.M.; et al. Combined DCE-MRI and DW-MRI for Predicting Breast Cancer Pathological Response After the First Cycle of Neoadjuvant Chemotherapy. *Investig. Radiol.* **2015**, *50*, 195–204. [CrossRef]
143. Erdem, G.; Erdem, T.; Karakas, H.M.; Mutlu, D.; Fırat, A.K.; Sahin, I.; Alkan, A. Diffusion-Weighted Images differentiate benign from malignant thyroid nodules. *J. Magn. Res. Imaging* **2010**, *31*, 94–100. [CrossRef]
144. Schob, S.; Voigt, P.; Bure, L.; Meyer, H.J.; Wickenhauser, C.; Behrmann, C.; Höhn, A.; Kachel, P.; Dralle, H.; Hoffmann, K.T.; et al. Diffusion-Weighted Imaging Using a Readout-Segmented, Multishot EPI Sequence at 3 T Distinguishes between Morphologically Differentiated and Undifferentiated Subtypes of Thyroid Carcinoma—A Preliminary Study. *Transl. Oncol.* **2016**, *9*, 403–410. [CrossRef]
145. Aydın, H.; Kızılgöz, V.; Tatar, I.; Damar, C.; Güzel, H.; Hekimoğlu, B.; Delibaşı, T. The role of proton MR spectroscopy and apparent diffusion coefficient values in the diagnosis of malignant thyroid nodules: Preliminary results. *Clin. Imaging* **2012**, *36*, 323–333. [CrossRef]
146. Zhai, G.; Kim, H.; Sarver, D.; Samuel, S.; Whitworth, L.; Umphrey, H.; Oelschlager, D.K.; Beasley, T.M.; Zinn, K.R. Early therapy assessment of combined anti-DR5 Antibody and Carboplatin in triple-negative breast cancer xenografts in mice using diffusion- weighted imaging and 1H MR Spectroscopy. *J. Magn. Res. Imaging* **2014**, *39*, 1588–1594. [CrossRef]
147. Simões, R.V.; Martinez-Aranda, A.; Martín, B.; Cerdán, S.; Sierra, A.; Arús, C. Preliminary characterization of an experimental breast cancer cells brain metastasis mouse model by MRI/MRS. *Magn. Reson. Mater. Phys.* **2008**, *21*, 237–249. [CrossRef]
148. Jennings, D.; Hatton, B.N.; Guo, J.; Galons, J.P.; Trouard, T.P.; Raghunand, N.; Marshall, J.; Gillies, R.G. Early response of prostate carcinoma xenografts to docetaxel chemotherapy monitored with diffusion MRI. *Neoplasia* **2002**, *4*, 255–262. [CrossRef]
149. Penet, M.F.; Pathak, A.P.; Raman, V.; Ballesteros, P.; Artemov, D.; Bhujwalla, Z.M. Noninvasive multiparametric imaging of metastasis-permissive microenvironments in a human prostate cancer xenograft. *Cancer Res.* **2009**, *69*, 8822–8829. [CrossRef]
150. Shi, R.Y.; Yao, Q.Y.; Zhou, Q.Y.; Lu, Q.; Suo, S.T.; Chen, J.; Zheng, W.J.; Dai, Y.M.; Wu, L.M.; Xu, J.R. Preliminary study of diffusion kurtosis imaging in thyroid nodules and its histopathologic correlation. *Eur. Radiol.* **2017**, *27*, 4710–4720. [CrossRef]
151. McPhail, L.D.; Chung, Y.L.; Madhu, B.; Clark, S.; Griffiths, J.R.; Kelland, L.R.; Robinson, S.P. Tumor dose response to the vascular disrupting agent, 5,6-dimethylxanthenone-4-acetic acid, using in vivo magnetic resonance spectroscopy. *Clin. Cancer Res.* **2005**, *11*, 3705–3713. [CrossRef]
152. Chung, Y.L.; Troy, H.; Banerji, U.; Jackson, L.E.; Walton, M.I.; Stubbs, M.; Griffiths, J.R.; Judson, I.R.; Leach, M.O.; Workman, P.; et al. Magnetic resonance spectroscopic pharmacodynamic markers of the heat shock protein 90 inhibitor 17-allylamino,17-demethoxygeldanamycin (17AAG) in human colon cancer models. *J. Natl. Cancer Inst.* **2003**, *95*, 1624–1633. [CrossRef]
153. Jensen, L.R.; Huuse, E.M.; Bathena, T.F.; Goab, P.E.; Bofin, A.M.; Pedersen, T.B.; Lundgren, S.; Gribbestad, I.S. Assessment of early docetaxel response in an experimental model of human breast cancer using DCE-MRI, ex vivo HR MAS, and in vivo 1H MRS. *NMR Biomed.* **2010**, *23*, 56–65. [CrossRef]

154. Castagnoli, L.; Iorio, E.; Dugo, M.; Koschorke, A.; Faraci, S.; Canese, R.; Casalini, P.; Nanni, P.; Vernieri, C.; Di Nicola, M.; et al. Intratumor lactate levels reflect HER2 addiction status in HER2-positive breast cancer. *J. Cell Physiol.* **2019**, *234*, 1768–1779. [CrossRef]
155. Esmaeili, M.; Bathen, T.F.; Engebraten, O.; Mælandsmo, G.M.; Gribbestad, I.S.; Moestue, S.A. Quantitative 31P HR-MAS MR spectroscopy for detection of response to PI3K/mTOR inhibition in breast cancer xenografts. *Magn. Res. Med.* **2014**, *71*, 1973–1981. [CrossRef]
156. Meisamy, S.; Bolan, P.J.; Baker, E.H.; Bliss, R.L.; Gulbahce, E.; Everson, L.I.; Nelson, M.T.; Emory, T.H.; Tuttle, T.M.; Yee, D.; et al. Neoadjuvant chemotherapy of locally advanced breast cancer: Predicting response with in vivo 1H MR Spectroscopy—A pilot study at 4 T. *Radiology* **2004**, *233*, 424–431. [CrossRef]
157. Ward, K.M.; Aletras, A.H.; Balaban, R.S. A new class of contrast agents for mri based on proton chemical exchange dependent saturation transfer (CEST). *J. Magn. Res.* **2000**, *143*, 79–87. [CrossRef]
158. Rivlin, M.; Horev, J.; Tsarfaty, I.; Navon, G. Molecular imaging of tumors and metastases using chemical exchange saturation transfer (CEST) MRI. *Sci. Rep.* **2013**, *3*, 3045. [CrossRef]
159. Vinogradov, E.; Sherry, A.D.; Lenkinski, R.E. CEST: From basic principles to applications, challenges and opportunities. *J. Magn. Res.* **2013**, *229*, 155–172. [CrossRef]
160. Jones, K.M.; Pollard, A.C.; Pagel, M.K. Clinical applications of chemical exchange saturation transfer (CEST) MRI. *J. Magn. Reson. Imaging* **2018**, *47*, 11–27. [CrossRef]
161. Rivlin, M.; Navon, G. CEST MRI of 3-o-methyl-d-glucose on different breast cancer models. *Magn. Res. Med.* **2018**, *79*, 1061–1069. [CrossRef]
162. Liu, G.; Li, Y.; Sheth, V.R.; Pagel, M.D. Imaging in vivo extracellular ph with a single paramagnetic chemical exchange saturation transfer magnetic resonance imaging contrast agent. *Mol. Imaging* **2012**, *11*, 47–57. [CrossRef]
163. Longo, D.L.; Bartoli, A.; Consolino, L.; Bardini, P.; Arena, F.; Schwaiger, M.; Aime, S. In Vivo Imaging of Tumor Metabolism and Acidosis by Combining PET and MRI-CEST pH Imaging. *Cancer Res.* **2016**, *76*, 6463–6470. [CrossRef]
164. Jia, G.; Abaza, R.; Williams, J.D.; Zynger, D.L.; Zhou, J.; Shah, Z.K.; Patel, M.; Sammet, S.; Wei, L.; Bahnson, R.R.; et al. Amide Proton Transfer MR Imaging of prostate cancer: A preliminary study. *J. Magn. Res. Imaging* **2011**, *33*, 647–654. [CrossRef]
165. Walker, R.; Kessar, P.; Blanchard, R.; Dimasi, M.; Harper, K.; DeCarvalho, V.; Yucel, E.K.; Patriquin, L.; Eustace, S. Turbo STIR magnetic resonance imaging as a whole-body screening tool for metastases in patients with breast carcinoma: Preliminary clinical experience. *J. Magn. Res. Imaging* **2000**, *11*, 343–350. [CrossRef]

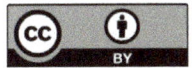

© 2019 by the authors. Licensee MDPI, Basel, Switzerland. This article is an open access article distributed under the terms and conditions of the Creative Commons Attribution (CC BY) license (http://creativecommons.org/licenses/by/4.0/).

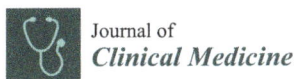

Review

Radiolabeled PET/MRI Nanoparticles for Tumor Imaging

Ernesto Forte [1,†], Dario Fiorenza [1,†], Enza Torino [2,3,4,*], Angela Costagliola di Polidoro [2,3], Carlo Cavaliere [1], Paolo A. Netti [2,3,4], Marco Salvatore [1] and Marco Aiello [1]

1. IRCCS SDN, Via Gianturco 113, 80143 Naples, Italy; eforte@sdn-napoli.it (E.F.); dfiorenza@sdn-napoli.it (D.F.); ccavaliere@sdn-napoli.it (C.C.); direzionescientifica@sdn-napoli.it (M.S.); maiello@sdn-napoli.it (M.A.)
2. Department of Chemical Engineering, Materials and Industrial Production, University of Naples Federico II, P.le Tecchio 80, 80125 Naples, Italy; an.costaglio@gmail.com (A.C.d.P.); nettipa@unina.it (P.A.N.)
3. Istituto Italiano di Tecnologia, IIT—Center for Advanced Biomaterials for Health Care, CABHC@CRIB, Largo Barsanti e Matteucci, 80125 Naples, Italy
4. Interdisciplinary Research Center on Biomaterials, CRIB, University of Naples Federico II, P.le Tecchio 80, 80125 Naples, Italy
* Correspondence: enza.torino@unina.it
† Both authors equally contributed to this manuscript.

Received: 19 November 2019; Accepted: 24 December 2019; Published: 29 December 2019

Abstract: The development of integrated positron emission tomography (PET)/magnetic resonance imaging (MRI) scanners opened a new scenario for cancer diagnosis, treatment, and follow-up. Multimodal imaging combines functional and morphological information from different modalities, which, singularly, cannot provide a comprehensive pathophysiological overview. Molecular imaging exploits multimodal imaging in order to obtain information at a biological and cellular level; in this way, it is possible to track biological pathways and discover many typical tumoral features. In this context, nanoparticle-based contrast agents (CAs) can improve probe biocompatibility and biodistribution, prolonging blood half-life to achieve specific target accumulation and non-toxicity. In addition, CAs can be simultaneously delivered with drugs or, in general, therapeutic agents gathering a dual diagnostic and therapeutic effect in order to perform cancer diagnosis and treatment simultaneous. The way for personalized medicine is not so far. Herein, we report principles, characteristics, applications, and concerns of nanoparticle (NP)-based PET/MRI CAs.

Keywords: multimodal imaging; hybrid imaging; positron emission tomography/magnetic resonance imaging (PET/MRI), nanotechnology; nanoparticles; in vivo imaging; 3D reconstruction

1. Introduction

The growing technological development improved diagnostic imaging techniques allowing early disease detection and diagnosis [1–4]. Even if different imaging modalities are extensively used in clinical practice such as magnetic resonance imaging (MRI), computed tomography (CT), positron emission tomography (PET), single-photon emission tomography (SPECT), each one presents strong points and limits. Nuclear medicine imaging techniques (PET and SPECT) are highly sensitive (pM range) and quantitative but suffer from poor resolution (mm range) [5,6]; CT is widely available and can detect several pathologies through rapid examinations and easy three-dimensional (3D) reconstructions but radiation dose to the patient is a noticeable concern and it is limited in soft-tissue resolution [7]; MRI gives high resolution, anatomical information, and good soft-tissue contrast but has low sensitivity (mM) [8–10]. Table 2 summarizes imaging modalities and related features. Since no single imaging modality allows gathering all the necessary morphological and functional information, the combination of two or more imaging techniques, also called *multimodal imaging* or *hybrid imaging*, can offer synergistic advantages over any modality alone [11], overcoming its drawbacks and strengthening the peculiarities. The traditional approach was directed to the integration of a structural imaging modality (CT, MRI) with a functional highly sensitive imaging modality (PET/SPECT). Thus, firstly, PET/CT and SPECT/CT were introduced in clinical settings. The first PET/CT scanner was developed in 1998 by Townsend and colleagues [12] and was commercialized in 2001. It consists of a PET component independent from CT, and a single bed moves axially into the scanner while the patient sequentially performs CT and PET scans [13]. To date, PET/CT scanners completely replaced standalone PET scanners [14], exploiting anatomical reference and attenuation estimation from CT data. The success of PET/CT scanners inspired the feasibility of a PET/MRI scanner [15]. Three different configuration options were developed over the years [16]: the first consists of a sequential acquisition, similarly to PET/CT, where the patient undergoes firstly a MRI scan and later a PET scan; even if the MRI and PET components must be minimally modified, two consecutive acquisitions are performed without simultaneity. Temporal mismatches between PET metabolic data and MRI morphological information such as patient motion are the main weak points [7]. Nearly 15 years ago, some researchers working in preclinical settings analyzed the possibility of integrating a modified PET scanner into an MRI system. In Tubingen, Germany, an MRI-compatible PET scanner was inserted into a 3T clinical MRI scanner [8]; this system is suitable for preclinical studies or human brain imaging. The third option considers a first fully integrated whole-body PET/MRI system, with MRI-compatible photodiodes (avalanche photodiodes) and MR-based attenuation correction, and it became commercially available in 2010. It is worth noting that, in addition to anatomical information, MRI also provides functional information such as diffusion-weighted imaging (DWI), blood level oxygen-dependent (BOLD) imaging in functional MRI (fMRI), T_1/T_2 mapping, perfusion imaging and spectroscopy, and dynamic contrast-enhanced (DCE) imaging. PET and MRI can take reciprocal advantages: MRI anatomical data are useful for correction of the partial volume effect caused by PET [17], enable motion correction, improve arterial input function characterization for PET kinetic modeling, and are used as priors in PET iterative reconstruction; on the other hand, PET provides molecular information and highly sensitive quantification [18]. Furthermore, the simultaneous acquisition of fMRI data and metabolic PET information can investigate the coupling between metabolic demand and functional activity of the brain, since oxygen and glucose metabolism are strongly related to cerebral blood flow that delivers O_2 and glucose to tissues [19]. High resolution and high tissue contrast, as well as multiparametric, functional, and quantitative imaging, supply complementary information for breast, head and neck [20], liver, musculoskeletal, and brain tumors [21] and heart [22] imaging. Hybrid imaging spread goes hand in hand with molecular imaging development, where molecular imaging stands for "in vivo" visualization, characterization, and measurement of biological processes at the molecular and cellular levels [23,24]. So far, various molecular imaging modalities were exploited not only for disease diagnosis, stratification, and treatment assessment [25] but also for image-guided therapy. Molecular imaging involves administration of imaging probes and detection of signals produced from the probes [26] and plays a key role in understanding important pathophysiological principles of diseases. In this context, personalized medicine aims to identify the adequate treatment and control its therapeutic efficacy. Suitable imaging probes are currently being developed and represent an exciting challenge for chemists and imaging scientists [27]. In this review, we focus on nanoparticle (NP)-based PET/MRI multimodal tracers in oncological imaging. A few of them were broadly tested in preclinical studies and show promising results in tumor detection, staging, and grading.

1.1. MRI Contrast Agents

In imaging, the term "contrast" refers to the capability of distinguishing between two adjacent structures; a contrast agent (CA) increases image contrast and highlights organs or blood vessels. The most common CAs used in X-ray or CT are iodinated and produce a direct effect on the image since they attenuate the X-ray beam, thereby increasing the signal intensity [20]; MRI CAs produce an indirect effect as they influence the relaxation times T_1 and T_2 of the neighboring water molecules. MRI CAs can act by reducing T_1 or T_2: the former are called T_1-weighted CAs since they reduce the T_1 relaxation time and brighten the resulting image, the latter are called T_2-weighted CAs since they reduce T_2 relaxation time and darken the resulting image [21]. T_1-weighted CAs are paramagnetic lanthanide compounds like gadolinium (Gd^{3+}) and manganese (Mn^{2+}) chelates, while T_2-weighted CAs are superparamagnetic agents like iron-oxide NPs [22]. CAs acting on both T_1 and T_2 relaxation times are called "dual mode" and are NP-based. MRI CAs available for the clinical practice are reported in Table 1.

The first requirement for a very efficient CA is a high relaxivity; this parameter indicates the efficiency in reducing T_1 or T_2 relaxation time of the surrounding water protons. Paramagnetic metal ions like Gd^{3+} cannot be used as CAs in their ionic form since their accumulation in specific tissues, for example, kidneys, liver, spleen, bone marrow, and the lymphatic system [28], causes toxicity. This challenge can be addressed by using chelators which hide the Gd ion through coordination bonds and are less likely to release it, conferring thermodynamic and kinetic stability and, therefore, less likely to induce toxicity. In particular, CAs based on Gd chelates are strongly associated with nephrogenic systemic fibrosis (NSF) in patients with renal impairment; the disease observed seems to be due to Gd release by chelating molecules in renal compartments [24]. In addition, recently, they were demonstrated to also accumulate in brain and kidneys in healthy patients [29,30].

Table 1. Magnetic resonance imaging contrast agents.

Brand Name	Active Substance	Chemical Name	Molecular Structure	Company	Current Status
Omniscan	Gadodiamide	Gd-DTPA-BMA	Linear, non-ionic	GE Healthcare	Suspended
OptiMARK	Gadoversetamide	Gd-DTPA-BMEA	Linear, non-ionic	Mallinckrodt	Suspended
Magnevist	Gadopentetic acid	Gd-DTPA	Linear, ionic	Bayer	Suspended
MultiHance	Gadobenic acid	Gd-BOPTA	Linear, ionic	Bracco	Only for liver scans
Primovist	Gadoxetic acid	Gd-EOB-DTPA	Linear, ionic	Bayer	In use
ProHance	Gadoteridol	Gd-HP-DO3A	Cyclic, non-ionic	Bracco	In use
Gadovist	Gadobutrol	Gd-BT-Do3A	Cyclic, non-ionic	Bayer	In use
Dotarem	Gadoteric acid	Gd-DOTA	Cyclic, ionic	Guerbet	In use

To improve diagnostic efficacy and reduce the nephrotoxic effects, an ideal CA should be stable, biocompatible, not toxic, and specific; it should remain within the system for a sufficient time to produce desired effects, such as tumor accumulation for oncological imaging, but should also be excreted from the body to minimize unwanted effects of foreign materials within body. In addition, higher relaxivity suggests a lower CA dose in patients. Most CAs currently used (typically small Gd^{3+} ion chelates) lack in specificity because they are confined in the vascular space and do not accumulate in a specific tissue. It is not a coincidence that, in the last decade, CAs were refined by optimizing the relaxivity and developing amplification strategies aimed at increasing probe accumulation at the target site [25]. Moreover, the recent development of molecular and cellular imaging led to the recognition of NPs as MRI CAs.

Table 2. Molecular imaging modalities.

Imaging Technique	Source of Imaging	Spatial Resolution	Tissue Penetration Depth	Sensitivity	Agent	Ref.
Magnetic resonance imaging (MRI)	Radio wave	25–100 µm	No limit	mM to µM (low)	Para-(Gd^{3+}) or superparamagnetic (Fe_3O_4) materials	[31]
Single-photon emission computed tomography (SPECT)	γ-ray	6–7 mm	No limit	pM (high)	Radionuclides ($^{99m}Tc, ^{201}Tl, ^{111}In, ^{131}I, ^{123}I, ^{67}Ga$)	[32]
Positron emission tomography (PET)	γ-ray	1–2 mm	No limit	pM (high)	Radionuclides ($^{18}F, ^{11}C, ^{13}N, ^{15}O, ^{124}I, ^{64}Cu, ^{68}Ga$)	[33]
Computed tomography (CT)	X-ray	50–200 µm	No limit	n.c.	High-atomic-number atoms (iodine, barium sulfate)	[34]
Ultrasonography (US)	Ultrasounds	50–500 µm	mm to cm	n.c.	Microbubbles	[35]
Optical fluorescence imaging	Visible or near-infrared light	In vivo 2–3 mm in vitro µm	<1 cm	nM to pM (medium)	Fluorescent dyes, quantum dots	[36,37]

n.c., not well characterized.

1.2. Nanoparticles

In its first applications, hybrid PET/MRI was realized through the simultaneous administration of a mixture of MRI and PET probes, resulting in a cocktail of imaging agents causing high risk for the patient [38]. Additionally, this mixture could not guarantee an exact spatial and temporal correlation of the two imaging modalities due to the different biodistribution, pharmacodynamic and pharmacokinetic properties of the imaging agent. To overcome these limitations, nanoparticles (NPs) were proposed as delivery systems for different imaging agents to obtain bimodal probes for the simultaneous monitoring of both modalities. NPs are defined as particles with at least one dimension lying between 1 and 100 nm [39,40]. In recent years, very different NPs such as proteins, polymers, dendrimers, micelles, liposomes, viral capsids, metal oxides (iron-oxide NPs), zeolites, and mesoporous silicas were investigated, and very different shapes, such as spheres, cylinders (nanorods), and tubes were explored [24].

An NP-based PET/MRI bimodal probe constitutes three essential components: a carrier, a PET tracer usually represented by a positron emitter radioisotope characterized by high sensitivity (e.g., ^{18}F-fluorodeoxyglucose), and an MRI component (e.g., gadopentetic acid (Gd-DTPA)), providing high tissue contrast and resolution. The MRI component can either work as a carrier itself (iron-oxide or gadolinium-oxide NPs) or can be a moiety bound to or entrapped in the carrier (e.g., Gd ions grafted onto NPs and polymeric matrices or biologically derived nanosized systems like apoferritin cages [41] and low-density lipoprotein (LDL) particles [42], respectively). Some possible configurations are reported in Figure 1.

As carriers, NPs offer a number of different design options, and the tailoring of their properties can be exploited to directly impact the in vivo fate of the resulting probe. Particle size, charge, core and surface properties, shape, and multivalency are the main features to be finely tuned in order to achieve a proper in vivo distribution, confer a targeting ability, and reduce toxicity of the NPs [43]. The hydrodynamic size determines the NP fate in the body, since vectors with a mean diameter smaller than 5 nm are usually eliminated by renal excretion, whereas larger particles (100 nm) are easily taken up by macrophages [44,45]. NP shape influences the internalization into cells that is relevant in cell tracking and labeling; for example, rod-like particles present higher internalization rates compared to spherical particles [46]. This phenomenon can be explained considering its similarity to rod-like bacterium internalization in nonphagocytic cells [47].

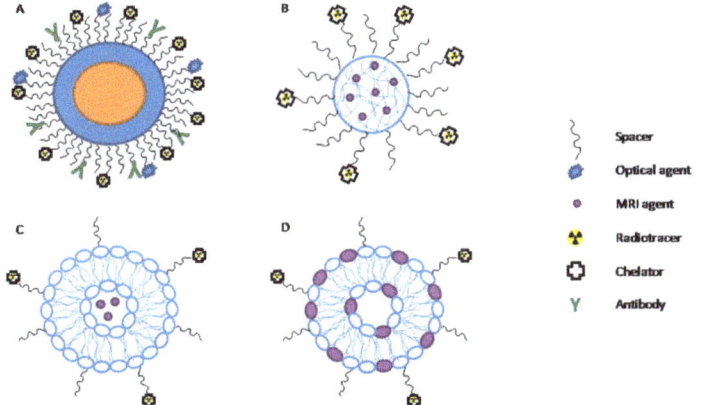

Figure 1. Multimodal nanoparticles. (**A**) Multimodal nanoparticle composed by a core (representing the magnetic resonance imaging (MRI) component) and a shell functionalized with an antibody. The positron emission tomography (PET) radiotracer is chelated and bound to the spacer. (**B**) A polymeric nanoparticle entrapping paramagnetic moieties is represented, where the PET radiotracer is chelated and bound to the spacer. (**C**) Liposomal formulation entraps paramagnetic moieties in the aqueous inner core, while the PET component is covalently linked to the spacer. (**D**) Liposomal formulation with paramagnetic ion inserted in the bilayer.

After NP injection into the bloodstream, they are rapidly coated by plasma proteins in a process called opsonization. The NPs are then recognized by plasma membrane receptors found on monocytes and macrophages and are, thus, taken up by the body's main defense system, the reticuloendothelial system (RES), also known as the mononuclear phagocyte system (MPS). The liver, spleen, and bone marrow are rich in macrophages, thus becoming the most accessible organs to NPs [48]. For these reasons, NPs should be coated by adequate materials, to avoid nonspecific uptake by the RES [48–50] (stealth effect). In general, hydrophilic and neutral surfaces do not tend to interact with blood components (serum proteins); therefore, they are optimal for minimizing opsonization and clearance [51,52]. Since neutral polymers have no functional groups (amine, carboxyl, or hydroxyl) for ligand linkage, a further step of functional group activation is often mandatory. Another coating strategy employs hydrophilic bifunctional materials such as biphosphonate [53] or aluminum hydroxide [54]. NPs with biocompatible coating layers such as polymers (polyethylene glycol (PEG)), dendrimers, polysaccharides (dextran and chitosan), and polypeptides (serum albumin) can have enhanced properties including better stability in terms of agglomeration, biocompatibility, and solubility in water, along with low toxicity. The most used coating polymers are dextran, chitosan and, above all, PEG [41]. PEG is a hydrophilic, water-soluble, biocompatible polymer widely used to reduce opsonization and increase circulation time from seconds or minutes up to hours [55]. It is important to notice that surface modifications may have an impact on the superparamagnetic properties of iron-oxide NPs; for this reason, coating materials must be carefully chosen [56]. In particular, the nature and the thickness of the coating affect relaxivity. A more hydrophilic coating material results in more water molecules being retained for interacting with the magnetic centers; on the other hand, a thicker coating results in more protons being shielded from the magnetic field [57].

NP delivery to malignant cells can be achieved through both passive and active targeting. Passive targeting is due to the enhanced permeability and retention effect (EPR); since tumor vessels have larger fenestrations, the vascular permeability is higher, and NPs can easily extravasate in tumor tissue. Moreover, the inefficient lymphatic drainage contributes to NP retention in the tumor interstitial space [58]. Even though non-targeted NPs can accumulate in the tumor region due to the EPR effect, the lack of efficient lymphatic drainage generates an increase in interstitial pressure and, consequently, a drop in pressure gradient between the vessel and the extracellular space, causing nanoparticle stacking around the vessel wall [44,59]. For these reasons, there is a need for the development of NPs capable of efficiently and specifically targeting tumor cells [27]. The high NP surface-to-volume ratio helps to overcome this limitation since the NP surface can be functionalized through target-specific moieties that allow an active targeting of cancer cells.

Finally, multivalence refers to the ability to bind different imaging probes, targeting ligands, and therapeutic formulations. This feature is very important for multimodal and molecular imaging where a significant number of targeting probes are needed to track a specific biological path.

1.3. Radiolabeled Nanoparticles

Tracers currently used in clinical practice are labeled using positron emitters with a relatively low half-life time ranging from 2.037 to 109.8 min. Most of the radionuclides used for labeling are produced via a cyclotron. It generates a beam of accelerated protons and deuterons that are used to irradiate a target (e.g., $^{14}N_2$ gas, ^{20}Ne gas, ^{18}O water or gas), thereby giving the desired radioisotope through a nuclear reaction. Table 3 shows the main radionuclides with related half-life time, the average energy of positron (β^+), and means of production.

Table 3. Principal radionuclides and related features.

Radionuclide	Half-Life Time *	Electronic Emission Energy β+	Production
^{11}C	20.385 min	386 keV	Cyclotron
^{13}N	9.965 min	492 keV	Cyclotron
^{15}O	122.24 s	735 keV	Cyclotron
^{18}F	109.77 min	250 keV	Cyclotron
^{64}Cu	12.701 h	655 keV	Cyclotron or reactor
^{68}Ga	67.629 min	836 and 353 keV **	Generator

* The values were obtained from the database of the National Nuclear Data Center (NNDC) at Brookhaven National Laboratory, Upton NY, USA. ** Mean energy of the β spectrum.

In PET clinical applications, ^{18}F is one of the most suitable radionuclides for radiotracer synthesis since 97% of isotope decay is via positron emission [60], with a fairly low energy of positron emission (maximum 0.635 MeV) and an optimal half-life of 109.8 min, which is considered acceptable for chemical syntheses and favorable when investigating biological processes with a time frame longer than 100 min [61]. ^{18}F-based radiotracers are essentially synthesized through two reactions: nucleophilic substitution or electrophilic substitution. Frequently, ^{18}F is introduced to replace hydrogen in biomolecules. However, in terms of size, the van der Waals radius of ^{18}F (1.47 Å) is closer to oxygen (1.52 Å) than that of hydrogen (1.20 Å) [62]; thus, ^{18}F is generally obtained starting from water enriched with ^{18}O through a nuclear reaction like $^{18}O(p, n)^{18}F$.

PET radiotracers for cancer diagnosis can be grouped based on their target mechanism as follows:

- Radiotracers for the evaluation of glucose metabolism, such as fluorodeoxyglucose (FDG);
- Radiotracers for cell proliferation, such as ^{18}F-fluorothymidine (FLT);
- Radiotracers for the evaluation of vascular perfusion, which include ^{15}O-water and ^{13}N-ammonia;
- Radiotracers for the evaluation of hypoxia, such as ^{18}F-fluoromisonidazole (FMISO).

Other widely used radionuclides are ^{68}Ga and ^{64}Cu. In particular, ^{64}Cu is gaining increasing interest for its theranostic potential [63]; during its decay, it emits both positron and Auger electrons allowing for both PET imaging and internal targeted radiation therapy. Indeed, Auger-emitting radionuclides that localize in the nucleus of tumor cells demonstrate a potential for cancer therapy. However, their biological effect is critically dependent on their sub-cellular (and sub-nuclear) localization [64] and on the DNA topology [65].

The chemical structures of the most common radiotracers are reported in Figure 2.

NP radiolabeling with the abovementioned tracers can be achieved through different techniques. In the literature, the four following main strategies are reported [66]:

1. Complexation reactions of metallic radioisotope ions through coordination chemistry with the use of chelators;
2. Direct NP bombardment;
3. NP synthesis from radioactive and non-radioactive precursors;
4. Post-synthesis NP radiolabeling without the use of chelators.

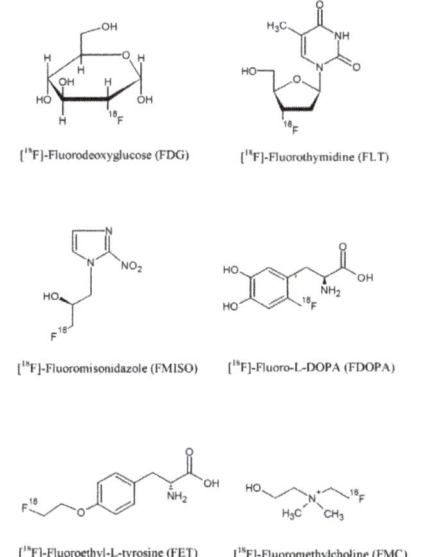

Figure 2. Chemical structure of fluorine-based radiopharmaceuticals.

The coordination chemistry approach is the most used since radioisotopes can be chelated by different molecules that are covalently bound directly to the NP surface. A strong linkage between the chelator coordinating the radioisotope and the NP surface is desired to assure the stability of the radiolabeling. It is worth noting that many exogenous chelators can currently only coordinate with certain radioisotopes, meaning that an effective chelator-based radiolabeling requires the selection of the best chelator for the isotope of interest [67]. In addition, the choice of the chelating agent should be such to minimize in vivo transchelation.

New chelators for metallic radioisotopes were recently synthesized, including tetradentate acyclic chelators such as PTMS, esadentate acyclic chelators such as ethylenediaminetetraacetic acid EDTA or DTPA, and macrocyclic chelators such as 1,4,7-triazacyclononane-N,N',N"-triacetic acid (NOTA) and 1,4,7,10-Tetraazacyclododecane-1,4,7,10-tetraacetic acid DOTA [68], whose chemical structures are presented in Figure 3.

Recently, Laverman et al. reported the possibility of ^{18}F chelation through an "Al–^{18}F" complex, which carries out a coordination bond with the macrocyclic chelator NOTA [69].

Direct bombardment is achieved by direct irradiation of inorganic NPs with protons and neutrons to obtain radiolabeled NPs. Perez-Campana et al. demonstrated the nuclear reaction ^{16}O(p, α)^{13}N on Al_2O_3 NPs, where the radioisotope is incorporated in the inorganic NPs without any modification of the particle surface and morphology. Moreover, they demonstrated the stability of the radiolabeling by monitoring the in vivo signal after NP intravenous (i.v.) injection [70]. The main limitation of this approach is related to its application to functionalized NPs; the irradiation procedure may induce damages to the organic molecules conjugated onto the NP surface, causing the loss of their biological activity.

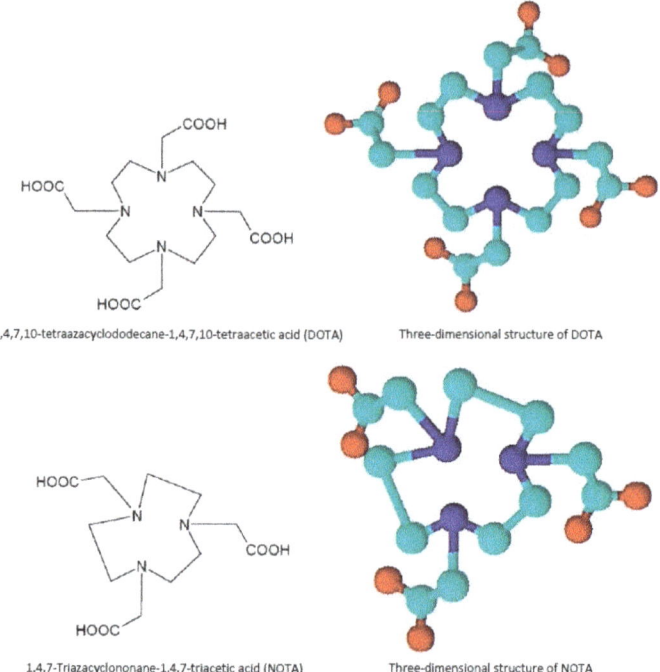

Figure 3. DOTA and NOTA chelators: chemical and three-dimensional structures. 1,4,7-triazacyclononane-N,N',N''-triacetic acid (NOTA) and 1,4,7,10-Tetraazacyclododecane-1,4,7,10-tetraacetic acid (DOTA).

An alternative approach is the synthesis of radioactive NPs starting from radioactive and non-radioactive precursors. ^{64}Cu is the most widely used radioisotope for this strategy thanks to which both organic and inorganic NPs can be obtained as liposomal ^{64}Cu, [^{64}Cu] CuS, or [^{64}Cu] CuFe$_3$O$_4$ [71–73]. However, high temperatures and elevated incubation times are required for their production; thus, radiocontamination problems may arise.

Finally, post-synthesis NP radiolabeling seems to be a very promising chelator-free approach. However, both NP properties and chemical and physical interactions between NPs and the radioisotope have to be carefully taken into account. As an example, Chakravarty et al. produced a probe for dual MRI/PET imaging by ^{69}Ge radiolabeling of superparamagnetic iron-oxide NPs (SPIONs). They were realized by exploiting the unique interaction between the NP surface and the radiotracer contact, overcoming all the limitations associated with the complex ^{69}Ge coordination chemistry of traditional chelator-based methods [74].

Moreover, by exploiting the ability of some radiotracers to emit α and β particles, radiolabeled NPs can be used for radiation therapy in theranostic applications. These radiotracers, indeed, generate ionization in the atoms (mostly in water molecules), with the formation of free radicals and consequent damage to cellular DNA. As an example, liposomes containing α-emitters are widely described in the literature for their ability to improve the radionuclide circulation time and mediate its interaction with the biological environment [75–77]. Through this approach, it is possible to improve the ratio between radiation dose to tumor and normal tissues. Secondly, because of a better time to circulate, these formulations cause larger concentrations to diffuse within the tumor tissue and may, therefore, provide a less heterogeneous tumor dose [75].

1.4. PET/MRI Nanoparticles and Preclinical Applications

NPs were extensively studied at a preclinical level as imaging probes for dual MRI/PET tumor imaging. According to the chemical composition of the core, NPs can be classified into inorganic and organic [78]. Inorganic NPs recently gained significant attention due to their unique physical and chemical properties. In particular, their chemical inertness, good stability, and the easiness of surface functionalization make inorganic NPs attractive for imaging of malignant tumors. However, their toxicity remains the main concern; it was demonstrated that iron-oxide NPs entering into cells through endocytosis show high toxicity because of their accumulation in endo-lysosomal compartments [59]. The most used carriers of this category are iron-oxide NPs and silica NPs. Common nanoconstructs are shown in Figure 4.

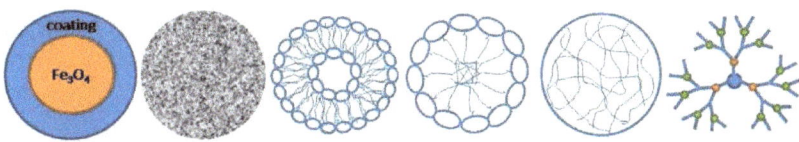

Figure 4. Typical nanocarriers: (from left) superparamagnetic iron-oxide nanoparticles, silica-based nanoparticles, liposomes, micelles, polymeric nanoparticles, and dendrimers.

1.4.1. Iron-Oxide Nanoparticles

Magnetic iron-oxide NPs, typically magnetite Fe_3O_4 and maghemite, $\gamma\ Fe_2O_3$, are broadly employed in MRI imaging especially for the liver, spleen, and bone marrow due, to their ability to shorten T_2 and T_2^* relaxation times. According to their size, they can be categorized into *micrometer-sized paramagnetic iron oxide* (MPIO) (several micrometers), *superparamagnetic iron oxide* (SPIO) (hundreds of nanometers), *ultrasmall superparamagnetic iron oxide* (USPIO) (below 50 nm) [79], and *mono crystalline iron oxide* (MION) (representing a subset of USPIO ranging from 10 to 30 nm) [78,80].

The most common method for SPIO and USPIO synthesis is the reduction and coprecipitation reaction of ferrous and ferric salts in a basic aqueous media [81–83]. Resulting NPs are generally polydisperse and poorly crystalline; therefore, other preparation methods are often preferred, such as thermal decomposition and microwave synthesis [17]. Bare NPs are prone to agglomeration due to their high surface energy. In order to improve both colloidal and chemical stability, many polymeric coating materials were proposed, such as dextran, carboxymethylated dextran, carboxydextran, chitosan, starch, PEG, heparin, albumin, arabinogalactan, glycosaminoglycan, sulfonated styrene–divinylbenzene, organic siloxane, polyvinyl alcohol, poloxamers, and polyoxamines [84,85]. In addition, the polymeric corona is able to protect iron-oxide NPs, preventing erosion at acidic pH, lowering cytotoxicity [63]. The coating can be performed during the co-precipitation process, with the synthesis of the NPs occurring simultaneously to its coating [86,87] or post-synthesis, with the coating realized after the synthesis of the NPs [88,89]. Surface coating is a key factor for NP bioconjugation to biological ligands such as peptides or antibodies; therefore, it represents clinical potential for cancer imaging. Nevertheless, iron-oxide NPs have some important drawbacks. First of all, they act as negative contrast and, after administration, there is a loss of signal that makes medical evaluation less easy compared to T_1 CA brightness. Moreover, the high susceptibility causes distortion artefacts and reduces the contrast-to-noise ratio [79]. Gd-based T_1 agents are the most extensively and clinically used. Alloy materials were investigated to obtain more efficient T_2 CAs because they are endowed with higher magnetic anisotropy [69], crystallinity, and relaxivity; thus, various bimetallic ferrite NPs named *magnetic engineered iron-oxide NPs*, such as $CoFe_2O_4$, $MnFe_2O_4$, and $NiFe_2O_4$, were tested [90].

There are several commercially available superparamagnetic iron-oxide NP formulations such as Feridex (Berlex,, Hanover, NJ, USA), Endorem (Guerbet, Villepinte, EU), and Resovist (Schering, EU, Japan). They are mostly used for liver and spleen tumors diagnosis [91], and the coating polymers are dextran for Feridex and Endorem, and an alkali-treated low-molecular-weight carboxydextran for Resovist [92]. Many preclinical studies were conducted to assess the iron-oxide NP potential as PET/MRI probes for cancer imaging exploiting both passive targeting (for lymph node mapping) and active targeting strategies (mainly through RGD (Arg–Gly–Asp) conjugation).

Thorek and coworkers [93] prepared ^{89}Zr radiolabeled iron-oxide NPs (ferumoxytol) to visualize the axillary and brachial lymph node drainage in healthy wild-type mice. In detail, the iron-oxide core was surrounded by a semisynthetic polysaccharide coating of polyglucose sorbitol carboxymethylether, and desferrioxamine was used as a chelator. In the same study [93], after intraprostatic administration in Hi-Myc transgenic mice bearing invasive prostatic adenocarcinoma, PET/MRI imaging delineated draining nodes in the abdomen and the inguinal region, in addition to prostatic ones.

In 2019, Madru et al. [94] proposed a new, time-efficient, chelator-free conjugation of ^{64}Cu on PEGylated SPIONs for PET/MRI detection and localization of sentinel lymph nodes (SLNs) in C57BL/6J mice. The stability of radiolabeling up to 24 h and NP accumulation in the SLN were demonstrated through a biodistribution study. Lymph nodes metastases are important markers for cancer staging and treatment, and their localization can be useful in presurgical planning.

Xie and colleagues [95] encapsulated iron-oxide NPs, after modification with dopamine, into human serum albumin (HSA) matrices and labeled them with Cy5.5 dye and ^{64}Cu-DOTA. NPs were injected into a U87MG xenograft mouse model; PET and NIRF imaging showed a higher signal-to-noise ratio compared to MRI because of their higher sensitivity. On the other hand, MRI scans post NP injection showed a clear inhomogeneous distribution thanks to their high spatial resolution. These findings were confirmed by histological studies. The HSA shell conferred prolonged circulation time and lower macrophage uptake rate. Such NPs are suitable for theranostic applications if co-loaded with drug molecules.

An active targeting probe was developed by Lee and coworkers [96] who conjugated RGD to ^{64}Cu radiolabeled iron-oxide NPs. As a coating material, polyaspartic acid was chosen since it exposes both carboxyl groups interacting with NPs and amine groups useful for DOTA and RGD conjugation. Imaging was performed on a U87MG mouse model, and both PET and MRI confirmed that the accumulation of NPs was mediated by $\alpha_v\beta_3$ integrin binding. Kim and colleagues [97] injected ^{68}Ga labeled iron-oxide NPs into BALB/c nude mice bearing colon cancer (HT-29) cells, using oleanolic acid as a tumor-targeting molecule. This ligand was shown to inhibit colon cancer cell proliferation, as well as induce apoptosis and cancer cell death. Binding assays and histological studies confirmed the tumor uptake of NPs thanks to oleanolic acid affinity for HT-29 cancer cells. PET/MRI scans provided high-quality images and precise quantification of the tumor area.

1.4.2. Silica-Based Nanoparticles

Silica-based NPs are widely applied in drug delivery, bio-imaging, and cell targeting as they are considered an ideal biocompatible matrix to integrate imaging probes. There are two major classes of silica-based NPs: solid (SiNPs) and mesoporous (MSNs). SiNPs are extensively used as optical imaging agents, while MSNs are often used in CT, MRI, PET, molecular, and multimodal imaging. MSNs are synthesized by a surfactant templated sol–gel method [98] and have attractive properties such as an extremely large surface area, a tunable structure in terms of size, morphology, and porosity, and ease of functionalization through synthetic approaches [99]. In bimodal PET/MRI imaging, MSNs are used as a coating material for metallic NPs or as carrier for MRI CAs and PET radioisotopes. CAs can be encapsulated in channels and protected from the environment, together with drugs or genes for theranostic purpose. A porous silica shell improves MRI contrast enhancement since the pores allow intimate contact between water molecules and the iron-oxide NPs [100]. We report two examples of MSNs in PET/MRI for cancer imaging. Burke and colleagues [101] described silica-coated iron-oxide-based nanorods radiolabeled with ^{68}Ga. In detail, nanorods were coated with various ratios of a siloxane-terminated tetraazamacrocycle (siloxane-DO3A) and a siloxane PEG derivative. Nanorods offer some advantages over nanospheres such as improved T_2 MRI contrast and direct uptake in the liver via phagocytosis. Moreover, thanks to the silica coating, a macrocyclic chelator for highly stable radiolabeled nanoconstructs was not required. Huang and coworkers [102] reported a mesoporous silica-based triple modal imaging nanoprobe to map and track tumor metastatic sentinel lymph nodes (T-SLNs). In this system, three imaging probes including near-infrared (NIR) dye ZW800, T_1 CA Gd-DTTA, and the positron-emitting radionuclide ^{64}Cu were integrated into MSNs via different conjugation strategies. PET and MRI imaging probes were located on the surface and in the mesoporous channel of NPs. A faster uptake rate and higher uptake of the multifunctional MSN probes were observed in T-SLNs compared with normal SLNs, confirming the feasibility of these MSN probes as CAs to map SLNs and identify tumor metastasis. Images revealed that NP accumulation in T-SLNs was much higher than in normal controlateral SLNs (N-SLNs), where almost no signal was observed.

1.4.3. Organic Nanoparticles

Over the last decade, a number of organic NPs, such as dendrimers, polymeric micelles, liposomes, and proteins were used in various applications for cancer diagnosis. These organic NPs carry imaging moieties such as radionuclides and show potential for tumor diagnosis [78]. Liposomes are spherical phospholipid bilayers similar to a cell membrane. Phospholipids are amphiphilic molecules as they have a hydrophilic head group and two hydrophobic tails; thus, they present an inner aqueous compartment that can encapsulate hydrophilic molecules, while hydrophobic agents can be inserted in the lipid shell. Liposomes can be classified by size or by the number of bilayers. In fact, they can also present more than one bilayer; these multilamellar constructs are characterized by an onion structure where each bilayer of phospholipids is separated from the adjacent by a water layer [82]. Among the various protocols for preparing liposomes with different size and number of layers, the most established are based upon sonication and extrusion [82]. Functional moieties can be attached on the bilayer membrane surface. They are biocompatible, non-toxic, and biodegradable, and they are extensively used for drug delivery. After PEGylation, the blood circulation time of liposomes can be prolonged for sustained release or targeted delivery of imaging and therapeutic agents [44]. Liposomes can exploit the EPR effect or active targeting with antibodies, peptides, and vitamins to reach cancer cells [103]. To date, several liposomal formulations were approved for cancer therapy, mainly loaded with doxorubicin, and treatment of infections such as fungal infections; a few anticancer-loaded liposomes are currently undergoing clinical trials [104].

In MRI imaging, liposomes can be used as a coating material to prevent iron-oxide NPs from aggregating and to target tumor cells. They are an excellent platform for multimodal imaging and theranostic application. As an example, Malinge et al. [85] realized magnetic liposomes by incorporation of iron-oxide NPs in the liposomal aqueous core. Liposomes were radiolabeled through a ^{68}Ga-based radiotracer allowing a dual-modality tracking of particle in vivo distribution through MRI and PET imaging; in addition, glucose was grafted onto the NP surface. On U87MG-bearing mice, the magnetic characteristic of the liposomes and the superficial presence of the glucose enabled a dual tumor-targeting mechanism. Through an external magnet, particles were driven in the tumoral region, and the Warburg mechanism allowed their preferential interaction with tumoral cells. In addition, this study confirmed the role of the lipid bilayer in regulating the exchange of water molecules from the external environment to the aqueous core and the consequent increase of the iron-oxide NPs relaxivity r_2, improving MRI performance. In another study, Li and colleagues [105] constructed a multifunctional theranostic liposomal drug delivery system; liposomes encapsulated doxorubicin and were conjugated with Gd-DOTA for MRI and IRDye for near-infrared fluorescence. Liposomes were also radiolabeled with ^{99m}Tc and ^{64}Cu for SPECT and PET imaging. After intratumoral injection, MR images displayed, with high resolution, the micro-intratumoral distribution of the liposomes in squamous cell carcinoma of head and neck tumor xenografts in nude rats. NIR fluorescent, SPECT, and PET images confirmed MRI findings. In addition, these multifunctional liposomes have the potential for the accurate monitoring and in vivo delivery of liposomal chemotherapeutic drugs or therapeutic radionuclides such as ^{186}Re/^{188}Re. Mitchell et al. [106] prepared liposomal formulations with short *n*-ethylene glycol spacers of varying length; multifunctional imaging was gained through a chelator (DOTA) in the head group of lipids, thereby chelating Gd^{3+} for MRI, ^{111}In for SPECT, and ^{64}Cu for PET. Compared to conventional PEG shielded liposomes (DSPE-PEG2000), this system showed good cellular internalization in tumor cells and similar distribution and blood half-lives. Abou and colleagues [107] radiolabeled preformed paramagnetic (Gd) liposomes with ^{89}Zr (positron emitter). The authors used a chelator-free strategy thanks to the radiometal affinity for the lipid phosphate head groups; this dual mode CA was conjugated with octreotide to selectively target neuroendocrine tumors via human somatostatin receptor subtype 2 (SSTr2). MR and PET images revealed significantly greater accumulation of octreotide liposomes to SSTr2-expressing cells compared to control liposomes.

Like liposomes, micelles are also characterized by a core/shell structure but, unlike liposomes, the core can also be hydrophobic while the shell is hydrophilic. Micelles can be made of nonionic surfactants (surfactant micelles) or of amphiphilic block copolymers (polymeric micelles). In polymeric micelles, the length of the hydrophilic block exceeds that of the hydrophobic one, thus resulting in spherical shapes [88]. Polymeric micelles were greatly investigated for delivering hydrophobic drugs; moreover, they have a smaller size compared to liposomes, and the hydrophilic shell reduces interactions with macrophages [108]. Because of the hydrophilic nature of CAs, they can be bound to the hydrophilic blocks or covalently conjugated to the hydrophobic lipid chain in order to be incorporated into micelles [109]. A special group of polymeric micelles can be synthesized by the conjugation of water-soluble copolymers with lipids constituting the hydrophobic blocks (such as polyethylene glycol–phosphatidyl ethanolamine, PEG–PE). The main feature that makes PEG–lipid micelles attractive for diagnostic imaging applications is their size [88]; in fact, due to the lipid bilayer curvature limitation, it is not possible to prepare liposomes that are smaller than a certain minimal diameter (usually, 70–100 nm) [110]. Such a vector was realized by Trubetskoy and colleagues [111]; Gd-DTPA-PE and ^{111}In-DTPA-SA were incorporated into 20-nm PEG–PE micelles to visualize lymph nodes during percutaneous lymphography using gamma scintigraphy and MRI imaging in rabbits. A recent study by Starmans et al. [112] provided a PET/MRI dual imaging polymeric micellar system consisting of self-assembling amphiphilic diblock copolymers functionalized with ^{89}Zr deferoxamine and Fe^{3+} deferoxamine. In vivo PET and MRI images clarified tumor visualization thanks to the EPR effect. However, both liposomes and micelles are unstable, especially in the presence of serum, and, for this reason, many authors crosslink them to achieve better stability [94,95].

Dendrimers are a group of highly branched spherical polymers with a tree-like internal structure. They are characterized by an inner core surrounded by a number of branches called *generations*. Depending on the number of generations, they vary in size and molecular weight. CAs or drugs can be encapsulated in the inner spaces or anchored on the external terminations [113]. To date, dendrimers as dual modal agents are used for MRI and fluorescence [114,115], optical imaging and nuclear medicine [116], CT, and MRI [117].

However, few studies on positron-emitting radionuclide-labeled dendrimers were reported [118,119], and when such dendrimer platforms are used to develop PET/MRI or SPECT/MRI agents, it is challenging to achieve precise control of radioisotope loading into specific chelating moieties [120]. Indeed, to our knowledge, studies about dendritic formulations for combined PET/MRI remain to be published.

In recent years, the biomimetic approach gained increasing interest in the scientific community, and many scientists are trying to mimic what naturally occurs in the body in order to obtain more biocompatible and biodegradable materials for medical applications. The crucial idea behind the biomimetic approach is that a biopolymer naturally occurring in living organs can be modified for diagnostic and therapeutic purposes, improving probe efficiency and reducing immunogenicity and inflammatory potential. Biological polymers such as alginate, hyaluronic acid, and chitosan, as well as proteins, antibodies, enzymes, lipoproteins, and viral capsids (protein cages), are becoming very attractive for diagnostic and therapeutic applications [121].

Maham et al. synthesized engineered platforms for drug delivery systems of different types and shapes (NPs, microspheres, films, minirods, hydrogels) using gelatin, albumin, collagen, elastin, ferritin/apoferritin, gliadin, casein, zein (corn protein), whey protein, and soy protein [103] highlighting promises and challenges.

Vecchione et al. [122] proposed a fully biocompatible platform for dual MRI/PET imaging with improved relaxometric properties. The core–shell nanocarriers made of chitosan and hyaluronic acid entrapped Gd-DTPA, boosting its relaxometric properties up to five times, and carried the adsorbed ^{18}F-FDG without any modification of both FDA-approved CAs.

Fan and coworkers [123] produced a water-soluble melanin NP formulation; this system, after PEGylation, naturally bound ^{64}Cu and Fe^{3+} for PET and MRI imaging, and its surface was functionalized with RGD. Shukla et al. [124] proposed a virus-based synthesis, where bacteriophages and plant viruses were used as a scaffold to carry ^{18}F and iron oxide or Gd^{3+}. These virus-based NPs resulted homogenous and monodisperse, representing a promising delivery system for CAs. However, there are still several open concerns related to their immunogenicity and loading efficiency. In Table 4, a comprehensive overview of nanoparticulate constructs used in PET/MRI imaging and related properties is provided.

Table 4. Overview of multimodal PET/MRI nanoparticles.

Nanostructure	MRI Component	PET Component	Chelator	Other	Biological Target	Ref.
Bacteriophages/plant viruses	Iron oxide/Gd^{3+}	^{18}F			Passive targeting	[124]
Hyaluronic acid + chitosan	Gd-DTPA	^{18}F-FDG	No chelator		Passive targeting	[122]
Iron oxide + ligands ($-NH_2$ $-COOH$)	Iron oxide	^{11}C	No chelator		Passive targeting	[125]
Iron oxide + micelle + PEG	Iron oxide	^{64}Cu	DOTA		Passive targeting	[126]
Iron oxide + dextran	Iron oxide	^{64}Cu	DTCBP		Passive targeting	[53]
Iron oxide + HSA	Iron oxide	^{64}Cu	DOTA	Cy5.5	Passive targeting	[95]
Iron oxide + mannose	Iron oxide	^{68}Ga	NOTA		Passive targeting	[127]
Iron oxide + micelle + PEG	Iron oxide	^{68}Ga	NOTA		Oleanolic acid	[97]
Iron oxide + PASP	Iron oxide	^{64}Cu	DOTA		RGD *	[96]
Iron oxide + PEG	Iron oxide	^{64}Cu	NOTA	Au	Anti EGFR affibody	[128]
Iron oxide + PLGA + lipids + PEG	Iron oxide	^{64}Cu	DOTA		Passive targeting	[129]
Iron oxide + polyglucose	Iron oxide	^{89}Zr	Desferrioxamine		Passive targeting	[93]
Iron oxide + PEG	Iron oxide	^{64}Cu	No chelator		Passive targeting	[94]
Iron oxide + silica + PEG	Iron oxide	^{68}Ga	DO3A		Passive targeting	[101]
Liposome	Iron oxide	^{68}Ga	NODA	Glucose	External magnetic field + Warburg effect	[130]
Liposome	Gd-DTPA	^{89}Zr	no chelator		Octreotide	[107]
Liposome	Gd^{3+}	^{64}Cu	DOTA	IRDye–doxorubicin–^{99m}Tc	Passive targeting	[105]
Liposome + nEG spacer	Gd^{3+}	^{64}Cu	DOTA	^{111}I-fluorescein	Passive targeting	[106]
Melanine NP + PEG	Fe^{3+}	^{64}Cu	No chelator		RGD *	[123]
Mesoporous silica NP	Gd^{3+}	^{64}Cu	DOTA	ZW800	Passive targeting	[102]
Micelle	Fe^{3+}	^{89}Zr	Desferrioxamine		Passive targeting	[112]
MnMEIO/iron oxide + Al(OH)$_3$	MnMEIO/iron oxide	^{18}F/^{64}Cu	No chelator/DTCBP		Passive targeting	[54]
MnMEIO + SA	MnMEIO	^{124}I	No chelator		Passive targeting	[131]
Silica NP	Gd^{3+}	^{68}Ga	DOTAGA/NODAGA		Passive targeting	[132]

* HSA = human serum albumin; RGD = Arg–Gly–Asp; PEG = polyethylene glycol; PLGA = polylactic-co-glycolic acid; nEG = n-ethylene glycol spacers; MnMEIO = Mn-doped magnetism engineered iron oxide; PASP = polyaspartic acid; DTCBP = dithiocarbamatebisphosphonate; EGFR = epidermal growth factor receptor; NOTA = 1,4,7-triazacyclonane-1,4,7-triacetic acid; DOTA = 1,4,7,10-tetraazacyclododecane-1,4,7,10-tetraacetic acid; DOTAGA = 1,4,7,10-tetraazacyclododecane-1-glutaric anhydride-4,7,10-triacetic acid; NODAGA = 2,2′-(7-(1-carboxy-4-((2,5-dioxopyrrolidin-1-yl)oxy)-4-oxobutyl)-1,4,7-triazonane-1,4-diyl) diacetic acid; DO3A = 1,4,7-tris(carboxymethylaza)cyclododecane-10-azaacetylamide. FDG = fluorodeoxyglucose.

2. Conclusions and Perspectives

Molecular imaging and multimodal imaging are current topics extensively investigated by researchers and scientists. Since each diagnostic modality presents advantages and drawbacks, no single technique is able to provide a comprehensive overview of morphological, functional, and metabolic processes underlying tumors. Thus, a deep analysis was conducted on hybrid imaging, and several multimodal scanners are now routinely used in clinical practice among which PET/CT and PET/MRI are the most popular. The complementary information simultaneously obtained by PET and MRI offers new insights into disease diagnosis and treatment. As an example, dynamic contrast-enhanced MRI and PET with perfusion tracers are used to assess the tumor perfusion. A dual CA in a single probe allows a really simultaneous acquisition, and the co-localization of the two CAs guarantees a temporal and spatial correlation of the two imaging modalities. NPs can be used in PET/MRI as CAs for cancer imaging and, in order to gather anatomical and pathological information, their features must be properly adjusted: size, shape, charge, coating, and multivalency. Nevertheless, active targeting opened new pathways through the possibility of NP accumulation at the pathological site and, therefore, quantification is possible also on low-sensitivity techniques such as MRI. The impact of this approach can also be huge in the theranostic field since cancer imaging, diagnosis, and characterization can be used to gather important information about drug release, efficient therapy, and monitoring of response to treatment. Ideal candidates for a specific treatment could be so individuated, and personalized medicine can offer better results and faster healing. Even though, in the last few years, a variety of multimodal probes were produced, only few of them are approved for clinical use. Many challenges must be solved to promote NP clinical translation for both diagnostic and theranostic purposes. A multidisciplinary approach is necessary in order to focus on diagnostic applications and understand biomolecular processes at the basis of several pathologies. We expect that prevention, early diagnosis, patient management, and treatment could be improved such that a single performance can provide a comprehensive examination from which all essential parameters can be derived. In this perspective, multimodality plays a key role, and NPs can display their potential.

Author Contributions: E.F., D.F., A.C.d.P., E.T., C.C., and M.A. wrote the manuscript with the support of P.A.N., M.S. All authors have read and agreed to the published version of the manuscript.

Funding: This research was supported by "Ricerca Corrente" Grant from Italian Ministry of Health (IRCCS SDN).

Conflicts of Interest: The authors declare no conflict of interest.

References

1. Orlacchio, A.; Ciarrapico, A.M.; Schillaci, O.; Chegai, F.; Tosti, D.; D'Alba, F.; Guazzaroni, M.; Simonetti, G. PET-CT in oncological patients: Analysis of informal care costs in cost-benefit assessment. *Radiol. Med.* **2014**, *119*, 283–289. [CrossRef] [PubMed]
2. Schillaci, O.; Scimeca, M.; Toschi, N.; Bonfiglio, R.; Urbano, N.; Bonanno, E. Combining Diagnostic Imaging and Pathology for Improving Diagnosis and Prognosis of Cancer. *Contrast Media Mol. Imaging* **2019**. [CrossRef] [PubMed]
3. Vaquero, J.J.; Kinahan, P. Positron Emission Tomography: Current Challenges and Opportunities for Technological Advances in Clinical and Preclinical Imaging Systems. *Annu. Rev. Biomed. Eng.* **2015**, *17*, 385–414. [CrossRef] [PubMed]
4. Liu, H.; Chen, Y.; Wu, S.; Song, F.H.; Zhang, H.; Tian, M. Molecular imaging using PET and SPECT for identification of breast cancer subtypes. *Nucl. Med. Commun.* **2016**, *37*, 1116–1124. [CrossRef]
5. Grueneisen, J.; Nagarajah, J.; Buchbender, C.; Hoffmann, O.; Schaarschmidt, B.M.; Poeppel, T.; Forsting, M.; Quick, H.; Umutlu, L.; Kinner, S. Positron Emission Tomography/Magnetic Resonance Imaging for Local Tumor Staging in Patients With Primary Breast Cancer A Comparison With Positron Emission Tomography/Computed Tomography and Magnetic Resonance Imaging. *Investig. Radiol.* **2015**, *50*, 505–513. [CrossRef]
6. Rampinelli, C.; de Marco, P.; Origgi, D.; Maisonneuve, P.; Casiraghi, M.; Veronesi, G.; Spaggiari, L.; Bellomi, M. Exposure to low dose computed tomography for lung cancer screening and risk of cancer: Secondary analysis of trial data and risk-benefit analysis. *BMJ Br. Med. J.* **2017**, *356*. [CrossRef]
7. Vannier, M. CT Clinical Perspective: Challenges and the Impact of Future Technology Developments. *Med. Phys.* **2009**, *36*. [CrossRef]

8. Garcia-Figueiras, R.; Baleato-Gonzalez, S.; Padhani, A.R.; Luna-Alcala, A.; Vallejo-Casas, J.A.; Sala, E.; Vilanova, J.; Koh, D.; Herranz-Carnero, M.; Vargas, H. How clinical imaging can assess cancer biology. *Insights Into Imaging* **2019**, *10*, 28. [CrossRef]
9. Vandenberghe, S.; Marsden, P.K. PET-MRI: A review of challenges and solutions in the development of integrated multimodality imaging. *Phys. Med. Biol.* **2015**, *60*, R115–R154. [CrossRef]
10. Bercovich, E.; Javitt, M.C. Medical Imaging: From Roentgen to the Digital Revolution, and Beyond. *Rambam Maimonides Med. J.* **2018**, *9*. [CrossRef]
11. Catana, C.; Procissi, D.; Wu, Y.; Judenhofer, M.S.; Qi, J.; Pichler, B.J.; Jacobs, R.E.; Cherry, S.R. Simultaneous in vivo positron emission tomography and magnetic resonance imaging. *Proc. Natl. Acad. Sci. USA* **2008**, *105*, 3705–3710. [CrossRef] [PubMed]
12. Beyer, T.; Townsend, D.W.; Brun, T.; Kinahan, P.E.; Charron, M.; Roddy, R.; Jerin, J.; Young, J.; Byars, L.; Nutt, R. A combined PET/CT scanner for clinical oncology. *J. Nucl. Med.* **2000**, *41*, 1369–1379. [PubMed]
13. Alessio, A.M.; Kinahan, P.E.; Cheng, P.M.; Vesselle, H.; Karp, J.S. PET/CT scanner instrumentation, challenges, and solutions. *Radiol. Clin. N. Am.* **2004**, *42*, 1017. [CrossRef]
14. Townsend, D.W.; Beyer, T.; Blodgett, T.M. PET/CT scanners: A hardware approach to image fusion. *Semin. Nucl. Med.* **2003**, *33*, 193–204. [CrossRef] [PubMed]
15. Catana, C.; Wu, Y.; Judenhofer, M.S.; Qi, J.; Pichler, B.J.; Cherry, S.R. Simultaneous acquisition of multislice PET and MR images: Initial results with a MR-compatible PET scanner. *J. Nucl. Med.* **2006**, *47*, 1968–1976. [PubMed]
16. Delso, G.; Ziegler, S. PET/MRI system design. *Eur. J. Nucl. Med. Mol. Imaging* **2009**, *36*, 86–92. [CrossRef]
17. Garcia, J.; Tang, T.; Louie, A.Y. Nanoparticle-based multimodal PET/MRI probes. *Nanomedicine* **2015**, *10*, 1343–1359. [CrossRef]
18. Nensa, F.; Beiderwellen, K.; Heusch, P.; Wetter, A. Clinical applications of PET/MRI: Current status and future perspectives. *Diagn. Interv. Radiol.* **2014**, *20*, 438–447. [CrossRef]
19. Aiello, M.; Salvatore, E.; Cachia, A.; Pappata, S.; Cavaliere, C.; Prinster, A.; Nicolai, E.; Salvatore, M.; Baron, J.-C.; Quarantelli, M. Relationship between simultaneously acquired resting-state regional cerebral glucose metabolism and functional MRI: A PET/MR hybrid scanner study. *Neuroimage* **2015**, *113*, 111–121. [CrossRef]
20. Covello, M.; Cavaliere, C.; Aiello, M.; Cianelli, M.S.; Mesolella, M.; Iorio, B.; Rossi, A.; Nicolai, E. Simultaneous PET/MR head-neck cancer imaging: Preliminary clinical experience and multiparametric evaluation. *Eur. J. Radiol.* **2015**, *84*, 1269–1276. [CrossRef]
21. Pace, L.; Nicolai, E.; Aiello, M.; Catalano, O.A.; Salvatore, M. Whole-body PET/MRI in oncology: Current status and clinical applications. *Clin. Transl. Imaging* **2013**, *1*, 31–44. [CrossRef]
22. Nappi, C.; Altiero, M.; Imbriaco, M.; Nicolai, E.; Giudice, C.A.; Aiello, M.; Diomiaiuti, C.; Pisani, A.; Spinelli, L.; Cuocolo, A. First experience of simultaneous PET/MRI for the early detection of cardiac involvement in patients with Anderson-Fabry disease. *Eur. J. Nucl. Med. Mol. Imaging* **2015**, *42*, 1025–1031. [CrossRef] [PubMed]
23. Weissleder, R.; Mahmood, U. Molecular imaging. *Radiology* **2001**, *219*, 316–333. [CrossRef] [PubMed]
24. Chen, K.; Chen, X. Design and Development of Molecular Imaging Probes. *Curr. Top. Med. Chem.* **2010**, *10*, 1227–1236. [CrossRef]
25. Cai, W.; Chen, X. Multimodality molecular imaging of tumor angiogenesis. *J. Nuclear Med.* **2008**, *49*, 113S–128S. [CrossRef]
26. Chen, K.; Conti, P.S. Target-specific delivery of peptide-based probes for PET imaging. *Adv. Drug Deliv. Rev.* **2010**, *62*, 1005–1022. [CrossRef]
27. Bouziotis, P.; Psimadas, D.; Tsotakos, T.; Stamopoulos, D.; Tsoukalas, C. Radiolabeled Iron Oxide Nanoparticles As Dual-Modality SPECT/MRI and PET/MRI Agents. *Curr. Top. Med. Chem.* **2012**, *12*, 2694–2702. [CrossRef]
28. Tweedle, M.F.; Wedeking, P.; Kumar, K. Biodistribution of radiolabeled, formulated gadopentetate, gadoteridol, gadoterate, and gadodiamide in mice and rats. *Investig. Radiol.* **1995**, *30*, 372–380. [CrossRef]
29. Kanda, T.; Oba, H.; Toyoda, K.; Kitajima, K.; Furui, S. Brain gadolinium deposition after administration of gadolinium-based contrast agents. *Jpn. J. Radiol.* **2016**, *34*, 3–9. [CrossRef]
30. McDonald, R.J.; McDonald, J.S.; Kallmes, D.F.; Jentoft, M.E.; Paolini, M.A.; Murray, D.L.; Williamson, E.E.; Eckel, L.J. Gadolinium Deposition in Human Brain Tissues after Contrast-enhanced MR Imaging in Adult Patients without Intracranial Abnormalities. *Radiology* **2017**, *285*, 546–554. [CrossRef]

31. Xiao, Y.D.; Paudel, R.; Liu, J.; Ma, C.; Zhang, Z.S.; Zhou, S.K. MRI contrast agents: Classification and application (Review). *Int. J. Mol. Med.* **2016**, *38*, 1319–1326. [CrossRef] [PubMed]
32. Ljungberg, M.; Pretorius, P.H. SPECT/CT: An update on technological developments and clinical applications. *Br. J. Radiol.* **2018**, *91*. [CrossRef] [PubMed]
33. Volterrani, D.; Erba, P.A.; Carrio, I.; Strauss, H.W.; Mariani, G. *Nuclear Medicine Textbook Methodology and Clinical Application*; Springer Nature Switzerland AG: Basel, Switzerland, 2019; Volume 2, ISBN 978-3-319-95563-6.
34. Lusic, H.; Grinstaff, M.W. X-ray-Computed Tomography Contrast Agents. *Chem. Rev.* **2013**, *113*, 1641–1666. [CrossRef] [PubMed]
35. Cheng, B.B.; Bandi, V.; Wei, M.Y.; Pei, Y.B.; D'Souza, F.; Nguyen, K.T.; Hong, Y.; Yuan, B. High-Resolution Ultrasound-Switchable Fluorescence Imaging in Centimeter-Deep Tissue Phantoms with High Signal-To-Noise Ratio and High Sensitivity via Novel Contrast Agents. *PLoS ONE* **2016**, *11*, e0165963. [CrossRef] [PubMed]
36. Kampschulte, M.; Langheinirch, A.C.; Sender, J.; Litzlbauer, H.D.; Althohn, U.; Schwab, J.D.; Alejandre-Lafont, E.; Martels, G.; Krombach, G.A. Nano-Computed Tomography: Technique and Applications. *RöFo-Fortschritte auf dem Gebiet der Röntgenstrahlen und der bildgebenden Verfahren* **2016**, *188*, 146–154. [CrossRef]
37. Kalimuthu, S.; Jeong, J.H.; Oh, J.M.; Ahn, B.C. Drug Discovery by Molecular Imaging and Monitoring Therapy Response in Lymphoma. *Int. J. Mol. Sci.* **2017**, *18*, 1639. [CrossRef]
38. Rosales, R. Potential clinical applications of bimodal PET-MRI or SPECT-MRI agents. *J. Label. Compd. Radiopharm.* **2014**, *57*, 298–303. [CrossRef]
39. Kim, B.Y.; Rutka, J.T.; Chan, W.C. Nanomedicine. *N. Engl. J. Med.* **2010**, *363*, 2434–2443. [CrossRef]
40. Chen, G.Y.; Roy, I.; Yang, C.H.; Prasad, P.N. Nanochemistry and Nanomedicine for Nanoparticle-based Diagnostics and Therapy. *Chem. Rev.* **2016**, *116*, 2826–2885. [CrossRef]
41. Aime, S.; Frullano, L.; Crich, S.G. Compartmentalization of a gadolinium complex in the apoferritin cavity: A route to obtain high relaxivity contrast agents for magnetic resonance imaging. *Angew. Chem. Int. Ed.* **2002**, *41*, 1017. [CrossRef]
42. Crich, S.G.; Lanzardo, S.; Alberti, D.; Belfiore, S.; Ciampa, A.; Giovenzanaz, G.B.; Lovazzano, C.; Pagliarin, R.; Aime, S. Magnetic resonance imaging detection of tumor cells by targeting low-density lipoprotein receptors with Gd-loaded low-density lipoprotein particles. *Neoplasia* **2007**, *9*, 1046–1056. [CrossRef] [PubMed]
43. Baetke, S.C.; Lammers, T.; Kiessling, F. Applications of nanoparticles for diagnosis and therapy of cancer. *Br. J. Radiol.* **2015**, *88*, 20150207. [CrossRef] [PubMed]
44. Peer, D.; Karp, J.M.; Hong, S.; FaroKhzad, O.C.; Margalit, R.; Langer, R. Nanocarriers as an emerging platform for cancer therapy. *Nat. Nanotechnol.* **2007**, *2*, 751–760. [CrossRef]
45. Sun, C.; Lee, J.S.H.; Zhang, M. Magnetic nanoparticles in MR imaging and drug delivery. *Adv. Drug Deliv. Rev.* **2008**, *60*, 1252–1265. [CrossRef] [PubMed]
46. Grimm, J.; Scheinberg, D.A. Will Nanotechnology Influence Targeted Cancer Therapy? *Semin. Radiat. Oncol.* **2011**, *21*, 80–87. [CrossRef] [PubMed]
47. Gratton, S.E.A.; Ropp, P.A.; Pohlhaus, P.D.; Luft, J.C.; Madden, V.J.; Napier, M.E.; DeSimone, J.M. The effect of particle design on cellular internalization pathways. *Proc. Natl. Acad. Sci. USA* **2008**, *105*, 11613–11618. [CrossRef]
48. Qiao, R.; Yang, C.; Gao, M. Superparamagnetic iron oxide nanoparticles: From preparations to in vivo MRI applications. *J. Mater. Chem.* **2009**, *19*, 6274–6293. [CrossRef]
49. Berry, C.C.; Curtis, A.S.G. Functionalisation of magnetic nanoparticles for applications in biomedicine. *J. Phys. D Appl. Phys.* **2003**, *36*, R198–R206. [CrossRef]
50. Blanco, E.; Shen, H.; Ferrari, M. Principles of nanoparticle design for overcoming biological barriers to drug delivery. *Nat. Biotechnol.* **2015**, *33*, 941–951. [CrossRef]
51. Neuberger, T.; Schopf, B.; Hofmann, H.; Hofmann, M.; von Rechenberg, B. Superparamagnetic nanoparticles for biomedical applications: Possibilities and limitations of a new drug delivery system. *J. Magn. Magn. Mater.* **2005**, *293*, 483–496. [CrossRef]
52. Choi, H.S.; Liu, W.; Misra, P.; Tanaka, E.; Zimmer, J.P.; Ipe, B.I.; Bawendi, M.G.; Frangioni, J.V. Renal clearance of quantum dots. *Nat. Biotechnol.* **2007**, *25*, 1165–1170. [CrossRef] [PubMed]

53. de Rosales, R.T.M.; Tavaré, R.; Paul, R.L.; Jauregui-Osoro, M.; Protti, A.; Glaria, A.; Varma, G.; Szanda, I.; Blower, P.J. Synthesis of 64CuII–bis (dithiocarbamatebisphosphonate) and its conjugation with superparamagnetic iron oxide nanoparticles: In vivo evaluation as dual-modality PET–MRI agent. *Angew. Chem. Int. Ed.* **2011**, *50*, 5509–5513. [CrossRef] [PubMed]
54. Cui, X.; Belo, S.; Krueger, D.; Yan, Y.; de Rosales, R.T.M.; Jauregui-Osoro, M.; Ye, H.; Su, S.; Mathe, D.; Kovács, N.; et al. Aluminium hydroxide stabilised MnFe2O4 and Fe3O4 nanoparticles as dual-modality contrasts agent for MRI and PET imaging. *Biomaterials* **2014**, *35*, 5840–5846. [CrossRef] [PubMed]
55. Owens, D.E.; Peppas, N.A. Opsonization, biodistribution, and pharmacokinetics of polymeric nanoparticles. *Int. J. Pharm.* **2006**, *307*, 93–102. [CrossRef] [PubMed]
56. Mikhaylova, M.; Kim, D.K.; Bobrysheva, N.; Osmolowsky, M.; Semenov, V.; Tsakalakos, T.; Muhammed, M. Superparamagnetism of magnetite nanoparticles: Dependence on surface modification. *Langmuir* **2004**, *20*, 2472–2477. [CrossRef] [PubMed]
57. LaConte, L.E.W.; Nitin, N.; Zurkiya, O.; Caruntu, D.; O'Connor, C.J.; Hu, X.; Bao, G. Coating thickness of magnetic iron oxide nanoparticles affects R-2 relaxivity. *J. Magn. Reson. Imaging* **2007**, *26*, 1634–1641. [CrossRef]
58. Jain, R.K.; Stylianopoulos, T. Delivering nanomedicine to solid tumors. *Nat. Rev. Clin. Oncol.* **2010**, *7*, 653–664. [CrossRef]
59. Stylianopoulos, T.; Jain, R.K. Design considerations for nanotherapeutics in oncology. *Nanomed. Nanotechnol. Biol. Med.* **2015**, *11*, 1893–1907. [CrossRef]
60. Dolle, F. Fluorine-18-labelled fluoropyridines: Advances in radiopharmaceutical design. *Curr. Pharm. Des.* **2005**, *11*, 3221–3235. [CrossRef]
61. Jacobson, O.; Chen, X.Y. PET Designated Flouride-18 Production and Chemistry. *Curr. Top. Med. Chem.* **2010**, *10*, 1048–1059. [CrossRef]
62. Ismail, F.M.D. Important fluorinated drugs in experimental and clinical use. *J. Fluor. Chem.* **2002**, *118*, 27–33. [CrossRef]
63. Sumer, B.; Gao, J. Theranostic nanomedicine for cancer. *Nanomedicine* **2008**, *3*, 137–140. [CrossRef] [PubMed]
64. Kassis, A.I. Molecular and cellular radiobiological effects of auger emitting radionuclides. *Radiat. Prot. Dosim.* **2011**, *143*, 241–247. [CrossRef] [PubMed]
65. Odonoghue, J.A.; Wheldon, T.E. Targeted radiotherapy using Auger electron emitters. *Phys. Med. Biol.* **1996**, *41*, 1973–1992. [CrossRef] [PubMed]
66. Sun, X.; Cai, W.; Chen, X. Positron Emission Tomography Imaging Using Radio labeled Inorganic Nanomaterials. *Acc. Chem. Res.* **2015**, *48*, 286–294. [CrossRef]
67. Ni, D.L.; Jiang, D.W.; Ehlerding, E.B.; Huang, P.; Cai, W.B. Radiolabeling Silica-Based Nanoparticles via Coordination Chemistry: Basic Principles, Strategies, and Applications. *Acc. Chem. Res.* **2018**, *51*, 778–788. [CrossRef]
68. Wadas, T.J.; Wong, E.H.; Weisman, G.R.; Anderson, C.J. Coordinating Radiometals of Copper, Gallium, Indium, Yttrium, and Zirconium for PET and SPECT Imaging of Disease. *Chem. Rev.* **2010**, *110*, 2858–2902. [CrossRef]
69. Laverman, P.; McBride, W.J.; Sharkey, R.M.; Eek, A.; Joosten, L.; Oyen, W.J.G.; Goldenberg, D.M.; Boerman, O.C. A Novel Facile Method of Labeling Octreotide with F-18-Fluorine. *J. Nucl. Med.* **2010**, *51*, 454–461. [CrossRef]
70. Perez-Campana, C.; Gomez-Vallejo, V.; Puigivila, M.; Martin, A.; Calvo-Fernandez, T.; Moya, S.E.; Ziolo, R.F.; Reese, T.; Llop, J. Biodistribution of Different Sized Nanoparticles Assessed by Positron Emission Tomography: A General Strategy for Direct Activation of Metal Oxide Particles. *ACS Nano* **2013**, *7*, 3498–3505. [CrossRef]
71. Zhou, M.; Zhang, R.; Huang, M.; Lu, W.; Song, S.; Melancon, M.P.; Tian, M.; Liang, D.; Li, C. A Chelator-Free Multifunctional Cu-64 CuS Nanoparticle Platform for Simultaneous Micro-PET/CT Imaging and Photothermal Ablation Therapy. *J. Am. Chem. Soc.* **2010**, *132*, 15351–15358. [CrossRef]
72. Wong, R.M.; Gilbert, D.A.; Liu, K.; Louie, A.Y. Rapid Size-Controlled Synthesis of Dextran-Coated, Cu-64-Doped Iron Oxide Nanoparticles. *Acs Nano* **2012**, *6*, 3461–3467. [CrossRef] [PubMed]
73. Lee, S.G.; Gangangari, K.; Kalidindi, T.M.; Punzalan, B.; Larson, S.M.; Pillarsetty, N.V.K. Copper-64 labeled liposomes for imaging bone marrow. *Nucl. Med. Biol.* **2016**, *43*, 781–787. [CrossRef] [PubMed]
74. Chakravarty, R.; Valdovinos, H.F.; Chen, F.; Lewis, C.M.; Ellison, P.A.; Luo, H.; Meyerand, M.E.; Nickles, R.J.; Cai, W. Intrinsically Germanium-69-Labeled Iron Oxide Nanoparticles: Synthesis and In-Vivo Dual-Modality PET/MR Imaging. *Adv. Mater.* **2014**, *26*, 5119–5123. [CrossRef] [PubMed]

75. Henriksen, G.; Schoultz, B.W.; Michaelsen, T.E.; Bruland, O.S.; Larsen, R.H. Sterically stabilized liposomes as a carrier for alpha-emitting radium and actinium radionuclides. *Nucl. Med. Biol.* **2004**, *31*, 441–449. [CrossRef]
76. Sofou, S.; Thomas, J.L.; Lin, H.Y.; McDevitt, M.R.; Scheinberg, D.A.; Sgouros, G. Engineered Liposomes for potential alpha-particle therapy of metastatic cancer. *J. Nucl. Med.* **2004**, *45*, 253–260.
77. Sofou, S.; Kappel, B.J.; Jaggi, J.S.; McDevitt, M.R.; Scheinberg, D.A.; Sgouros, G. Enhanced retention of the alpha-particle-emitting daughters of actinium-225 by liposome carriers. *Bioconjugate Chem.* **2007**, *18*, 2061–2067. [CrossRef]
78. Xing, Y.; Zhao, J.; Conti, P.S.; Chen, K. Radiolabeled Nanoparticles for Multimodality Tumor Imaging. *Theranostics* **2014**, *4*, 290–306. [CrossRef]
79. Bulte, J.W.M.; Kraitchman, D.L. Iron oxide MR contrast agents for molecular and cellular imaging. *NMR Biomed.* **2004**, *17*, 484–499. [CrossRef]
80. Thorek, D.; Czupryna, J.; Chen, A.; Tsourkas, A. Molecular Imaging of Cancer with Superparamagnetic Iron Oxide Particles. *Cancer Imaging Instrum. Appl.* **2008**, *2*, 85–95.
81. Jung, C.W.; Jacobs, P. Physical and chemical-properties of superparamagnetic iron-oxide mr contrast agents—Ferumoxides, ferumoxtran, ferumoxsil. *Magn. Reson. Imaging* **1995**, *13*, 661–674. [CrossRef]
82. Wang, Y.X.J.; Hussain, S.M.; Krestin, G.P. Superparamagnetic iron oxide contrast agents: Physicochemical characteristics and applications in MR imaging. *Eur. Radiol.* **2001**, *11*, 2319–2331. [CrossRef] [PubMed]
83. Wunderbaldinger, P.; Josephson, L.; Weissleder, R. Crosslinked iron oxides (CLIO): A new platform for the development of targeted MR contrast agents. *Acad. Radiol.* **2002**, *9*, S304–S306. [CrossRef]
84. Mornet, S.; Vasseur, S.; Grasset, F.; Duguet, E. Magnetic nanoparticle design for medical diagnosis and therapy. *J. Mater. Chem.* **2004**, *14*, 2161–2175. [CrossRef]
85. Laurent, S.; Forge, D.; Port, M.; Roch, A.; Robic, C.; Elst, L.V.; Muller, R.N. Magnetic iron oxide nanoparticles: Synthesis, stabilization, vectorization, physicochemical characterizations, and biological applications. *Chem. Rev.* **2008**, *108*, 2064–2110. [CrossRef] [PubMed]
86. Griffiths, S.M.; Singh, N.; Jenkins, G.J.; Williams, P.M.; Orbaek, A.W.; Barron, A.R.; Wright, C.J.; Doak, S.H. Dextran coated ultrafine superparamagnetic iron oxide nanoparticles: Compatibility with common fluorometric and colorimetric dyes. *Anal. Chem.* **2011**, *83*, 3778–3785. [CrossRef] [PubMed]
87. Babic, M.; Horák, D.; Trchová, M.; Jendelová, P.; Glogarová, K.; Lesný, P.; Herynek, V.; Hájek, M.; Syková, E. Poly (L-lysine)-modified iron oxide nanoparticles for stem cell labeling. *Bioconjugate Chem.* **2008**, *19*, 740–750. [CrossRef]
88. Maeng, J.H.; Lee, D.-H.; Jung, K.H.; Bae, Y.-H.; Park, I.-S.; Jeong, S.; Jeon, Y.-S.; Shim, C.-K.; Kim, W.; Kim, J.; et al. Multifunctional doxorubicin loaded superparamagnetic iron oxide nanoparticles for chemotherapy and magnetic resonance imaging in liver cancer. *Biomaterials* **2010**, *31*, 4995–5006. [CrossRef]
89. Liao, Z.; Wang, H.; Lv, R.; Zhao, P.; Sun, X.; Wang, S.; Su, W.; Niu, R.; Chang, J. Polymeric liposomes-coated superparamagnetic iron oxide nanoparticles as contrast agent for targeted magnetic resonance imaging of cancer cells. *Langmuir* **2011**, *27*, 3100–3105. [CrossRef]
90. Lee, J.-H.; Huh, Y.-M.; Jun, Y.-W.; Seo, J.-W.; Jang, J.-T.; Song, H.-T.; Kim, S.; Cho, E.-J.; Yoon, H.-G.; Suh, J.-S.; et al. Artificially engineered magnetic nanoparticles for ultra-sensitive molecular imaging. *Nat. Med.* **2007**, *13*, 95–99. [CrossRef]
91. Lawaczeck, R.; Menzel, M.; Pietsch, H. Superparamagnetic iron oxide particles: Contrast media for magnetic resonance imaging. *Appl. Organomet. Chem.* **2004**, *18*, 506–513. [CrossRef]
92. Blasiak, B.; van Veggel, F.C.; Tomanek, B. Applications of nanoparticles for MRI cancer diagnosis and therapy. *J. Nanomater.* **2013**. [CrossRef]
93. Thorek, D.L.J.; Ulmert, D.; Diop, N.-F.M.; Lupu, M.E.; Doran, M.G.; Huang, R.; Abou, D.S.; Larson, S.M.; Grimm, J. Non-invasive mapping of deep-tissue lymph nodes in live animals using a multimodal PET/MRI nanoparticle. *Nat. Commun.* **2014**, *5*, 3097. [CrossRef] [PubMed]
94. Madru, R.; Budassi, M.; Benveniste, H.; Lee, H.; Smith, S.D.; Schlyer, D.J.; Vaska, P.; Knutsson, L.; Strand, S.-E. Simultaneous Preclinical Positron Emission Tomography-Magnetic Resonance Imaging Study of Lymphatic Drainage of Chelator-Free Cu-64-Labeled Nanoparticles. *Cancer Biother. Radiopharm.* **2018**, *33*, 213–220. [CrossRef] [PubMed]
95. Xie, J.; Chen, K.; Huang, J.; Lee, S.; Wang, J.; Gao, J.; Li, X.; Chen, X. PET/NIRF/MRI triple functional iron oxide nanoparticles. *Biomaterials* **2010**, *31*, 3016–3022. [CrossRef] [PubMed]

96. Lee, H.-Y.; Li, Z.; Chen, K.; Hsu, A.R.; Xu, C.; Xie, J.; Sun, S.; Chen, X. PET/MRI dual-modality tumor imaging using arginine-glycine-aspartic (RGD)—Conjugated radiolabeled iron oxide nanoparticles. *J. Nucl. Med.* **2008**, *49*, 1371–1379. [CrossRef]
97. Kim, S.-M.; Chae, M.K.; Yim, M.S.; Jeong, I.H.; Cho, J.; Lee, C.; Ryu, E.K. Hybrid PET/MR imaging of tumors using an oleanolic acid-conjugated nanoparticle. *Biomaterials* **2013**, *34*, 8114–8121. [CrossRef]
98. Vivero-Escoto, J.L.; Huxford-Phillips, R.C.; Lin, W. Silica-based nanoprobes for biomedical imaging and theranostic applications. *Chem. Soc. Rev.* **2012**, *41*, 2673–2685. [CrossRef]
99. Nakamura, T.; Sugihara, F.; Matsushita, H.; Yoshioka, Y.; Mizukami, S.; Kikuchi, K. Mesoporous silica nanoparticles for 19 F magnetic resonance imaging, fluorescence imaging, and drug delivery. *Chem. Sci.* **2015**, *6*, 1986–1990. [CrossRef]
100. Patel, D.; Kell, A.; Simard, B.; Deng, J.; Xiang, B.; Lin, H.-Y.; Gruwel, M.; Tian, G. Cu2+-labeled, SPION loaded porous silica nanoparticles for cell labeling and multifunctional imaging probes. *Biomaterials* **2010**, *31*, 2866–2873. [CrossRef]
101. Burke, B.P.; Baghdadi, N.; Kownacka, A.E.; Nigam, S.; Clemente, G.S.; Al-Yassiry, M.M.; Domarkas, J.; Lorch, M.; Pickles, M.; Gibbs, P.; et al. Chelator free gallium-68 radiolabelling of silica coated iron oxide nanorods via surface interactions. *Nanoscale* **2015**, *7*, 14889–14896. [CrossRef]
102. Huang, X.; Zhang, F.; Lee, S.; Swierczewska, M.; Kiesewetter, D.O.; Lang, L.; Zhang, G.; Zhu, L.; Gao, H.; Choi, H.S.; et al. Long-term multimodal imaging of tumor draining sentinel lymph nodes using mesoporous silica-based nanoprobes. *Biomaterials* **2012**, *33*, 4370–4378. [CrossRef] [PubMed]
103. Elbayoumi, T.A.; Torchilin, V.P. Current trends in liposome research. *Methods Mol. Biol.* **2010**, *605*, 1–27. [PubMed]
104. Puri, A.; Loomis, K.; Smith, B.; Lee, J.-H.; Yavlovich, A.; Heldman, E.; Blumenthal, R. Lipid-Based Nanoparticles as Pharmaceutical Drug Carriers: From Concepts to Clinic. *Crit. Rev. Ther. Drug Carr. Syst.* **2009**, *26*, 523–580. [CrossRef] [PubMed]
105. Li, S.; Goins, B.; Zhang, L.; Bao, A. Novel Multifunctional Theranostic Liposome Drug Delivery System: Construction, Characterization, and Multimodality MR, Near-Infrared Fluorescent, and Nuclear Imaging. *Bioconjugate Chem.* **2012**, *23*, 1322–1332. [CrossRef]
106. Mitchell, N.; Kalber, T.L.; Cooper, M.S.; Sunassee, K.; Chalker, S.L.; Shaw, K.P.; Ordidge, K.L.; Badar, A.; Janes, S.M.; Blower, P.J.; et al. Incorporation of paramagnetic, fluorescent and PET/SPECT contrast agents into liposomes for multimodal imaging. *Biomaterials* **2013**, *34*, 1179–1192. [CrossRef]
107. Abou, D.S.; Thorek, D.L.J.; Ramos, N.N.; Pinkse, M.W.H.; Wolterbeek, H.T.; Carlin, S.D.; Beattie, B.J.; Lewis, J.S. Zr-89-Labeled Paramagnetic Octreotide-Liposomes for PET-MR Imaging of Cancer. *Pharm. Res.* **2013**, *30*, 878–888. [CrossRef]
108. Savic, R.; Luo, L.B.; Eisenberg, A.; Maysinger, D. Micellar nanocontainers distribute to defined cytoplasmic organelles. *Science* **2003**, *300*, 615–618. [CrossRef]
109. Trubetskoy, V.S. Polymeric micelles as carriers of diagnostic agents. *Adv. Drug Deliv. Rev.* **1999**, *37*, 81–88. [CrossRef]
110. Enoch, H.G.; Strittmatter, P. Formation and properties of 1000-A-diameter, single-bilayer phospholipid vesicles. *Proc. Natl. Acad. Sci. USA* **1979**, *76*, 145–149. [CrossRef]
111. Trubetskoy, V.S.; FrankKamenetsky, M.D.; Whiteman, K.R.; Wolf, G.L.; Torchilin, V.P. Stable polymeric micelles: Lymphangiographic contrast media for gamma scintigraphy and magnetic resonance imaging. *Acad. Radiol.* **1996**, *3*, 232–238. [CrossRef]
112. Starmans, L.W.; Hummelink, M.A.; Rossin, R.; Kneepkens, E.; Lamerichs, R.; Donato, K.; Nicolay, K.; Grüll, H. 89Zr-and Fe-Labeled Polymeric Micelles for Dual Modality PET and T1-Weighted MR Imaging. *Adv. Healthc. Mater.* **2015**, *4*, 2137–2145. [CrossRef]
113. Lee, D.-E.; Koo, H.; Sun, I.-C.; Ryu, J.H.; Kim, K.; Kwon, I.C. Multifunctional nanoparticles for multimodal imaging and theragnosis. *Chem. Soc. Rev.* **2012**, *41*, 2656–2672. [CrossRef]
114. Xu, H.; Regino, C.A.; Koyama, Y.; Hama, Y.; Gunn, A.J.; Bernardo, M.; Kobayashi, H.; Choyke, P.L.; Brechbiel, M.W. Preparation and preliminary evaluation of a biotin-targeted, lectin-targeted dendrimer-based probe for dual-modality magnetic resonance and fluorescence imaging. *Bioconjugate Chem.* **2007**, *18*, 1474–1482. [CrossRef]
115. Koyama, Y.; Talanov, V.S.; Bernardo, M.; Hama, Y.; Regino, C.A.; Brechbiel, M.W.; Choyke, P.L.; Kobayashi, H. A dendrimer-based nanosized contrast agent dual-labeled for magnetic resonance and optical fluorescence

imaging to localize the sentinel lymph node in mice. *J. Magn. Reson. Imaging* **2007**, *25*, 866–871. [CrossRef] [PubMed]
116. Kobayashi, H.; Koyama, Y.; Barrett, T.; Hama, Y.; Regino, C.A.; Shin, I.S.; Jang, B.-S.; Le, N.; Paik, C.H.; Choyke, P.L.; et al. Multimodal nanoprobes for radionuclide and five-color near-infrared optical lymphatic imaging. *ACS Nano* **2007**, *1*, 258–264. [CrossRef] [PubMed]
117. Wen, S.; Li, K.; Cai, H.; Chen, Q.; Shen, M.; Huang, Y.; Peng, C.; Hou, W.; Zhu, M.; Zhang, G.; et al. Multifunctional dendrimer-entrapped gold nanoparticles for dual mode CT/MR imaging applications. *Biomaterials* **2013**, *34*, 1570–1580. [CrossRef]
118. Almutairi, A.; Rossin, R.; Shokeen, M.; Hagooly, A.; Ananth, A.; Capoccia, B.; Guillaudeu, S.; Abendschein, D.; Anderson, C.J.; Welch, M.J.; et al. Biodegradable dendritic positron-emitting nanoprobes for the noninvasive imaging of angiogenesis. *Proc. Natl. Acad. Sci. USA* **2009**, *106*, 685–690. [CrossRef] [PubMed]
119. Kobayashi, H.; Wu, C.; Kim, M.-K.; Paik, C.H.; Carrasquillo, J.A.; Brechbiel, M.W. Evaluation of the in vivo biodistribution of indium-111 and yttrium-88 labeled dendrimer-1B4M-DTPA and its conjugation with anti-Tac monoclonal antibody. *Bioconjugate Chem.* **1999**, *10*, 103–111. [CrossRef] [PubMed]
120. Kumar, A.; Zhang, S.R.; Hao, G.Y.; Hassan, G.; Ramezani, S.; Sagiyama, K.; Lo, S.-T.; Takahashi, M.; Sherry, A.D.; Öz, O.K.; et al. Molecular Platform for Design and Synthesis of Targeted Dual Modality Imaging Probes. *Bioconjugate Chem.* **2015**, *26*, 549–558. [CrossRef] [PubMed]
121. MaHam, A.; Tang, Z.; Wu, H.; Wang, J.; Lin, Y. Protein-Based Nanomedicine Platforms for Drug Delivery. *Small* **2009**, *5*, 1706–1721. [CrossRef]
122. Vecchione, D.; Aiello, M.; Cavaliere, C.; Nicolai, E.; Netti, P.A.; Torino, E. Hybrid core shell nanoparticles entrapping Gd-DTPA and F-18-FDG for simultaneous PET/MRI acquisitions. *Nanomedicine* **2017**, *12*, 2223–2231. [CrossRef]
123. Fan, Q.; Cheng, K.; Hu, X.; Ma, X.; Zhang, R.; Yang, M.; Lu, X.; Xing, L.; Huang, W.; Gambhir, S.S.; et al. Transferring Biomarker into Molecular Probe: Melanin Nanoparticle as a Naturally Active Platform for Multimodality Imaging. *J. Am. Chem. Soc.* **2014**, *136*, 15185–15194. [CrossRef]
124. Shukla, S.; Steinmetz, N.F. Virus-based nanomaterials as positron emission tomography and magnetic resonance contrast agents: From technology development to translational medicine. *Wiley Interdiscip. Rev. Nanomed. Nanobiotechnol.* **2015**, *7*, 708–721. [CrossRef]
125. Sharma, R.; Xu, Y.; Kim, S.W.; Schueller, M.J.; Alexoff, D.; Smith, S.D.; Wang, W.; Schlyer, D. Carbon-11 radiolabeling of iron-oxide nanoparticles for dual-modality PET/MR imaging. *Nanoscale* **2013**, *5*, 7476–7483. [CrossRef]
126. Glaus, C.; Rossin, R.; Welch, M.J.; Bao, G. In vivo evaluation of 64Cu-labeled magnetic nanoparticles as a dual-modality PET/MR imaging agent. *Bioconjugate Chem.* **2010**, *21*, 715–722. [CrossRef]
127. Yang, B.Y.; Moon, S.-H.; Seelam, S.R.; Jeon, M.J.; Lee, Y.-S.; Lee, D.S.; Chung, J.-K.; Kim, Y.; Jeong, J.M. Development of a multimodal imaging probe by encapsulating iron oxide nanoparticles with functionalized amphiphiles for lymph node imaging. *Nanomedicine* **2015**, *10*, 1899–1910. [CrossRef]
128. Yang, M.; Cheng, K.; Qi, S.; Liu, H.; Jiang, Y.; Jiang, H.; Li, J.; Chen, K.; Zhang, H.; Cheng, Z. Affibody modified and radiolabeled gold-Iron oxide hetero-nanostructures for tumor PET, optical and MR imaging. *Biomaterials* **2013**, *34*, 2796–2806. [CrossRef]
129. Aryal, S.; Key, J.; Stigliano, C.; Landis, M.D.; Lee, D.Y.; Decuzzi, P. Positron Emitting Magnetic Nanoconstructs for PET/MR Imaging. *Small* **2014**, *10*, 2688–2696. [CrossRef]
130. Malinge, J.; Geraudie, B.; Savel, P.; Nataf, V.; Prignon, A.; Provost, C.; Zhang, Y.; Ou, P.; Kerrou, K.; Talbot, J.-N.; et al. Liposomes for PET and MR Imaging and for Dual Targeting (Magnetic Field/Glucose Moiety): Synthesis, Properties, and in Vivo Studies. *Mol. Pharm.* **2017**, *14*, 406–414. [CrossRef]

131. Choi, J.-S.; Park, J.C.; Nah, H.; Woo, S.; Oh, J.; Kim, K.M.; Cheon, G.J.; Chang, Y.; Yoo, J.; Cheon, J. A hybrid nanoparticle probe for dual-modality positron emission tomography and magnetic resonance imaging. *Angew. Chem. Int. Ed.* **2008**, *47*, 6259–6262. [CrossRef]
132. Truillet, C.; Bouziotis, P.; Tsoukalas, C.; Brugiere, J.; Martini, M.; Sancey, L.; Brichart, T.; Denat, F.; Boschetti, F.; Darbost, U.; et al. Ultrasmall particles for Gd-MRI and Ga-68-PET dual imaging. *Contrast Media Mol. Imaging* **2015**, *10*, 309–319. [CrossRef]

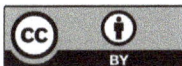

© 2019 by the authors. Licensee MDPI, Basel, Switzerland. This article is an open access article distributed under the terms and conditions of the Creative Commons Attribution (CC BY) license (http://creativecommons.org/licenses/by/4.0/).

MDPI
St. Alban-Anlage 66
4052 Basel
Switzerland
Tel. +41 61 683 77 34
Fax +41 61 302 89 18
www.mdpi.com

Journal of Clinical Medicine Editorial Office
E-mail: jcm@mdpi.com
www.mdpi.com/journal/jcm

www.ingramcontent.com/pod-product-compliance
Lightning Source LLC
LaVergne TN
LVHW070454100526
838202LV00014B/1723